The Year in Metabolism
1975-1976

The Year in Metabolism

Editor-in-Chief: NORBERT FREINKEL • Chicago, Illinois

Editorial Board

The Year in Metabolism

1975-1976

Edited by

Norbert Freinkel, M. D.

Kettering Professor of Medicine,
Professor of Biochemistry,
Director, Center for Endocrinology, Metabolism, and Nutrition,
Northwestern University Medical School,
Chicago, Illinois

PLENUM MEDICAL BOOK COMPANY
NEW YORK AND LONDON

Library of Congress Cataloging in Publication Data

Main entry under title:

The year in metabolism, 1976.

  Includes bibliographies and index.
  1. Metabolism, Disorders of. 2. Metabolism.
I. Freinkel, Norbert. [DNLM: 1. Metabolism—Period. W1 YE41]
RC627.54.Y4   616.3'9   76-44885
ISBN 978-1-4684-7658-3   ISBN 978-1-4684-7656-9 (eBook)
DOI 10.1007/978-1-4684-7656-9

© 1976 Plenum Publishing Corporation
Softcover reprint of the hardcover 1st edition 1976

227 West 17th Street, New York, N. Y. 10011

Plenum Medical Book Company is an imprint of Plenum Publishing Corporation

Contributors

G. D. Aurbach, M.D.
Chief, Metabolic Diseases Branch, National Institute of Arthritis, Metabolism, and Digestive Diseases, National Institutes of Health, Bethesda, Maryland 20014

Louis V. Avioli, M.D.
Shoenberg Professor of Medicine; Director, Division of Bone and Mineral Metabolism, Washington University School of Medicine, St. Louis, Missouri 63110

Stefan S. Fajans, M.D.
Professor of Internal Medicine;

Head, Division of Endocrinology and Metabolism; Director, Metabolism Research Unit, The University of Michigan, Ann Arbor, Michigan 48109

Philip Felig, M.D.
Professor and Vice Chairman, Department of Internal Medicine; Chief, Section of Endocrinology, Yale University School of Medicine, New Haven, Connecticut 06510

DeWitt S. Goodman, M.D.
Tilden-Weger-Bieler Professor,

Department of Medicine, College
of Physicians and Surgeons of
Columbia University, New York,
New York 10032

Jules Hirsch, M.D.
Professor and Senior Physician;
Chairman, Department of Human
Behavior and Metabolism, Rocke-
feller University, New York, New
York 10021

Charles S. Lieber, M.D.
Chief, Section of Liver Disease and
Nutrition, Veterans Administra-
tion Hospital, Bronx, New York
10468; Professor of Medicine and
Pathology, Mount Sinai School of
Medicine of the City University of
New York, New York, New York
10029

Leon E. Rosenberg, M.D.
Professor and Chairman, Department of Human Genetics, Yale
University, New Haven, Connecticut 06510

Bruce S. Schneider, M.D.
Assistant Professor, Rockefeller
University; Associate Physician,
Rockefeller University Hospital,
New York, New York 10021

J. Edwin Seegmiller, M.D.
Professor of Medicine, The
University of California San
Diego, La Jolla, California

Kay Tanaka, M.D.
Senior Research Scientist, Depart-
ment of Human Genetics, Yale
University School of Medicine,
New Haven, Connecticut 06510

Roger H. Unger, M.D.
Professor of Internal Medicine,
University of Texas Southwestern
Medical School; Veterans Admin-
istration Hospital, Dallas, Texas
75216

Hibbard E. Williams, M.D.
Professor of Medicine and Vice
Chairman, Department of Medi-
cine, University of California, San
Francisco; Chief, Medical Service,
San Francisco General Hospital,
San Francisco, California

Myron Winick, M.D.
R. R. Williams Professor of Nutri-
tion; Professor of Pediatrics;
Director, Institute of Human
Nutrition, College of Physicians
and Surgeons of Columbia
University, New York, New York
10032

Preface

It is unclear, and really no longer relevant, whether the information explosion that we now contend with has been fostered by the growth of specialization and subspecialization in medicine, or vice versa. What is clear is that the two are mutually supportive and constitute what would be in endocrine parlance a short-loop positive feedback system. As a result, for most areas of medicine, even the subspecialist in that area has a problem in maintaining currency, the more general specialist has substantial difficulty in doing so, and the generalist is tempted to abandon the effort altogether.

Nevertheless, for all, both the internal pressures of conscience and self-esteem and the external pressures generated by peer review, recertification, and subspecialty boards create the need for continuous self-education. We are, therefore, in an era in which the means of dissemination of new information deserves as much creative attention as does its acquisition.

Because of the complexity of their underlying physiology and biochemistry and the diversity of disease entities that they encompass, the
fields of endocrinology and metabolism have been prone to subspecialization as much as or more than any others. To meet the problems attendant
upon this fact, two major approaches, apart from traditional journals and
textbooks, have been developed; both generally appear on an annual
basis. In the first, abstracts of the preceding year's key papers in a given
area are presented. What this format gains in detail and comprehensive-
ness, it necessarily gives up with respect to integration, despite accompanying insightful editorial comment. Another type of annual publication
presents authoritative, in-depth reviews of selected topics within one or
more specialty or subspecialty areas. What this format gains in compre-
hensiveness and integration, it necessarily loses in breadth of subject
matter.

The present companion volumes, *The Year in Metabolism* and *The Year
in Endocrinology*, reflect our effort to approach the problem of information
acquisition in these fields, and to bridge the gap between the foregoing
types of annual publication, in a still different manner. In our idealized
vision, they would represent a transposition into the written word of what
might have been the content of several evenings' discussion of each topic
with an acknowledged authority in that area, who would, in a relaxed and
relaxing manner, describe what has appeared in the field during the past
year that he or she considers important, why it is important, how it relates
to what has gone before, and how it might influence what will come in the
future. Although we hope that these volumes can be turned to by readers
who are seeking a particular recent reference or a discussion of a highly
specific topic, our principal aim is to provide a source that readers would
turn to with the thought that an evening's reading of a particular chapter
would provide them with a quite comprehensive, integrated overview of
recent findings and trends within that topic area.

Most authors have accepted five-year appointments to the Editorial
Board. Such continuity should not only permit comprehensive coverage
in succeeding years of any aspects that have been slighted in a single year,
but should also facilitate the kind of fine-tuning of the product from year
to year that would increase its value and interest. Most importantly, the
continuity of authorship should maximize the likelihood that the faithful
reader will, over time, come to perceive the implicit or explicit philosophi-
cal approach of each author to his field. In a few cases, where it appears
appropriate, pairs of topics will be covered every other year in an alternat-
ing manner. Moreover, the intention is to include, when appropriate, a
special chapter on some subject of broad general interest and immediacy.

Idealized visions never come entirely to pass, particularly in the early
efforts to bring them to fruition, and we recognize that this is true of both

volumes in this new series, since errors of both omission and commission have quite clearly occurred. It is our hope that these "teething troubles" will diminish and disappear as the series gains maturity. The Editors also hope that the series will achieve its own popularity, without encroaching upon the deserved popularity of existing publications. It is our desire instead that *The Year in Metabolism* and *The Year in Endocrinology* provide an efficient and enjoyable bridge between those who are creating new knowledge at the bench or at the bedside and the professional consciousness of those for whom such knowledge is ultimately intended.

Sidney H. Ingbar, M.D.
Norbert Freinkel, M.D.

Contents

Chapter 1
Hormone Receptors, Cyclic Nucleotides, and Control of Cell Function
G. D. Aurbach

Chapter 2
Diabetes Mellitus
Stefan S. Fajans

Chapter 3
Glucagon
Roger H. Unger

Chapter 4
Recent Developments in Body Fuel Metabolism
Philip Felig

Chapter 5
Recent Endocrine and Metabolic Investigations Relevant to Obesity
Jules Hirsch and Bruce S. Schneider

Chapter 6
Disorders of Lipid and Lipoprotein Metabolism
DeWitt S. Goodman

Chapter 7
Metabolism of Amino Acids and Organic Acids
Leon E. Rosenberg and Kay Tanaka

Chapter 8
Disorders of Purine and Pyrimidine Metabolism
J. Edwin Seegmiller

Chapter 9
What's New—Vitamins and Minerals
Louis V. Avioli

Chapter 10
Nutrition, Growth, and Development
Myron Winick

Chapter 11
Metabolic Aspects of Renal Stone Disease
Hibbard E. Williams

Chapter 12
Metabolism and Metabolic Actions of Ethanol
Charles S. Lieber

Hormone Receptors, Cyclic Nucleotides, and Control of Cell Function

G. D. Aurbach

1.1. Introduction

It is now widely recognized that many polypeptide or amine hormones and neurotransmitters act through the intermediation of cyclic 3',5'-adenosine monophosphate (cAMP). These agonists bind to specific receptors at the outer surface or plasma membrane of the cell and, through a mechanism still under study, activate the enzyme adenylate cyclase, which catalyzes the formation of cAMP from ATP. The cAMP generated as a consequence becomes the "second messenger" that interacts with cyclic nucleotide receptors regulating intracellular enzymes that ultimately account for the physiological response. The concentration of cyclic nucleotides in cells can be regulated not only through biosynthesis, but also by enzymatic destruction (cyclic nucleotide phosphodiesterases) or elaboration into the extracellular space.

G. D. AURBACH • Metabolic Diseases Branch, National Institute of Arthritis, Metabolism, and Digestive Diseases, National Institutes of Health, Bethesda, Maryland 20014.

This type of mechanism, mediated by cell membrane-receptor and cyclic nucleotide, as well as phenomena in the cell regulated by cyclic guanylate, prostaglandin, and metal ion (calcium), are the subjects to be reviewed under this general heading in this volume and subsequent volumes of *The Year in Metabolism*. The plan is to emphasize particular areas of immediate interface with clinical medicine and topics of especially current interest. Obviously, it will not be possible to summarize more than a fraction of the field in any one volume. This limitation necessitates arbitrary restrictions on the scope of each year's presentation and on the completeness of literature citation. Nevertheless, the goal is to keep the reader apprised of research potentially relevant to clinical investigation. It is expected that related topics currently omitted from discussion will be reviewed in later volumes.

During the past year, significant advances have been made in the area of opiate receptors and β-adrenergic receptors, and in understanding a phenomenon that leads to a new concept of "immunopathic receptor disorders." In addition, further knowledge has been developed concerning the biochemistry of the adenylate cyclase reaction and how it relates to the actions of certain bacterial toxins and choleratoxin in particular. These topics, as well as receptor interactions of certain peptide hormones and the physiological and clinical significance of cyclic nucleotides in the extracellular fluids, are discussed in this chapter.

1.2. Receptor Systems

1.2.1. General Regulatory Mechanisms and Kinetics

Given a system dependent on ligand–receptor interaction and the premise that activity is proportional to receptor occupancy ($[HR]$ in the reaction below), then a change in any function—affinity (K), ligand (hormone, neurotransmitter, or drug) concentration ($[H]$), or total number of receptors (R_o)—will cause a change in response or activity:

$$[HR] = \frac{[R_0][H]}{1/K + [H]}$$

This reaction represents the simplest case in which response is directly coupled to $[HR]$; $[H]$ is the free-ligand (hormone) concentration; $[R_o]$ is the total receptor concentration. Whenever coupling is nonlinear, for example, with "spare receptors" (Stephenson, 1956) or negative or positive cooperativity (De Meyts *et al.*, 1973; Atkinson, 1965), a change in receptor number or affinity will not necessarily cause a proportional linear change in response. We can classify regulatory influences on receptors as acute or rapid versus slow. Regulation can obviously be exerted by change in affinity or change in number, and such alterations can be brought about by physiological influences or by pathophysiological processes.

1.2.1.1. Physiological Regulation of Receptors

One form of acute change in receptor function is effected by "negative cooperativity" (De Meyts, 1975). In this instance, rapid control is brought about by occupancy of the first few receptors. As more and more sites are filled, there is a progressive decrease in affinity of the receptors remaining unfilled.

Another type of regulation discovered by Roth and his associates (Roth *et al.*, 1975) is longer term and involves ligand regulation of receptor concentration ("down regulation"). It seems possible that this phenomenon may be fairly general. Exposure of receptor-bearing cells to a high concentration of hormone causes, within hours, a decrease in the number of receptors per cell. Monocytes bear insulin receptors, and incubation of human lymphocytes *in vitro* with insulin caused a loss in number of receptors per cell (Fig. 1). The magnitude and rate of loss of

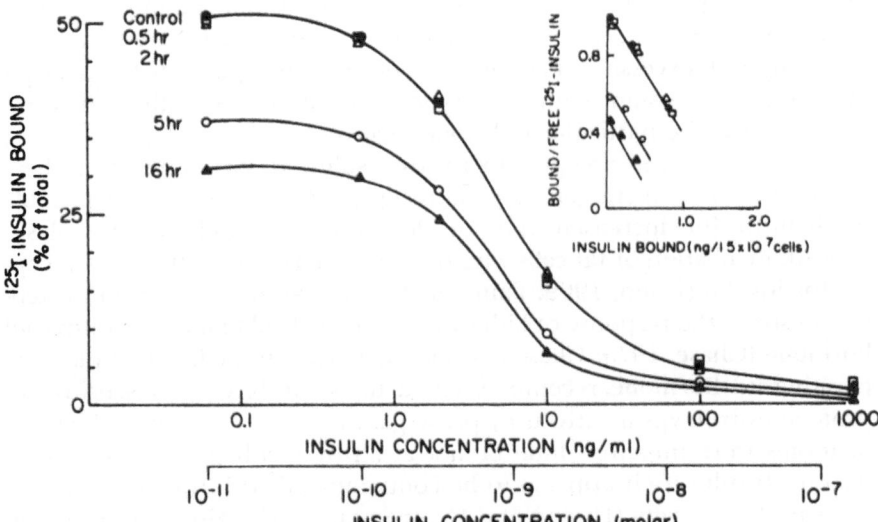

Fig. 1. Regulation of receptor number by hormone. Receptors were lost from lymphocytes cultured with insulin added at concentrations shown in tissue culture for 16 hr. At the end of incubation, cells showed a reduction in the number of receptors per cell; the degree of receptor loss was a function of the concentration of insulin added. (From Roth *et al.*, 1975, with permission.)

receptors were related to the insulin concentration in the medium. Removal of insulin from the medium allowed restoration of receptors, so that by 24 hr, the number of receptors per cell had reached a number comparable to that found before incubation with insulin. Inhibitors of protein synthesis impaired the reappearance of receptors on the cells. This experiment and other experiments indicated that the effect of insulin on receptor loss was mediated by destruction, not inhibition, of receptor synthesis. Similar types of regulatory phenomena have been observed with growth hormone, TRH, and catecholamines. IM-9 lymphocytes showed a 30% loss of growth-hormone receptors by 6 hr when incubated at 37°C with as little as 10^{-10} M growth hormone (Roth et al., 1975). As with insulin receptors, removal of ligand from the medium allowed resynthesis of receptors. Hinkle and Tashjian (1975) have observed loss of TRH receptor function on GH_3 cells incubated with TRH. Recently, it has been shown both in vivo and in vitro that β-adrenergic receptors on frog erythrocytes can be regulated by concentration of catecholamines (Mukherjee et al., 1975a; Mickey et al., 1975). It is also likely that β-receptors in the pineal gland are regulated by a similar mechanism (see Section 1.2.3). Roth (Roth et al., 1975) has pointed out that this type of mechanism might account for clinical states of resistance to growth hormone (acromegaly or the newborn) or to insulin (obesity). It will clearly be of importance to determine whether similar regulatory phenomena apply in other hormone-resistant states, including secondary hyperparathyroidism, pseudohypoparathyroidism, medullary carcinoma of the thyroid (excessive calcitonin secretion), nephrogenic diabetes insipidus, or other resistant endocrine syndromes associated with high secretory rates for the particular hormone involved.

Ligand-induced receptor loss with insulin, at least, appears to be a manifestation of increased rate of receptor degradation. One possible mechanism for increased rate of degradation would be proteolysis. Indeed, incubation of fat cells with trypsin apparently destroys the receptor for insulin (Kono, 1969; Fain and Loken, 1969), and trypsin proteolysis destroys the response of kidney tissue or skeletal tissue to parathyroid hormone (Chase, 1975; Chase and Obert, 1975). In the latter studies, the parathyroid hormone receptor seemed to be preferentially sensitive to proteolysis by trypsin. Effects of prostaglandins or calcitonin in the same materials were impaired little or not at all by incubation of tissue with trypsin. Insulin itself appears to be contaminated with trace amounts of protease-like activity (Huang and Cuatrecasas, 1975). However, pharmacological concentrations of insulin (approximately 1000 times the amount needed to reduce receptors in lymphocytes) were required to demonstrate proteolytic activity.

1.2.2. Opiate Receptors

Recent investigations are leading to exciting new concepts concerning the mechanism of action of opiates. Several laboratories have developed radioreceptor assays for opiates (Lowney *et al.*, 1974; Goldstein *et al.*, 1971; Pert and Synder, 1973; Simon *et al.*, 1973; Terenius, 1973; Lee *et al.*, 1973). Tritiated ligands (usually tritiated naloxone, dextrorphan, or etorphine) bind to the receptor with stereospecificity characteristic of biological properties of the opiates. In addition, evidence has accumulated that the actions of the opiates control cyclic nucleotide concentrations through interaction with the receptors identified with tritiated ligands. Even more exciting have been the reports that there are endogenous peptides in neural tissues, and possibly in other tissues, capable of interacting specifically with the opiate receptors found in brain, vas deferens, or ileum. Perhaps most provocative is the potential general corollary that many if not all drugs produced artificially or derived from plants and interacting with specific tissue receptors have physiological counterparts, yet to be identified, biosynthesized *in vivo* to act at precisely the same receptors that are influenced by exogenous administration of drugs.

Klee and co-workers (Klee and Nirenberg, 1974; Klee *et al.*, 1975; Sharma *et al.*, 1975a,b) have found morphine receptors on neuroblastoma X glioma hybrid cells. The concentration of receptors in the hybrid cells was much higher than the concentration found in either of the parent strains (indeed, the glioma parent contained no detectable receptors). The receptors identified on the hybrid cells with either [^{3}H]dihydromorphine or [^{3}H]naloxone were stereospecific and discriminated for the active levorotatory forms of morphine congeners. The cell hybrids also contained adenylate cyclase that was inhibitable by opiate drugs. Collier and Roy (1974) and Collier and Francis (1975) had found that morphine inhibits formation of cAMP in the brain, and that a morphine-abstinence syndrome in rats is associated with increase in brain cAMP content. A similar type of phenomenon has been observed with the hybrid cell lines *in vitro* (Klee *et al.*, 1975; Sharma *et al.*, 1975a,b). Morphine added to homogenates of hybrid cells caused inhibition of basal adenylate cyclase as well as of PGE$_1$-stimulated adenylate cyclase. The inhibition was overcome by adding naloxone. Of particular interest is that the hybrid cells cultured for several days in media containing morphine developed a biochemical change analogous to that seen in morphine-abstinence syndrome in the rat. The cells became "tolerant," in that adenylate cyclase activity increased to normal concentrations, and the cells were "dependent" on morphine, in that adenylate cyclase activity in the absence of opiate was abnormally high. In fact, addition of the opiate-receptor antagonist naloxone further increased the basal adenylate cyclase activity of "addicted" cells and dramatically enhanced the stimulation of adenylate cyclase by PGE_1. Development of "tolerance" analogous to the addicted state *in vivo* was associated with enhanced adenylate cyclase activity and increased production of cyclic AMP. The enhanced activity was stimulated even further by the narcotic antagonist naloxone, which induced the withdrawal syndrome. These changes in cells cultured *in vitro* are similar to findings on morphine-dependent animals *in vivo*. One report indicates that morphine increases cGMP concentrations in neuroblastoma glioma hybrid cells (Gullis *et al.*, 1975).

1.2.2.1. Endogenous Peptides Active at the Opiate Receptor

Several groups of investigators have raised the possibility that there is an endogenous neurotransmitter substance that acts as the natural ligand interacting with opiate receptors *in vivo*. Hughes (1975) prepared extracts of brains from pigs as well as laboratory animals, and tested them on preparations of guinea pig myenteric plexus or mouse vas deferens. The extracts contained a substance that inhibited contraction of these preparations in a fashion similar to the action of morphine. Moreover, the effects of the extract, like those of morphine, were specifically inhibited by naloxone. The chemical and physical properties of the substances suggested that it was of low molecular weight, possibly less than 700 daltons, and was probably peptide in nature. They also found that the distribution of this peptide in brain generally paralleled the distribution of morphine-receptor sites. Terenius and Wahlström (1975) similarly found that extracts of brain contain peptidelike material that inhibited binding to the opiate receptor in plasma membrane fractions of rat brain as well as guinea pig ileum. The active fraction seemed to have a molecular weight in the 1000–1200 dalton range. Pasternak *et al.* (1975) also found in rat and calf brain a morphinelike substance with a regional distribution analogous to that found for opiate receptors. Their assay was based on inhibition by morphinomimetic peptide of the specific binding of tritiated naloxone or tritiated dihydromorphine. They also observed that sodium ion, which reduces opiate-receptor binding, markedly decreases the ability of the morphinomimetic peptide fraction to inhibit binding of tritiated naloxone. Active extracts are found not only in the brain, but also in the pituitary. Teschemacher *et al.* (1975) and Cox *et al.* (1975) have isolated a peptide fraction from bovine pituitary glands that is bioactive on the myenteric plexus and also on opiate receptors, as determined by naloxone binding. They also found that the pituitary peptide fraction showed

Tyr · Gly · Gly · Phe · Met

Methionine Enkephalin

Tyr · Gly · Gly · Phe · Leu

Leucine Enkephalin

Fig. 2. Structures of methionine and leucine enkephalin.

reduced receptor activity in the presence of sodium—again, as is characteristic of opiate receptors.

A significant advance has been made recently by Hughes and his collaborators (Hughes *et al.*, 1975), who have determined the structure of enkephalin, the morphinomimetic fraction they extracted from brain. From this extract, they purified two pentapeptides that differ only in the C-terminal amino acid (Fig. 2); these peptides were called *methionine enkephalin* and *leucine enkephalin*. Methionine enkephalin was 2–5 times as potent as leucine enkephalin, and was at least 3 times more potent than morphine in inhibiting binding of tritiated naloxone to receptors in brain homogenates. Both peptides were active in inhibiting contractions of mouse vas deferens and guinea pig ileum. It is of interest that methionine enkephalin represents residues 61–65 in β-lipoprotein, a peptide found in pituitary extracts and related structurally to β-MSH and ACTH. It is of particular interest that Goldstein and his colleagues (Teschemacher *et al.*, 1975; Cox *et al.*, 1975) have found morphinomimetic peptide material in bovine pituitary and crude ACTH preparations. The exact relationship between the enkephalins and the peptides in the pituitary is yet to be established, although the latter appear to be somewhat higher in molecular weight (Teschemacher *et al.*, 1975).

The remarkable identification and isolation of natural peptides interacting with opiate receptors are obviously significant for the entire field of drug-receptor mechanisms, pharmacology, and therapeutics. This work will undoubtedly prompt a search for endogenous factors that might interact with any number of drug receptors. Peptides, as naturally occurring endogenous regulators, also provide the biological advantage of better control of receptor activation, since they can be rapidly degraded by peptidases. Further work will undoubtedly allow comparisons of the kinetics of morphine analogues and morphinomimetic peptides with the kinetics of receptors.

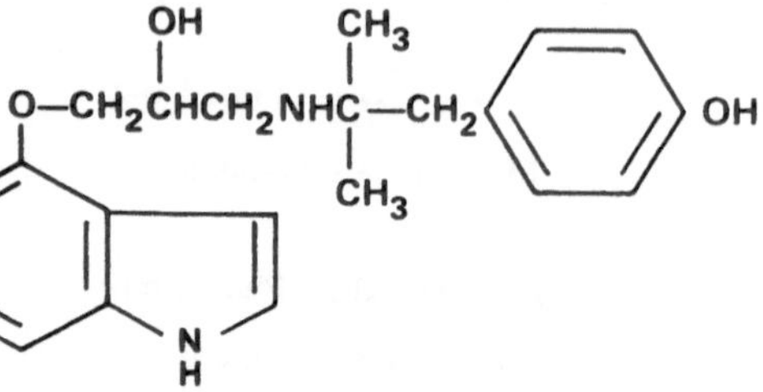

Hydroxybenzylpindolol

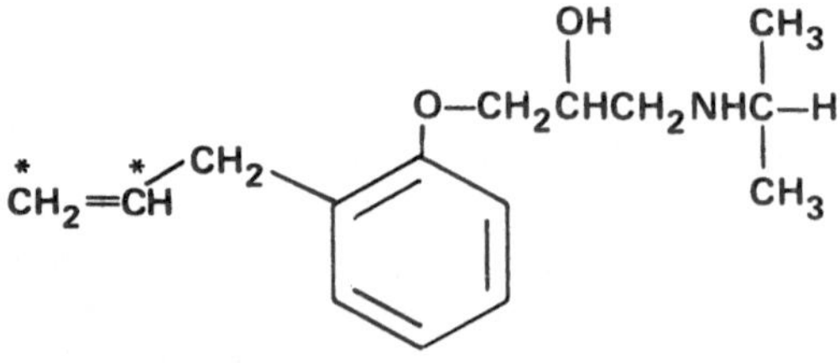

Alprenolol

Fig. 3. Structures of the β-adrenergic ligands hydroxybenzylpindolol and alprenolol. Alprenolol is available as [³H] alprenolol (*represents site of tritiation), specific activity 20–50 Ci/mmole. Hydroxybenzylpindolol can be iodinated to give [¹²⁵I] hydroxybenzyl-pindolol, specific activity 2200 Ci/mmole.

1.2.3. β-Adrenergic Receptors

The original studies of Sutherland and his co-workers (see Robison *et al.*, 1971, for a review) established that β-adrenergic catecholamines act through the intermediation of cAMP, and that interaction of catecholamines with β-receptors causes activation of the enzyme adenylate cyclase. During the past year, several groups have developed methods that allow direct identification of β-adrenergic receptors by radioligand binding. The radioactive ligands used were tritiated propranolol (Atlas *et al.*, 1974; Levitzki *et al.*, 1974), tritiated alprenolol (Lefkowitz *et al.*, 1974), and iodinated hydroxybenzylpindolol (Aurbach *et al.*, 1974). The structures of alprenolol and hydroxybenzylpindolol are shown in Fig. 3. In each of these four studies, receptor binding activity proved specific for the characteristic features of β-adrenergic receptors: (1) the response was stereospecific, with levorotatory (−)agonists the most potent by 1–2 orders of magnitude. (2) Interaction with the receptor was specifically blocked by β-adrenergic antagonists, and not by α-adrenergic blockers. (3) The order of potency of series of agonists in competing for ligand at the receptor site paralleled the potency of these agonists in activating adenylate cyclase. (4) Receptor interactions were characteristic of either β_1 or β_2 subclassifications according to the scheme of Lands *et al.* (1967). Both β_1- and β_2-type adrenergic receptors are most sensitive to isoproterenol; β_1 receptors respond about equally well to norepinephrine and epinephrine. β_2 receptors, however, are characteristically more sensitive to epinephrine than to norepinephrine. The turkey erythrocyte shows β_1-type responsiveness (the apparent affinities of epinephrine and norepinephrine are the same) in terms of adenylate cyclase activation and cAMP generation; comparative binding studies using iodohydroxybenzylpindolol as ligand also provide virtually identical affinity constants for epinephrine and norepinephrine for the receptor. The frog erythrocyte, on the other hand (Mukherjee *et al.*, 1975a,b), displays the β_2-type receptor, as is evident from both adenylate cyclase activation studies and direct receptor-binding studies. Lung and bronchial tissues are characteristically β_2-type (Lands *et al.*, 1967) and similarly display β_2 characteristics in terms of receptor binding and adenylate cyclase activity (Brown, Marx, and Aurbach, unpublished data). Alexander *et al.* (1975b) have also identified β-adrenergic receptors in cardiac tissue. This study may represent one exception, in that the heart is characteristically considered β_1-type in character (Lands *et al.*, 1967); yet Alexander *et al.* (1975b), in their studies, found epinephrine to be considerably more potent than norepinephrine on their cardiac β-receptor preparation. This apparent discrepancy remains to be explained. β-Receptors have also been identified in brain (Alexander *et al.*, 1975a), lymphocytes (Williams *et al.*, 1976), and rat reticulocytes (Spiegel *et al.*, 1975).

Recently, Maguire *et al.* (1976) have studied the β-adrenergic receptor in rat glioma cells and related cell clones in tissue culture. They used iodinated hydroxybenzylpindolol, and found a binding constant for this ligand of 250 pM, with approximately 4000 receptor sites/cell; k_1 (the forward reaction rate constant) was $10^8\,M^{-1}$ per min. The dissociation rate constant was 0.017/min. Brown *et al.* (1976a,b) have carried out extensive analyses of the chemical and kinetic properties of [^{125}I]hydroxybenzylpindolol. Hydroxybenzylpindolol is a high-affinity β-adrenergic blocker bearing a phenolic group that can be radioiodinated to high specific activities. Binding of this ligand to turkey cell membranes shows every aspect of specificity characteristic of the β-receptor. The structure of iodohydroxybenzylpindolol has been established by mass spectroscopy, and the kinetics of interaction of the ligand with the β-receptor on turkey erythrocytes have been studied in detail (Brown *et al.*, 1976a). The monoiodinated hydroxybenzylpindolol (the location of the iodine was established as being on the phenolic group) binds rapidly to the receptor and shows an affinity of $5\times10^{10}\,M^{-1}$. Competitive inhibition by agonists or antagonists of ligand binding directly paralleled biological effectiveness (Fig. 4). Interaction of the ligand with the receptor showed linear Scatchard plots, gave no evidence for negative cooperativity, indicated a single stereospecific site for interaction with the receptor, and on dilution dissociated rapidly (half-life approximately 3 min) from the receptor on turkey erythrocyte membranes. Formal analysis of kinetic studies with computer programs accounting for exact solution of differential equations involved gave constants in excellent agreement with the equilibrium constant and dissociation rate constants determined experimentally (Brown et al., 1976a). At 37°C, k_1 (the forward reaction rate constant) was 9×10^8/sec; k_2 was 0.009/sec.

All groups have found an extremely close correlation between binding constants for inhibitors, as determined by analysis of competitive inhibition of binding of radioactive ligand to receptor, and inhibition constants (K_i) for inhibition of catecholamine-stimulated adenylate cyclase (Mukherjee et al., 1975a,b; Atlas et al., 1974; Maguire et al., 1976; Brown et al., 1976b). Agonists, however, show up to a 10-fold difference between K_D (dissociation constant for inhibition of ligand binding) and apparent affinity in activating adenylate cyclase in membrane preparations. This difference is virtually abolished with turkey erythrocyte membranes by adding guanylylimidodiphosphate (see Section 1.3.2). This guanine nucleotide does not affect binding of agonists or antagonists in the turkey erythrocyte, but does enhance the degree of adenylate cyclase activation for any given amount of agonist bound. It is thus possible that in vivo there is a nucleotide subserving the same function as added guanylylimidodiphosphate in vitro. Indeed Brown et al. (1976) have shown that intact turkey erythrocytes incubated in vitro show apparent affinity constants for agonists in producing cAMP in intact cells that are identical to apparent affinities for activating cyclase from the membranes of the same cell when guanylylimidodiphosphate is included. It is implied, then, that in preparing membranes from intact cells, a component of the system that regulates adenylate cyclase (a component involving a nucleotide, possibly GTP) is lost, and that addition of guanylylimidodiphosphate effectively replaces this lost function. There is no loss of receptors. Membrane preparations show receptor numbers compatible with complete recovery of sites from the intact cell.

1.2.3.1. Regulation of β-Adrenergic Receptors

Negative cooperativity may be a control mechanism influencing β-adrenergic receptors in frog erythrocytes (Limbird et al., 1975). This mechanism is not found, however, in the high-affinity turkey erythrocyte system (Brown et al., 1976a). The latter study suggests that negative

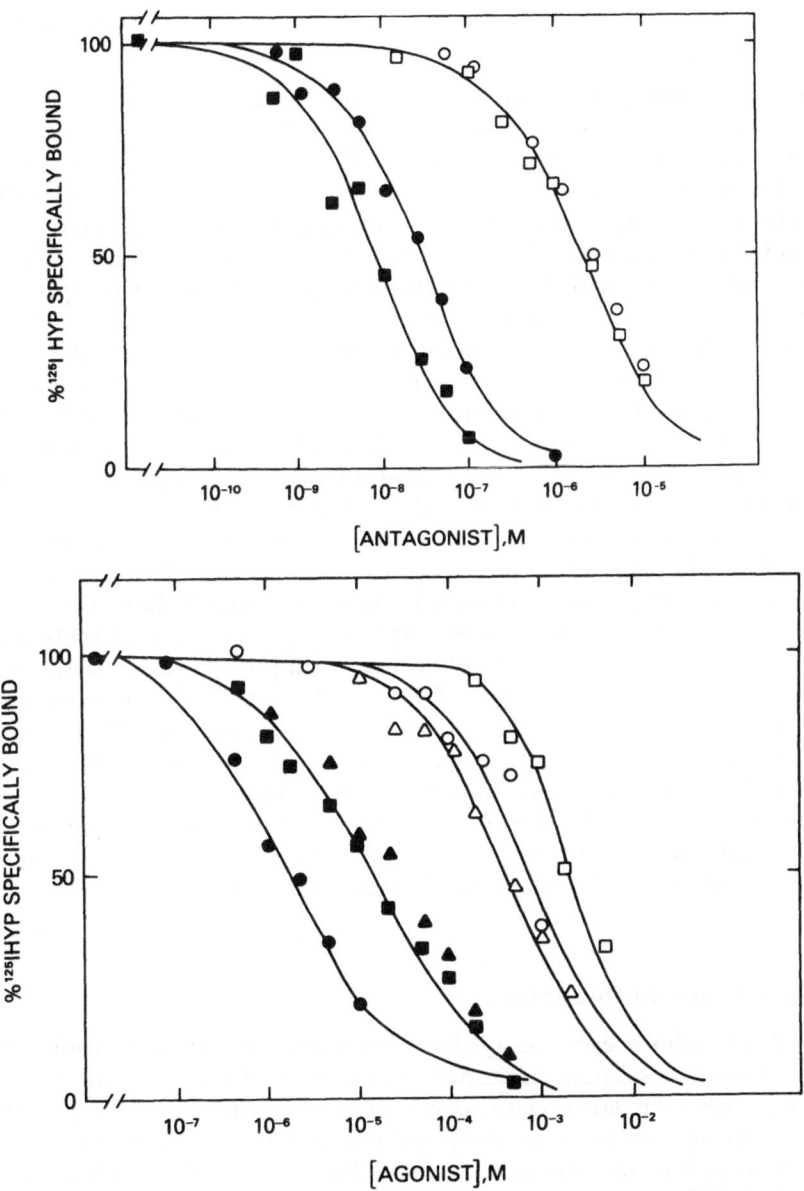

Fig. 4. Stereospecific interaction of β-adrenergic blockers (A) or agonists (B) with adrenergic receptor on turkey erythrocyte membranes. Levorotatory antipodes (solid symbols) are biologically the most active *in vivo,* as well as in interaction with receptor, represented here as inhibition of binding of specific ligand ^{125}I hydroxybenzylpindolol to receptor site. (A) (−)Propranol (solid squares) and (−)alprenolol (solid circles) are 100-fold more potent inhibitors of receptor–ligand complex than are the corresponding (+) antipodes (open symbols) of the same compounds. (B) Agonists isoproterenol (circles), epinephrine (triangles), and norepinephrine (squares) show orders of potency characteristic of β_1-type adrenergic receptor. Levorotatory antipodes (solid symbols) are 100-fold more potent than dextrorotatory antipodes (open symbols). (From Brown *et al.,* 1976b.)

cooperative interactions are not functions necessary for the biological properties of β-adrenergic receptors. On the other hand, there appear to be important physiological control mechanisms brought about through regulation of β-adrenergic receptors. One group (Mickey *et al.*, 1975; Mukherjee *et al.*, 1975b) has shown that catecholamines injected *in vivo* or added *in vitro* cause a decrease in the sensitivity of adenylate cyclase in frog erythrocytes, and this "subsensitivity" parallels loss of receptor sites from the cells. Only agonists were capable of producing this loss of receptors. Another very interesting report (Romero *et al.*, 1975) indicates that the normal diurnal light cycle in rats induces a change in β-adrenergic receptors in the rat pineal gland. It had been known that at the onset of darkness, there is an increased release of norepinephrine from synthetic nerves that induces a 30- to 50-fold increase in N-acetyltransferase of the rat pineal gland. Moreover, the sensitivity of pineal gland adenylate cyclase to stimulation with isoproterenol is maximal at the end of a long period of light exposure. With darkness, there is a progressive decrease in sensitivity of the pineal receptors. Romero *et al.* (1975) have now shown that this diurnal variation in sensitivity to isoproterenol correlates to a very high degree with the numbers of receptors on pineal cells, as determined by tritiated alprenolol binding (Fig. 5). The mechanism is presumably analogous to the regulatory phenomenon reported by Mickey *et al.* (1975); that is, high concentrations of endogenous catecholamine (associated with darkness in the rat) cause a decrease in the number of receptors on the pineal cell. With the onset of light exposure, there is a decrease in circulating norepinephrine released from sympathetic nerves, allowing an increased number (?biosynthesis) of receptors on the pineal cells.

1.2.4. Calcitonin Receptors

Valid radioreceptor assays have been developed for calcitonin utilizing ^{125}I-labeled salmon calcitonin (Marx *et al.*, 1972; Ardaillou, 1975). Studies with adenylate cyclase activation or receptor-binding analysis show that calcitonin receptors are concentrated in the region (corticomedullary junction) rich in sodium–potassium ATPase, a locus distinct from either parathyroid hormone or vasopressin receptors. Calcitonin-sensitive adenylate cyclase and calcitonin receptors show the same distribution anatomically and on sucrose-gradient centrifugation of plasma membranes; both functions are sensitive to inactivation by low concentrations of the nonionic detergent Lubrol PX (Marx and Aurbach, 1975). Fluoride-sensitive adenylate cyclase was stable to concentrations of detergent that abolished the sensitivity of adenylate cyclase to calcitonin. The same detergent was

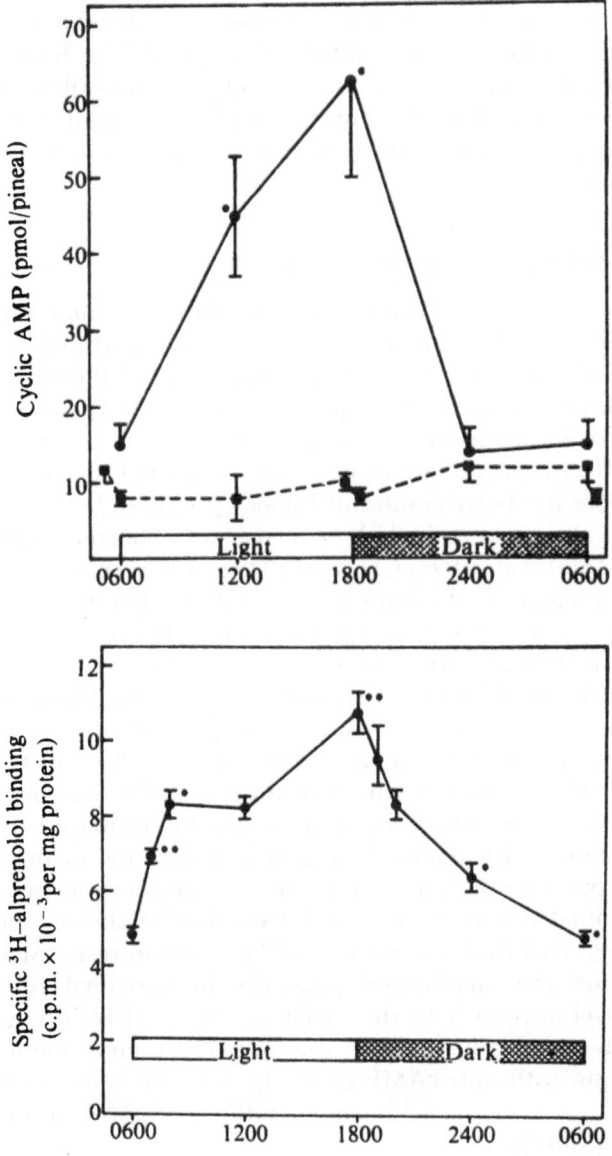

Fig. 5. Diurnal change in pineal β-adrenergic receptors regulated by light. (A) At times indicated, rats were injected with saline (dashed line) or isoproterenol (solid line), 5 mg/kg, and the AMP content was determined on pineal glands removed 10 min later. (B) Receptor binding of pineal glands taken under the same conditions as in A. (From Romero *et al.*, 1975, with permission.)

used at higher concentrations to partially solubilize adenylate cyclase from
pig kidney; the solubilized enzyme was stimulated by high concentrations
(10 μM) of porcine calcitonin (Queener et al., 1975). Solubilization of
calcitonin-sensitive activity was dependent on preincubation of membranes with sodium fluoride. Further studies on ligand specificity and
solubility properties are needed before this preparation can be fully
characterized.

1.2.5. Parathyroid Hormone Receptors

The problem of developing a physiologically valid radioreceptor
assay for parathyroid hormone (see Aurbach and Heath, 1974; Heath and
Aurbach, 1975) has never been satisfactorily solved. Although a number of
groups have attempted to develop valid binding assays, none has shown
complete biological specificity with putative receptor activity paralleling
biological effectiveness of analogues, strict hormonal specificity, and high
affinity. There has been significant further progress, however, in localizing anatomical regions in the kidney responsive to hormonal ligands. One
approach (Morel et al., 1975; Chabardès et al., 1975b) utilized microdissec-
tion of serial segments along the rabbit nephron. Parathyroid hormone–
sensitive adenylate cyclase was present in the early proximal tubule and at
another distinct locus, although less active, in the distal tubule (Fig. 6).
Conversely, vasopressin-sensitive adenylate cyclase was localized in medullary collecting tubules (Imbert et al., 1975). Catecholamine-sensitive adenylate cyclase was localized in the distal cortical collecting tubule (Chabardès et al., 1975a). The proximal locus for parathyroid hormone action
fits well with knowledge concerning the locus of parathyroid action gained
from several other disciplines. Agus et al. (1971) found by micropuncture
studies that parathyroid hormone influences ion transport predominantly
in the proximal tubule. Scurry and Pauk (1974) showed by stop-flow
studies in dogs that the increase in cAMP in urine in response to parathyroid hormone was manifested primarily in proximal tubular fluid.
Another novel approach to the problem was used by Chase (personal
communication), who has utilized the indirect Coombs' immunofluorescent technique with anti cAMP antibody. His preliminary experiments
also indicate that parathyroid hormone influences cAMP accumulation in
the proximal tubular cells.

Another set of investigations has been carried out to determine the
cytological localization of receptors for hormonal ligands as well as for
cAMP itself. Wilfong and Neville (1970) developed a method for preparing isolated brush border membranes from rat kidney. They showed that
parathyroid hormone–sensitive adenylate cyclase was not concentrated in

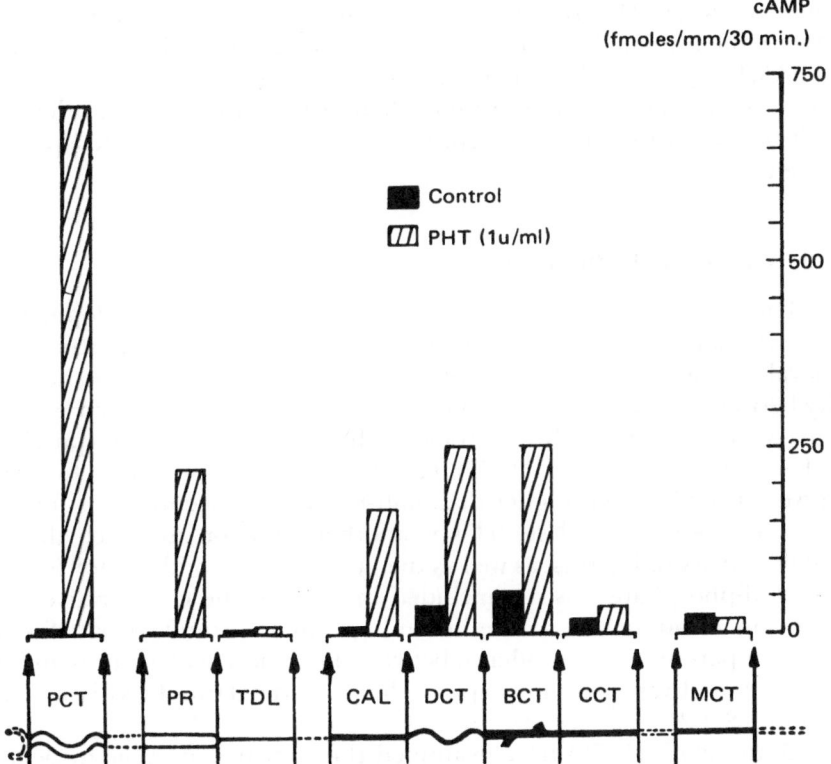

Fig. 6. Localization of parathyroid hormone–sensitive adenylate cyclase in nephron of rabbit. Adenylate cyclase activity with (hatched bars) or without (control, solid bars) addition of parathyroid hormone in kidney tubule segments: (PCT) proximal tubule; (TDL) thin descending limb; (CAL) cortical ascending limb; (DCT) distal collecting tubule; (BCT) branched collecting tubule; (CCT) cortical collecting tubule; (MCT) medullary collecting tubule. (From Chabardès *et al.*, 1975b, with permission.)

the brush border preparation. Shlatz *et al.* (1975) have succeeded in separating basal–lateral membranes from brush border membranes of the rat kidney proximal tubule. They found parathyroid hormone–sensitive adenylate cyclase in the contraluminal (basilar membrane) fraction, whereas the cAMP-dependent protein kinase is located in the luminal border (Kinne, *et al.*, 1975; Insel *et al.*, 1975). The preliminary experiments of Chase (personal communication) also suggest that the cytological localization for production of cAMP (adenylate cyclase) is distinct from the locus within the cell in which the cyclic nucleotide acts. Chase injected rats with either normal saline as a control or parathyroid hormone. Two minutes after injection, the kidney was perfused with formaldehyde, sectioned, and stained by the indirect Coombs' immunofluorescent technique for cAMP. He found a strong immunofluorescent localization of cAMP in the luminal border of proximal tubular cells. It is implied, then, that cAMP is produced in the basilar portion of the proximal tubular cell in response to parathyroid hormone, then diffuses through the cell to the brush border at the luminal surface, where the cAMP-regulated protein kinase exists.

1.2.6. Vasopressin Receptors

The work of Jard and his collaborators has led to the development of tritiated vasopressin and oxytocin analogues for use in binding studies. In general, studies with these compounds have shown considerable nonlinearity between receptor binding and biological function expressed as adenylate cyclase activity. These problems have been reviewed (Jard and Bockaert, 1975; Jard *et al.*, 1975). Half-maximal concentrations for binding were usually much higher than half-maximal concentrations for activation of adenylate cyclase. This is another situation in which the low specific activity of ligands, as well as the guanine nucleotide factor (guanylylimidodiphosphate was not included in most of the comparative measurements of adenylate cyclase in binding), may account in part for the lack of apparent correspondence between biological activity and binding. Localization of vasopressin receptors along the renal tubule is discussed in Section 1.2.4.2.

Dousa *et al.* (1975) have examined the enzymes of cyclic nucleotide metabolism in the renal medulla of rats with hypothalamic diabetes insipidus. The renal cortex response to parathyroid hormone was normal, as was the response of liver adenylate cyclase to glucagon. Medullary adenylate cyclase, on the other hand, was reduced relative to that of heterozygotes. Treatment of homozygotes with pitressin partially corrected the defect. There were no differences between heterozygotes and homozygotes in phosphodiesterase, cytochrome oxidase, or several other marker enzymes; similarly, these marker enzymes were not changed in concentration in homozygotes treated with pitressin. The results suggest that chronic vasopressin deficiency with impaired concentrating ability may further aggravate the metabolic abnormality in the Brattlaboro strain rat.

1.2.7. Insulin, Nonsuppressible Insulinlike Activity, Somatomedin, Nerve Growth Factor, and Epidermal Growth Factor Receptors

Insulin receptors have been detected in many tissues, including adipocytes, liver membranes, circulating leukocytes, thymic leukocytes, lymphoblastic cells cultured *in vitro,* and turkey erythrocytes. Studies on insulin receptors have been reviewed by Kahn and Roth (1975), Roth *et al.* (1975), and Cuatrecasas *et al.* (1975a). In general, receptor interactions in these various preparations show parallel reactivities for a series of insulin congeners as inhibitors of iodo–insulin binding and biological activity (glucose oxidation) in isolated cells *in vitro.* Several groups have studied insulin receptors in hereditary obese (OB-OB) mice, as well as in obese human beings (Soll *et al.,* 1975a,b; Archer *et al.,* 1975; Roth *et al.,* 1975; Chang *et al.,* 1975; Olefsky and Reaven, 1975; Amatruda *et al.,* 1975). These states of obesity are associated with high concentrations of endogenous insulin, and it is apparent that high circulating-insulin concentrations cause a decrease ("down regulation") in insulin receptors on insulin-sensitive tissues. Reduction of circulating-insulin concentrations allows recovery toward normal in the number of receptors on cells from obese man or animal. In man, circulating leukocytes (monocytes in particular, Schwartz *et al.,* 1975) represent a readily available test tissue. The liver cell membrane was the test material for studies with obese mice (Soll *et al.,* 1975a,b). Dietary restriction with weight reduction allowed reduction in circulating-insulin concentrations and an increase in the number of receptors on circulating leukocytes in man (Archer *et al.,* 1975). Kern *et al.* (1975) have also shown that hyperinsulinemia is associated with decreased numbers of liver membrane receptors for insulin in hereditary diabetic mice. All these studies, then, suggest that insulin resistance attendant on hyperinsulinemia is associated with a decrease in numbers (and possibly affinity as well) of receptors from liver. Studies with adipocytes conflict, however. Amatruda and his associates (Amatruda *et al.,* 1975) found that the number of insulin receptors on adipose cells was not decreased in human obesity. Fat cells are larger in obesity, and they concluded that the number of receptors per cell remains constant, the change being merely in the number of receptors per unit of surface area. Olefsky and Reaven (1975), however, found decreased receptors on adipocytes from obese rats. Another report (Hepp *et al.,* 1975) showed that the number of insulin receptors *increases* in the diabetic Chinese hamster. This animal is markedly *deficient* in insulin, and is analogous to the juvenile diabetic. The latter findings support further the physiological relevance of regulation by insulin itself of the concentration of insulin receptors on target cells.

Jarrett and Smith (1975) have carried out very interesting studies to cytologically identify receptor sites for insulin on adipocytes. They prepared a ferritin–insulin ligand that seemed to bind specifically to the cell surface, as detected by electron microscopy. They found cytological evidence for approximately 170,000 sites/cell, which corresponded to the number they obtained with [^{125}I]insulin. This number seems inordinately high relative to other studies, however, and there is need for further proof of specificity.

1.2.7.1. Insulin and Nonsuppressible Insulinlike Activity Receptors

Studies on insulin receptors provide new understanding concerning hypoglycemic syndromes produced by noninsulin-secreting tumors. Nonsuppressible insulinlike activity (NSILA) has been identified as a plasma component with insulinlike properties (stimulation of glucose oxidation *in vitro*, production of hypoglycemia *in vivo*), but physically distinct from insulin and without reactivity toward antiinsulin antibodies. Recently, Megyesi *et al.* (1975) studied the interaction of radioiodinated NSILA with rat liver membranes, and concluded that the membranes contain NSILA receptors distinct from insulin receptors. Nevertheless, each ligand can react with receptors for the other: insulin reacts with the NSILA receptor at lower affinity than NSILA; the insulin receptor reacts with NSILA, but with lower affinity than for insulin itself.

Of particular interest to clinical medicine is the finding by Roth *et al.* (1975) that some of the noninsulin-secreting tumors of mesenchymal origin that produce hypoglycemia apparently secrete a factor that interacts with the NSILA receptor; the humoral material elaborated by these tumors is presumably NSILA or a closely related molecule. These findings may explain the perplexing observations of many concerning tumor-induced hypoglycemia that is apparently humoral in character, but is not explainable by insulin; attempts to identify insulin by radioimmunoassay as the causative agent in this syndrome had not been fruitful.

1.2.7.2. Somatomedin, Nerve Growth Factor, and Epidermal Growth Factor Receptors

Somatomedins (also known as sulfation factor) are a group of circulating proteins released in response to growth hormone (reviewed by van Wyk *et al.*, 1975). One form of somatomedin (somatomedin A) is probably structurally related to, if not identical to, NSILA. Somatomedin, like NSILA, shows partial reactivity with insulin receptors on liver membranes, which also have separate unique receptors for somatomedin (van Wyk *et al.*, 1975). Somatomedin A interacts with NSILA receptors (Megyesi *et al.*, 1975). Two other growth factors, epidermoid growth factor and nerve growth factor, have no or very little reactivity toward NSILA or insulin receptors (Megyesi *et al.*, 1975), but have unique receptors (Hollenberg and Cuatrecasas, 1975; Banerjee *et al.*, 1975) identified on responsive tissues *in vitro*.

1.2.8. Metabolic Defects Involving Receptors

1.2.8.1. Receptor Deficiency

Although constitutional lack of primary receptors might be a possible explanation for hormone resistance associated with high endogenous hormone secretion (e.g., pseudohypoparathyroidism, nephrogenic diabetes insipidus, Laron-type dwarfism), a deficiency in number of receptors has so far been established only as a secondary phenomenon (see Sections 1.2.1 and 1.2.5). Another type of receptor defect has been identified as an autoimmune phenomenon (immunopathic receptor disorder) in certain endocrinopathies.

1.2.8.2. Immunopathic Receptor Disorders

It is now clear that certain clinical metabolic abnormalities can be caused by interaction of antibodies with receptors. Antibodies were identified (Kriss et al., 1964; Meek et al., 1964) in the pathophysiology of hyperthyroidism evolving from the classic reports of McKenzie (1958) and Adams and Purves (1956). Recent work indicates that in Graves' disease, an antithyroid antibody interacts with the thyrotropin receptor on thyroid cells and stimulates adenylate cyclase (Smith and Hall, 1974; Manley et al., 1974; Mehdi and Nussey, 1975; Yamashita and Field, 1972). A thyrotropin-type receptor in retroorbital tissue might be the basis for the pathophysiology of malignant exophthalmos. Indeed, it has been shown that serum taken from patients with malignant exophthalmos can enhance binding of the thyrotropin β-chain to retroorbital tissue from guinea pigs and activate adenylate cyclase (Winand and Kohn, 1974; Bolonkin et al., 1975). Myasthenia gravis appears to be another disease caused by an autoimmune phenomenon involving receptors. Immunization of animals with cholinergic receptors causes in the recipient a syndrome similar to myasthenia gravis, and circulating antibodies can be detected that react with skeletal muscle cholinergic receptors (Patrick and Lindstrom, 1973; Patrick et al., 1973). Recent investigations indicate that patients with myasthenia gravis show circulating antibodies to cholinergic receptors in human or rat muscle (Lennon, et al., 1975; Almon et al., 1974). The circulating antibody detected in these cases inhibits binding of radioactive ligand (tritiated carbomyl choline or iodinated α-bungarotoxin). The inhibition is not completely competitive, and only about 60% of the binding of the radioactive ligand is inhibited. This observation suggests the possibility that antibody is directed at a region near the receptor molecule, but not exclusively at the active site itself. On the other hand, a distinct type of mechanism to explain this disease has been proposed by Goldstein and Schlesinger (1975). They have found that injection of a synthetic peptide representing positions 29–41 of bovine thymopoietin causes a neuromuscular block resembling myasthenia gravis in mice. They interpret these findings as possibly implicating thymopoietin in the pathophysiology of the disorder. They suggest that antibodies rather, than blocking cholinergic receptors, directly stimulate the release of thymopoietin, which in turn is the putative causative agent.

More recently, still another immune disease involving receptors has been discovered by Flier and his colleagues (Flier *et al.*, 1975). They found a state of severe insulin resistance in several women with acanthosis nigricans. Insulin concentrations in the plasma of these patients were increased 10- to 100-fold, and some required 1000 times the usual dose of insulin to control blood sugar. The apparent receptor concentration on circulating monocytes in these subjects was markedly reduced. The investigators further found that there is an antibody in the serum of these patients that reacts with insulin receptors. Incubation of monocytes (circulating monocytes normally contain insulin receptors) with serum from the insulin-resistant acanthosis nigricans patients caused marked loss or inactivation of receptors on cultured lymphocytes. The antireceptor activity of the patients' serum was apparently limited to insulin receptors; growth-hormone receptors on the same cells incubated with patients' serum were normal. An etiological role of the antireceptor antibody in this disease is further supported by extremely high concentrations of the antibody in patients most severely affected. Serum from one subject at dilutions as high as 1:600 caused almost complete inhibition of binding of iodinated insulin to receptors on cultured lymphocytes.

The several studies suggesting that autoimmune phenomena may directly influence receptor function and cause disease states, as indicated in Graves' disease, myasthenia gravis, and insulin resistance, raise the possibility that similar immunopathic receptor disorders may be relatively widespread in the pathophysiology of diseases in diverse systems in medicine. As specific test systems are developed for diverse ligand receptor systems, this hypothesis will undoubtedly be examined further.

1.3. Regulation of Adenylate Cyclase

1.3.1. General

The classic studies of Sutherland and his collaborators (see Robison *et al.*, 1971, for a review) proved that many hormones act by stimulating the enzyme adenylate cyclase. In fact, one model included the possible concept that the adenylate cyclase enzyme itself might be the hormone receptor. One subunit of the enzyme might represent the receptor, the other the catalytic subunit. This model was modified as evidence accrued that receptor occupancy was not necessarily directly linked to adenylate cyclase activity, and that phospholipids (see Levey *et al.*, 1975, for a review), guanine nucleotides, and metals are further important modifiers of enzyme activity. Orly and Schramm (1975) found that long-chain fatty acids also enhance responsiveness to catecholamines in membranes from turkey erythroyctes. The mechanism for this effect has not been elucidated.

1.3.2. Guanine Nucleotides and Regulation of Adenylate Cyclase

The investigations begun originally by Rodbell and his associates (Rodbell *et al.*, 1971; Salomon *et al.*, 1975; Rodbell *et al.*, 1975) indicate that purine nucleotides are important in modulating hormone-regulated adenylate cyclase activity. Kinetic evidence from adenylate cyclase assays, direct binding studies with guanine nucleotides (Rodbell *et al.*, 1975; Spiegel and Aurbach, 1974; Lefkowitz, 1975), and certain studies with direct binding of hormone ligand (Brown *et al.*, 1976a; Spiegel *et al.*, 1976; Glossmann, 1975) indicate that the action of guanine nucleotides is mediated by interaction of nucleotides with a unique site distinct from that of the receptor or from the catalytic site for ATP. In turkey erythrocyte membranes, purine nucleotides enhance activation of adenylate cyclase by catecholamines, with no detectable effect on affinity or number of binding sites of the receptor (Brown *et al.*, 1976b; Spiegel *et al.*, 1976). Moreover, binding studies as well as kinetic analysis for adenylate cyclase reaction itself show that GTP and analogues have much higher affinities for the guanine nucleotide site than does ATP (Rodbell *et al.*, 1975; Spiegel and Aurbach, 1974; Lefkowitz, 1975). Guanine nucleotides seem to enhance the affinity of ATP for the catalytic site. Kinetic studies show reduced K_m for ATP when GTP (Hanoune *et al.*, 1975) or GMPPNP (Aurbach *et al.*, 1975) are added. The catalytic site for ATP (that is, adenylate cyclase enzyme itself) can apparently be separated from the guanine nucleotide regulatory site. Recent studies on guanine nucleotide regulation of adenylate cyclase have utilized analogues of GTP, particularly guanylylimidodiphosphate [Gpp(NH)p], a compound resistant to hydrolysis by the usual nucleoside triphosphatases. In the presence of guanylylimidodiphosphate, there is a marked enhancement of catecholamine-stimulated adenylate cyclase activity observed in turkey as well as frog erythrocyte membranes (Spiegel and Aurbach, 1974; Schramm and Rodbell, 1975; Schramm, 1975; Lefkowitz and Caron, 1975). In the turkey erythrocyte membrane, isoproterenol causes a 3–4-fold increase in adenylate cyclase activity, but in the presence of 10^{-5} M Gpp(NH)p, isoproterenol causes a 40-fold stimulation of the enzyme in a standard assay for 10 min (Spiegel and Aurbach, 1974). Moreover, the apparent K_D for isoproterenol activation of adenylate cyclase is reduced by an order of magnitude in the presence of 10^{-5} M Gpp(NH)p (Spiegel and Aurbach, 1974; Aurbach et al., 1975; Schramm, 1975). Guanylylimidodiphosphate also causes a similar apparent increase in potency for the glucagon-activated adenylate cyclase system of the hepatic adenylate cyclase system, and also causes apparent enhanced sensitivity of rabbit blood cell adenylate cyclase to prostaglandins (Hosey and Tao, 1975) and of ACTH to adrenal adenylate cyclase (Glossmann and Gips, 1975).

The introduction by Rodbell and his associates of the use of guanylylimidodiphosphate was important as a point of departure in studying the mechanism by which guanine nucleotides regulate adenylate cyclase. The action of guanylylimidodiphosphate, although it is similar to that of GTP, differs significantly. In the course of the adenylate cyclase reaction in the presence of Gpp(NH)p, the enzyme becomes persistently activated (Schramm and Rodbell, 1975; Pfeuffer and Helreich, 1975; Lefkowitz and Caron, 1975; Cuatrecasas et al., 1975b; Aurbach et al., 1975; Spiegel et al., 1976). In this state, the enzyme remains activated even under conditions in which the agonist has been dissociated, or even when the specific hormone antagonist is added. The fully activated or "holocatalytic" state of the enzyme formed in the presence of isoproterenol and Gpp(NH)p in avian erythrocyte membranes is also more readily solubilized (Pfeuffer and Helmreich, 1975; Schramm and Rodbell, 1975) than is enzyme in the basal state. Moreover, even though the enzyme has been converted to this persistently activated state, there is no change in number or affinity of the β-adrenergic receptors (Spiegel et al., 1976). Studies have been carried out on the rate of binding of guanylylimidodiphosphate to the guanine nucleotide site on the plasma membrane (Rodbell et al., 1975; Lefkowitz, 1975; Pfeuffer and Helmreich, 1975; Spiegel and Aurbach, 1974; Glossmann, 1975). Radioactive guanylylimidodiphosphate binds to this site with high affinity, and other nucleotides compete for binding with affinities paralleling their apparent effectiveness in modulating adenylate cyclase activity. However, binding of labeled Gpp(NH)p to the membrane-bound adenylate cyclase system occurs much more rapidly than development of the "holocatalytic" state. Moreover, binding is not dependent on the presence of hormone agonist, whereas development of the "holocatalytic" state is. Experiments of this type from several laboratories indicate that binding of guanine nucleotide alone is not sufficient for activation of adenylate cyclase, but that a further temperature- and time-

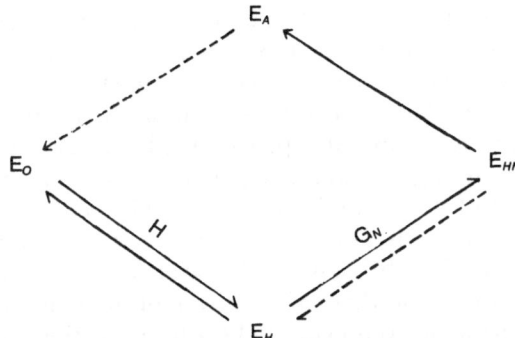

Fig. 7. Distinct activity states of adenylate cyclase enzyme in turkey erythrocyte membranes. State E_O represents basal enzyme activity. In the presence of agonist, the enzyme is converted to state E_H. Addition of guanine nucleotide to state E_H yields state E_{HN}, which contains bound agonist plus bound guanine nucleotide. In a temperature-dependent reaction, state E_{HN} is gradually converted to state E_A, the fully activated or holocatalytic form of the enzyme. The holocatalytic state is "irreversibly" activated, and is not inhibited by addition of propranolol.

dependent reaction is required for development of the persistently activated state. All this information suggests that sites with high affinity for guanine nucleotides are involved in regulating hormonal-activated adenylate cyclase. For catecholamine-activated adenylate cyclase, the sequence of events appears to be (Fig. 7): (1) binding of catecholamine agonist to receptor to produce state E_H; (2) binding of guanine nucleotide to a specific site on a G-binding protein to produce state E_N; (3) conversion of state E_{HN} by a temperature- and time-dependent process to produce state E_A, the active or "holocatalyic" state of adenylate cyclase.

1.3.3. Toxins

The induction of cholera in animals as well as in man is associated with an increase in adenylate cyclase activity of intestinal mucosa (Sharp and Hyney, 1971; Kimberg *et al.*, 1971; Chen *et al.*, 1971). Moreover, cholera toxin added to a variety of cell systems *in vitro* causes activation of adenylate cyclase in the cells, and in addition enhances the sensitivity of adenylate cyclase to catecholamines (Field, 1974; Bennett and Cuatrecasas, 1975a,b) or to glucagon (Bennett *et al.*, 1975). Recent studies (Bitensky *et al.*, 1975b) indicate the NAD is involved in the activation of adenylate cyclase in response to cholera toxin. The observations by Flores and Sharp (1975) imply strongly that NAD interacts with the same site that is influenced by guanine nucleotides, or with a closely related one. They found that activation of rat liver adenylate cyclase by cholera toxin *in vivo* or in homogenates *in vitro* blocked the stimulatory effect of guanyly-limidodiphosphate. Conversely, maximal concentrations of guanylylimi-dodiphosphate blocked the stimulatory effect of cholera toxin. The activation of adenylate cyclase in cell-free membrane preparations requires NAD (Gill, 1975; Flores and Sharp, 1975). The observations of the latter two groups strongly suggest an analogy between the mechanism of action of cholera toxin and that of diphtheria toxin (Gill *et al.*, 1973). Diphtheria toxin, like cholera toxin, is a protein composed of two chains. On entering the cell membrane, diphtheria toxin dissociates into its A and B subunits; the A chain is an enzyme that causes covalent attachment of part of the NAD molecule to a site requiring GTP on elongation factor II, a ribosomal protein required for protein synthesis. Cholera toxin consists of A and B chains, and it is the A chain that is involved in activation of adenylate cyclase (van Heyningen and King, 1975; Gill and King, 1975). The B components of the toxin apparently are involved with binding of the toxin to the cell, a phenomenon involving interaction with gangliosides (Cuatrecasas, 1973). The A chain may be an enzyme analogous to the enzymatic chain of diptheria toxin, and it is possible that the mechanism of action of cholera toxin is as follows: (1) binding of cholera toxin to the external surface of the plasma membrane, a process involving interaction with gangliosides; (2) reduction of disulfide bonds in the toxin molecule, allowing dissociation into A and B chains; (3) catalysis by the A chain thus activated of formation of a covalent link between the NAD molecule and a site on a guanine nucleotide–binding protein in the adenylate cyclase complex; (4) occupation of the guanine nucleotide–binding site by the covalently linked fragment of NAD, causing full activation of adenylate cyclase analogous to the activated state ("irreversibly" activated to "holocatalytic" state, see above) produced by incubating the adenylate cyclase enzyme with guanylylimidodiphosphate.

The scheme for the mechanism of cholera toxin action described above would account reasonably well for the observations of Gill and of Flores and Sharp. It is possible that other toxins act in a similar fashion, and it has been observed (Hewlett *et al.*, 1974) that *Escherichia coli* toxin is also capable of activating adenylate cyclase in adipocytes. Wolff and Cook (1975b), moreover, have shown that lipopolysaccharides from *E. coli, Serratia marcescens,* or *Salmonella typhosa* are capable of increasing adenylate cyclase activity after a latent period in mouse adrenal tumor cells in tissue culture. The response to these toxins was not inhibited by gangliosides, as was found with cholera toxin. Moreover, the effect was attributable to lipopolysaccharides, and not enterotoxin. It seemed likely in this latter study that liposaccharides from these organisms activated adenylate cyclase through a mechanism distinct from that produced by cholera toxin.

1.4. Cyclic 3′,5′-Adenosine Monophosphate Concentration in Tissue and Protein Kinase Activation

1.4.1. General

The metabolism of almost all tissues is regulated at least in part by cyclic nucleotides, but activation of adenylate cyclase it not the sole mechanism by which ligands regulate cyclic nucleotide concentration. The concentration of cAMP in the cell is a function of synthesis (adenylate cyclase reaction), degradation (cyclic nucleotide phosphodiesterase), and extrusion from the cell. Hormonal ligands can control adenylate cyclase or phosphodiesterase, and certain drugs (probenecid, vincristine) inhibit elaboration (?transport) of cyclic nucleotides from cells into the extracellular compartment. The concentration of cyclic nucleotides, and in particular that bound to cAMP-receptor protein, controls protein kinase enzymes in cells, and this enzymatic activity in turn regulates metabolic functions of the cell.

1.4.2. Protein Kinases

There is considerable evidence that accumulation of cAMP in tissues in response to hormones produces a physiological effect through the intermediation of protein kinases. This group of enzymes catalyzes the transfer of the γ-phosphate of ATP to a hydroxyamino acid (usually serine) in the acceptor protein. Kinase activation by cAMP has been implicated in activation of phosphorylase, inactivation of glycogen synthetase, activation of adipocyte lipase, and activation of ion transport in avian erythrocytes (see the reviews of Beavo *et al.*, 1975; Corbin *et al.*, 1975; and Rudolph and Greengard, 1974). Pittman *et al.* (1975) have also described activation through protein kinase of cholesterol esterase in adipocytes. The work of Krebs and his associates has established that cAMP-sensitive kinases are composed of subunits of two types: The receptor subunit is a protein that specifically finds cAMP receptor subunits and catalytic subunits. On interaction with cAMP, the receptor subunit with cAMP bound to it dissociates from the catalytic unit as follows:

$$RC + cAMP \rightleftharpoons R \cdot cAMP + C$$

The molecular weight of the entire enzyme complex is 170,000, and this represents a tetramer composed of 2 R and 2 C subunits (Beavo *et al.*, 1975). The holoenzyme can be regulated not only by cAMP, but also by magnesium·ATP, which is required for recombination of the C+R subunits; by an inhibitor protein (Beavo *et al.,* 1975); and possibly by auto-phosphorylation as well (Rosen *et al.,* 1975).

The array of factors that potentially activate kinase activity may account for the fact that in several tissues, changes in physiological effects of hormones can be brought about without a detectable increase in total cAMP concentration. Beavo *et al.* (1975) have calculated that under normal physiological conditions, the concentration of cAMP in muscle is normally about half-maximally effective in terms of kinase activity. Hence, a fall in cAMP concentration will produce a highly significant reduction in kinase activity, whereas even a 10-fold increase in concentration can produce only a doubling of kinase activity. The combination of high concentrations of kinase relative to the dissociation constant for the cyclic AMP receptor protein plus the regulation by magnesum·ATP (which exists at high concentrations in muscle) contributes to the relatively low sensitivity of kinase itself to changes in total cAMP concentration *in vivo.* On the other hand, the parameter controlled by kinase enzyme activity could be regulated sensitively with small changes in cAMP concentration. Corbin *et al.* (1975) have developed methods to determine the degree of activation of kinase *in vivo* in response to hormones. Epinephrine added to intact rat adipose tissue causes an increase in the fraction of protein kinase in the free catalytic subunit form. Addition of 10^{-7} M epinephrine to adipose tissue causes an increase in protein kinase activity and a doubling in the rate of glycerol release. These changes are brought about without a significant increase in total cAMP concentration. Under similar conditions, the further addition of insulin significantly reduces the active protein kinase and glycerol release, again without change in total cAMP concentration (Corbin *et al.,* 1975).

1.4.3. Regulation of Cyclic Nucleotide Phosphodiesterase Activity

Another enzyme important in controlling the concentrations of cAMP in tissues is cyclic nucleotide phosphodiesterase. The activity of this enzyme can also be controlled by ligands. In rat heart, there appear to be three different forms of cyclic nucleotide phosphodiesterase: (1) a form inhibitable by cAMP itself; (2) a cyclic guanine nucleotide phosphodiesterase, which is regulated by calcium; and (3) a phosphodiesterase regulated directly by cyclic guanosine 3′,5′-monophosphate (Appleman and Terasaki, 1975). Moreover, it is apparent that one way in which calcium may be able to regulate tissue metabolism is through stimulation of cyclic nucleotide phosphodiesterases (Wang *et al.,* 1975). The effect of calcium on cyclic nucleotide phosphodiesterases seems to be effected through interaction with a specific calcium-binding protein that is part of the phosphodiesterase complex (Kakiuchi *et al.*, 1975; Wang *et al.*, 1975). Boudreau and Drummond (1975) found three forms of cyclic nucleotide phosphodiesterase in superior cervical ganglia extracts. One form showed a low K_m for cGMP, and two other forms were most sensitive for cAMP as substrate. One of the latter was stimulated by cGMP. Thus, it is apparent that cyclic nucleotide phosphodiesterases can be regulated by cyclic nucleotides themselves, by ions, or by other factors.

1.4.3.1. Cyclic Nucleotide Phosphodiesterase in the Physiology of Vision

Another area in which regulation of phosphodiesterase activity appears to be important is in the physiology of vision. Bitensky and his collaborators (Bitensky *et al.*, 1975a) have studied activation of phosphodiesterase in amphibian rod outer segments and have reviewed (Bitensky *et al.*, 1975a) findings from a number of laboratories in this area. The phosphodiesterase of the outer rod segments is specifically inhibited by ATP in the presence of light. The preferred substrate for the phosphodiesterase appears to be cGMP. Activation of the phosphodiesterase in the presence of light requires a nucleoside triphosphate. Neither α,β-methylene ATP nor β,γ-methylene ATP was an effective substitute for nucleoside triphosphates. This observation suggested that photoactivation of the phosphodiesterase might involve phosphorylation from the γ-phosphate of ATP (Bitensky *et al.*, 1975a).

Insulin can also regulate phosphodiesterase (Loten and Sneyd, 1970), and this effect probably accounts for the reduced cAMP content of tissues exposed to insulin under certain conditions. Kono *et al.* (1975) have presented evidence that a phosphodiesterase enzyme disulfide group may be alternately oxidized and reduced (with consequent activation or deactivation, respectively, of the enzyme) in reponse to insulin.

1.5. Cyclic Nucleotides in the Extracellular Fluids

1.5.1. General

Many, perhaps all, cells that form cyclic nucleotides in response to particular stimuli elaborate the nucleotides into the extracellular space. This was discovered in the original studies of Sutherland and his collaborators (Davoren and Sutherland, 1963; Hardman *et al.*, 1966), who found cAMP in urine of mammals and in media containing pigeon erythrocytes stimulated with catecholamines. Subsequently, cAMP has been identified in media from many cell types, and in blood plasma, central spinal fluid, milk, bile, gastric juice, and seminal fluid. Plasma cAMP content increases after stimulation with glucagon (Broadus *et al.*, 1970b), increases in adrenal vein plasma after injection of ACTH (Peytreman *et al.*, 1973), increases in the general circulation after injection of β-adrenergic catecholamines (Ball *et al.*, 1972; Issekutz, 1975; Strange and Mjøs, 1975), and increases (presumably) in renal vein plasma after injection of parathyroid hormone (Kaminsky *et al.*, 1970; Tomlinson *et al.*, 1976).

1.5.2. Plasma Cyclic Nucleotides—Production Rates and Clearance

The group at Vanderbilt has carried out classic studies on plasma clearance of cAMP and cGMP in man (Broadus *et al.*, 1970a; Ball *et al.*, 1972). Both cyclic nucleotides appear to distribute in a space exceeding the extracellular fluid volume, and both show $T_{1/2}$'s of approximately 30 min in man. Renal excretion of the cyclic nucleotide into the urine accounts for only 20% of the clearance of cyclic nucleotides from the miscible pool in man. In the dog, the kidney accounts for 3% of the total clearance of cyclic nucleotide from plasma (Blonde *et al.*, 1974). Only about ⅔ of the renal clearance is accounted for by excretion; the remainder appears to represent enzymatic destruction of the nucleotide within the kidney.

The major sites of production of cyclic nucleotides under basal conditions have not been clearly established. Although parathyroid hormone, catecholamines, ACTH, and glucagon in large doses are capable of increasing the plasma cAMP concentration, none of the corresponding receptor tissues—liver, kidney, or adrenal—seems to be the major source for plasma cAMP under resting conditions (Blonde *et al.*, 1974; Wehmann *et al.*, 1974). Strange and Mjøs (1975) have confirmed the earlier findings of Liljenquist *et al.* (1974) and Broadus *et al.* (1970b) that glucagon causes striking increases in the plasma concentration of cAMP. Moreover, Strange and Mjøs (1975) showed that hepatectomy obliterates the response to glucagon in increasing cAMP, but does not significantly influence the rise in plasma cAMP following injection of isoproterenol. Epinephrine has a much more striking effect on cAMP concentration than does norepinephrine (Issekutz, 1975). Moreover, the response to epinephrine is accentuated after treatment of dogs with methylprednisolone. Calculation of plasma cAMP production rates from results with tritiated cAMP clearance indicated that the increase in plasma cAMP is a result of production, not of decreased destruction via phosphodiesterase activity (Issekutz, 1975). Methylprednisolone causes a decrease in basal concentrations of cAMP in plasma; there was an associated slight increase in blood glucose, as well as in insulin secretion. Since insulin has been shown to decrease hepatic production of cAMP (Exton *et al.,* 1972), it was suggested that the decrease in plasma cAMP in the methylprednisolone-treated dogs might be caused by the increased rate of insulin secretion. Although the corticosteroid-treated dogs showed lower basal concentrations of cAMP in plasma, the response to epinephrine was exaggerated strikingly, whereas the effects of norepinephrine on plasma cAMP were affected little at all. These studies suggest that epinephrine is the endogenous catecholamine primarily responsible for releasing cAMP into plasma. These studies, of course, did not prove the precise source of plasma cAMP in response to catecholamines. Also, it was unfortunate that there were no direct comparisons between the effects of glucagon and catecholamines on plasma cAMP in these studies, nor were responses tested with stereospecific β- or α-blockers (see "1.2.3. β-Adrenergic Receptors"). Further studies in this area should be of value in elucidating the source of production of plasma cAMP.

1.5.3. Cyclic 3′,5′-Adenosine Monophosphate in Cerebrospinal Fluid

Earlier reports had indicated that cAMP occurs in cerebrospinal fluid, and that probenecid or exercise causes an increase in the CSF content of cAMP (Cramer *et al.,* 1972). Sebens and Korf (1975) have examined CSF cAMP further in rabbits. They showed that cAMP in the CSF must reflect that generated within the CNS, in that cAMP did not appear to be cleared from plasma into the spinal fluid. Histamine as well as norepinephrine, isoproterenol, or dopamine given intracysternally caused an increase in cAMP in CSF. L-Dopa given parenterally was without effect on cAMP in CSF. Intravenous administration of isoproterenol, on the other hand, did cause an increase in the cAMP content of CSF (Sebens and Korf, 1975). The latter confirmed the findings of Cramer *et al.* (1972) that probenecid increases accumulation of cAMP in CSF; this effect of probenecid presumably was mediated by a decrease in the clearance of cAMP from CSF. However, this latter point has not been established by experimental test. The authors correctly conclude that accumulation of cAMP in the spinal fluid does not necessarily reflect specific interaction of any particular neurotransmitter with any unique receptor cell. The multiple classes of cells responding to an array of neurotransmitters within the CNS limit the interpretation of any changes in cAMP concentration in CSF.

1.5.4. Urinary Excretion of Cyclic 3′,5′-Adenosine Monophosphate

Plasma cAMP in man is cleared in part by glomerular filtration into the urine, and the renal clearance of plasma cAMP is equal to the clearance of inulin. Kaminsky *et al.* (1970) showed that the amount derived from plasma clearance in man represents only 50–60% of the total cAMP in the urine. The remaining 40–50% represents nephrogenously generated cAMP, and this nephrogenous contribution is for the most part under the control of parathyroid hormone (Chase and Aurbach, 1967; Chase *et al.*, 1969; Kaminsky *et al.*, 1970). Induction of hypercalcemia with consequent suppression of parathyroid hormone secretion decreases the nephrogenous component by about 80% in the rat. Similarly, the nephrogenous component increases dramatically on injection of parathyroid hormone. On the other hand, it is not possible to suppress the nephrogenous contribution completely by infusing calcium. This perhaps is not unexpected, in that catecholamines, calcitonin, vasopressin, and possibly other factors such as prostaglandins are capable of influencing the nephrogenous components; these factors are not known to be suppressed or inhibited by hypercalcemia.

1.5.5. Parathyroid Hormone and Renal Clearance of Cyclic 3′,5′-Adenosine Monophosphate

The discovery that parathyroid hormone was the major factor regulating urinary cAMP excretion in the rat (Chase and Aurbach, 1967) prompted the development of urinary cAMP response as an index of clinical physiological–pathophysiological status. In the rat, induction of hypercalcemia and consequent inhibition of parathyroid hormone secretion causes an 80% reduction in the rate of excretion of cAMP into the urine. It was postulated that this phenomenon could be developed into a clinically useful test for hyperparathyroidism. Indeed, a number of studies have shown that excretion of cAMP into the urine is higher than normal in hyperparathyroidism (Kaminsky *et al.*, 1970; Murad, 1973; Neelon *et al.*, 1973; Mallette *et al.*, 1974; Bartley *et al.*, 1975), and that infusion of calcium causes a decrease in urinary cAMP excretion (Kaminsky *et al.*, 1970; Murad, 1973). However, since only 40–50% of urinary cAMP represents that under the control of parathyroid hormone, induction of hypercalcemia causes only a 30–40% decrease in the rate of excretion of cAMP. On the other hand, several groups of investigators have shown that excretion of cyclic AMP is increased in hyperparathyroidism, and returns to the normal or low range following parathyroidectomy. Usually, results on clinical subjects have been expressed as the cAMP:creatinine ratio in the urine, or sometimes simply as the rate of excretion of cAMP. Since creatinine clearance can vary from one subject to another, and since only a fraction of urinary cAMP represents that regulated by parathyroid hormone, Bower et al. (1974) and Broadus (personal communication) have simultaneously determined creatinine clearance and cAMP clearance. With this information, cAMP excretion can be segregated according to nephrogenous or systemic origin. Nephrogenous cAMP correlates very highly with parathyroid activity. Indeed, even correcting the urinary cAMP:creatinine ratio for serum creatinine [(urinary cAMP/urinary creatinine) × plasma creatinine], which expression is equivalent to cAMP excretion/100 ml glomerular filtrate] provides an expression that correlates virtually as well as clearance ratios (cAMP clearance/creatinine clearance) for diagnostic purposes (Broadus, personal communication). Application of a correction factor for creatinine clearance is particularly important in any clinical situation associated with abnormal renal function (renal impairment leads to a significant increase in basal plasma cAMP concentration, as well as to a reduction in creatinine clearance, producing a bifold aberration in the parameter cAMP:creatinine ratio), or in any wasting disease associated with reduced creatinine production. For example, the cAMP:creatinine ratio is abnormally high in hyperthyroidism (Guttler et al., 1975; Lin et al., 1973). However, the high ratio in hyperthyroidism is totally accounted for by the reduced creatinine formation and excretion in hyperthyroidism (Guttler et al., 1975). The latter authors also observed an increase in sensitivity to infused catecholamines in hyperthyroidism in terms of urinary cAMP excretion. This observation parallels the enhanced sensitivity of catecholamines found in the hyperthyroid state. Moreover, they found that hyperthyroid subjects excreted greater amounts of cAMP per 24 hr than normal subjects. This seemed attributable to the activity and consequent secretion of catecholamines, since in the basal state, hyperthyroid subjects excrete only normal amounts of cAMP (Lin et al., 1973). In general, the results of all these studies support further the validity of utilizing cAMP excretion per 100 ml GF or cAMP:creatinine clearance ratios, rather than total cAMP excretion or cAMP:creatinine ratios on urine determinations only.

1.5.5.1. Pseudohypoparathyroidism

Pseudohypoparathyroidism is characterized by resistance to exogenous parathyroid hormone, and those cases given intravenous parathyroid hormone show little or no increase in urinary cAMP excretion (Chase et al., 1969). Tomlinson et al. (1976) have reported a rapid infusion test for parathyroid responsiveness. Normal subjects show a rise in plasma cAMP reaching a peak in 10 min. Subjects with pseudohypoparathyroidism respond little or not at all.

Pak *et al.* (1975) have suggested tests to differentiate resorptive and renal hypercalciuric states. Renal hypercalciuric subjects showed high fasting cAMP:creatinine ratios, which fell to normal when a calcium load was given. Absorptive hypercalciuria was associated with normal basal ratios, and there was an appropriate slight decrease in ratio when calcium was given by mouth. As expected, hyperparathyroid subjects showed high basal ratios of cAMP:creatinine in urine, and the ratio did not change with calcium challenge. There was, however, considerable overlap between groups in absolute results for basal values as well as responses to calcium. Moreover, the effect of potential changes in clearance ratios ($C_{cAMP}/C_{creatinine}$) was not evaluated.

1.5.6. Other Factors and Hormones That Affect Urinary Cyclic 3′,5′-Adenosine Monophosphate Excretion

Kuchel and his associates (Kuchel *et al.*, 1975) have studied cAMP metabolism in idiopathic edema. They found that these subjects had abnormally high concentrations of cAMP in plasma under basal conditions, and showed an excessive increase in plasma cAMP following assumption of the upright position. At the same time, clearance of cAMP into the urine was decreased. It was postulated that this abnormality reflected enhanced sensitivity to β-adrenergic stimulation, since it is known that catecholamines cause an increase in plasma cAMP, as well as a decrease in the clearance of cAMP into the urine (Ball *et al.*, 1972).

Murad *et al.* (1975) have examined further the excretion of cAMP and cGMP in normal children as compared to those with cystic fibrosis. Earlier studies (Linarelli, 1972) had shown that cAMP:creatinine ratios were high in young children, and gradually fell with progressive age toward ratios found in adult subjects. Murad *et al.* (1975) showed that cAMP excretion, when corrected for body surface area, is the same in children as in adults. In this same study, the authors found that older children with cystic fibrosis excreted higher amounts of cGMP than did normal subjects. This observation, however, has no immediately apparent explanation.

References

Adams, D., and Purves, H. D., 1956, Abnormal responses in the assay of thyrotropin, *Proc. Univ. Otago Med. School* **34:**11.

Agus, Z. S., Puschett, J. B., Senesky, D., and Goldberg, M., 1971, Mode of action of parathyroid hormone and cyclic adenosine 3′,5′-monophosphate on renal tubular phosphate reabsorption in the dog, *J. Clin. Invest.* **50:**617.

Alexander, R. W., Davis, J. N., and Lefkowitz, R. J., 1975a, Direct identification and characterisation of β-adrenergic receptors in rat brain, *Nature* **258**:437.

Alexander, R. W., Williams, L. T., and Lefkowitz, R. J., 1975b, Identification of cardiac β-adrenergic receptors by (−)[³H]alprenolol binding, *Proc. Nat. Acad. Sci. U.S.A.* **72**:1564.

Almon, R. R., Andrew, C. G., and Appel, S. H., 1974, Serum globulin in myasthenia gravis: Inhibition of α-bungarotoxin binding to acetylcholine receptors, *Science* **186**:55.

Amatruda, J. M., Livingston, J. N., and Lockwood, D. H., 1975, Insulin receptor: Role in the resistance of human obesity to insulin, *Science* **188**:264.

Appleman, M. M., and Terasaki, W. L., 1975, Regulation of cyclic nucleotide phosphodiesterase, *Adv. Cyclic Nucleotide Res.* **5**:153.

Archer, J. A., Gorden, P., and Roth, J., 1975, Defect in insulin binding to receptors in obese man: Amelioration with calorie restriction, *J. Clin. Invest.* **55**:166.

Ardaillou, R., 1975, Kidney and calcitonin, *Nephron* **15**:250.

Atkinson, D. E., 1966, Regulation of enzyme activity, *Ann. Rev. Biochem.* **35**:85.

Atlas, D., Steer, M. L., and Levitzki, A., 1974, Stereospecific binding of propranolol and catecholamines to the β-adrenergic receptor, *Proc. Nat. Acad. Sci. U.S.A.* **71**:4246.

Aurbach, G. D., and Heath, D. A., 1974, Parathyroid hormone and calcitonin regulation of renal function, *Kidney Intl.* **6**:331.

Aurbach, G. D., Fedak, S. A., Woodard, C. J., Palmer, J. S., Hauser, D., and Troxler, F., 1974, β-Adrenergic receptor: Stereospecific interaction of iodinated β-blocking agent with high affinity site, *Science* **186**:1223.

Aurbach, G. D., Spiegel, A. M., and Gardner, J. D., 1975, β-Adrenergic receptors, cyclic AMP, and ion transport in the avian erythrocyte, *Adv. Cyclic Nucleotide Res.* **5**:117.

Ball, J. H., Kaminsky, N. I., Hardman, J. G., Broadus, A. E., Sutherland, E. W., and Liddle, G. W., 1972, Effects of catecholamines and adrenergic-blocking agents on plasma and urinary cyclic nucleotides in man, *J. Clin. Invest.* **51**:2124.

Banerjee, S. P., Cuatrecasas, P., and Snyder, S. H., 1975, Nerve growth factor receptor binding, *J. Biol. Chem.* **250**:1427.

Bartley, P. C., Willgoss, D., and Lloyd, H. M., 1975, Urinary excretion of cyclic AMP in primary hyperparathyroidism, *Aust. N. Z. J. Med.* **5**:36.

Beavo, J. A., Bechtel, P. J., and Krebs, E. G., 1975, Mechanism of control for cAMP-dependent protein kinase from skeletal muscle, *Adv. Cyclic Nucleotide Res.* **5**:241.

Bennett, V., and Cuatrecasas, 1975a, Mechanism of action of *Vibrio cholerae* enterotoxin: Effects on adenylate cyclase of toad and rat erythocyte plasma membranes, *J. Membrane Biol.* **22**:1.

Bennett, V., and Cuatrecasas, P., 1975b, Mechanism of activation of adenylate cyclase by *Vibrio cholerae* enterotoxin, *J. Membrane Biol.* **22**:29.

Bennett, V., O'Keefe, E., and Cuatrecasas, P., 1975, Mechanism of action of cholera toxin and the mobile receptor theory of hormone receptor–adenylate cyclase interactions, *Proc. Nat. Acad. Sci. U.S.A.* **72**:33.

Bitensky, M. W., Miki, N., Keirns, J. J., Keirns, M., Baraban, J. M., Freeman, J., Wheeler, M. A., Lacy, J., and Marcus, F. R., 1975a, Activation of photoreceptor disk membrane phosphodiesterase by light and ATP, *Adv. Cyclic Nucleotide Res.* **5**:213.

Bitensky, M. W., Wheeler, M. A., Mehta, H., and Miki, N., 1975b, Cholera toxin activation of adenylate cyclase in cancer cell membrane fragments, *Proc. Nat. Acad. Sci. U.S.A.* **72**:2572.

Blonde, L., Wehmann, R. E., and Steiner, A. L., 1974, Plasma clearance rates and renal clearance of ^{3}H-labeled cyclic AMP and ^{3}H-labeled cyclic GMP in the dog, *J. Clin. Invest.* **53**:163.

Bolonkin, D., Tate, R. L., Luber, J. H., Kohn, L. D., and Winand, R. J., 1975, Experimental exophthalmos: Binding of thyrotropin and an exophthalmogenic factor derived from thyrotropin to retro-orbital tissue plasma membranes, *J. Biol. Chem.* **250**:6516.

Boudreau, R. J., and Drummond, G. I., 1975, The effect of Ca^{++} on cyclic nucleotide phosphodiesterases of superior cervical ganglion, *J. Cyclic Nucleotide Res.* **1**:219.

Bower, R. H., Babka, J. C., and Sode, J., 1974, Nephrogenous cyclic adenosine monophosphate (cAMP) in the diagnosis of hyperparathyroidism, *Program of the 56th Meeting of The Endocrine Society*, Abstract No. 297, p. A-204.

Broadus, A. E., Kaminsky, N. I., Hardman, J. G., Sutherland, E. W., and Liddle, G. W., 1970a, Kinetic parameters and renal clearances of plasma adenosine 3',5'-monophosphate and guanosine 3',5'-monophosphate in man, *J. Clin. Invest.* **49**:2222.

Broadus, A. E., Kaminsky, N. I., Northcutt, R. C., Hardman, J. G., Sutherland, E. W., and Liddle, G. W., 1970b, Effects of glucagon on adenosine 3',5'-monophosphate and guanosine 3',5'-monophosphate in human plasma and urine, *J. Clin. Invest.* **49**:2237.

Brown, E. M., Aurbach, G. D., Hauser, D., and Troxler, F., 1976a, β-Adrenergic receptor interactions: Characterization of iodohydroxybenzylpindolol as a specific ligand, *J. Biol. Chem.* **251**:1232.

Brown, E. M., Fedak, S. A., Woodard, C. J., Aurbach, G. D., and Rodbard, D., 1976b, β-Adrenergic receptor interactions: Direct comparison of receptor and biological activity, *J. Biol. Chem.* **251**:1239.

Brown, E. M., Gardner, J. D., and Aurbach, G. D., Direct determination of ligand interactions with β-adrenergic receptors on intact turkey erythrocytes: Correlation of binding with biological activity, *Endocrinology* (in press).

Chabardès, D., Imbert-Teboul, M., Montégut, M., Clique, A., Morel, F., 1975a, Catecholamine-sensitive adenylate cyclase activity in different segments of rabbit nephron, *Pflügers Arch.* **361**:9.

Chabardès, D., Imbert, M., Clique, A., Montégut, M., and Morel, F., 1975b, PTH sensitive adenyl cyclase activity in different segments of the rabbit nephron, *Pflügers Arch.* **354**:229.

Chang, K. J., Huang, D., and Cuatrecasas, P., 1975, The defect in insulin receptors in obese-hyperglycemic mice: A probable accompaniment of more generalized alterations in membrane glycoproteins, *Biochem. Biophys. Res. Commun.* **64**:566.

Chase, L. R., 1975, Selective proteolysis of the receptor for parathyroid hormone in renal cortex, *Endocrinology* **96:**70.

Chase, L. R., and Aurbach, G. D., 1967, Parathyroid function and the renal excretion of 3′,5′-adenylic acid, *Proc. Nat. Acad. Sci. U.S.A.* **58:**518.

Chase, L. R., and Obert, K. A., 1975, Selective proteolysis of the receptor for parathyroid hormone in skeletal tissue, *Metabolism* **24:**1067.

Chase, L. R., Melson, G. L., and Aurbach, G. D., 1969, Pseudohypoparathyroidism: Defective excretion of 3′,5′-AMP in response to parathyroid hormone, *J. Clin. Invest.* **48:**1832.

Chen, L. C., Rohde, J. E., and Sharp, G. W. G., 1971, Intestinal adenyl cyclase activity in human cholera, *Lancet* **1:**939.

Collier, H. O. J., and Francis, D. L., 1975, Morphine abstinence is associated with increased brain cyclic AMP, *Nature* **255:**159.

Collier, H. O. J., and Roy, A. C., 1974, Morphine-like drugs inhibit the stimulation by E prostaglandins of cyclic AMP formation by rat brain homogenate, *Nature* **248:**24.

Corbin, J. D., Keely, S. L., Soderling, T. R., and Park, C. R., 1975, Hormonal regulation of adenosine 3′,5′-monophosphate–dependent protein kinase, *Adv. Cyclic Nucleotide Res.* **5:**265.

Cox, B. M., Opheim, K. E., Teschemacher, H., and Goldstein, A., 1975, A peptide-like substance from pituitary that acts like morphine. 2. Purification and properties, *Life Sci.* **16:**1777.

Cramer, H., Goodwin, F. K., Post, R. M., and Bunney, W. E., Jr., 1972, Effects of probenecid and exercise on cerebrospinal fluid cyclic AMP in affective illness, *Lancet* **1:**1346.

Cuatrecasas, P., 1973, Interaction of *Vibrio cholerae* enterotoxin with cell membranes, *Biochemistry* **12:**3547.

Cuatrecasas, P., Hollenberg, M. D., Chang, K.-J., and Bennett, V., 1975a, Hormone receptor complexes and their modulation of membrane function, *Recent Prog. Horm. Res.* **31:**37.

Cuatrecasas, P., Jacobs, S., and Bennett, V., 1975b, Activation of adenylate cyclase by phosphoramidate and phosphonate analogs of GTP: Possible role of covalent enzyme–substrate intermediates in the mechanism of hormonal activation, *Proc. Nat. Acad. Sci. U.S.A.* **72:**1739.

Davoren, P. R., and Sutherland, E. W., 1963, The effect of 1-epinephrine and other agents on the synthesis and release of adenosine 3′,5′-phosphate by whole pigeon erythrocytes, *J. Biol. Chem.* **238:**3009.

De Meyts, P., 1976, Insulin and growth hormone receptors in human cultured lymphocytes and peripheral blood monocytes, *in: Methods in Molecular Biology*, M. Dekker, New York (in press).

De Meyts, P., Roth, J., Neville, D. M., Jr., Gavin, J. R., III, and Lesniak, M. A., 1973, Insulin interactions with its receptors: Experimental evidence for negative cooperativity, *Biochem. Biophys. Res. Commun.* **55:**154.

Dousa, T. P., Hui, Y. F. S., and Barnes, L. D., 1975, Renal medullary adenylate cyclase in rats with hypothalamic diabetes insipidus, *Endocrinology* **97:**802.

Exton, J. H., Lewis, S. B., Ho, R. J., and Park, C. R., 1972, The role of cyclic AMP in the control of hepatic glucose production by glucagon and insulin, *Adv. Cyclic Nucleotide Res.* **1:**91.

Fain, J. N., and Loken, S. C., 1969, Response of trypsin-treated brown and white fat cells to hormones: Preferential inhibition of insulin action, *J. Biol. Chem.* **244:**3500.

Field, M., 1974, Mode of action of cholera toxin stabilization of catecholamine-sensitive adenylate cyclase in turkey erythrocytes, *Proc. Nat. Acad. Sci. U.S.A.* **71:**3299.

Flier, J. S., Kahn, C. R., Roth, J., and Bar, R. S., 1975, Antibodies that impair insulin receptor binding in an unusual diabetic syndrome with severe insulin resistance, *Science* **190:**63.

Flores, J., and Sharp, G. W. G., 1975, Effects of cholera toxin on adenylate cyclase: Studies with guanylylimidodiphosphate, *J. Clin. Invest.* **56:**1345.

Gill, D. M., 1975, Involvement of nicotinamide adenine dinucleotide in the action of cholera toxin *in vitro*, *Proc. Nat. Acad. Sci. U.S.A.* **72:**2064.

Gill, D. M., and King, C. A., 1975, The mechanism of action of cholera toxin in pigeon erythrocyte lysates, *J. Biol. Chem.* **250:**6424.

Gill, D. M., Pappenheimer, A. M., Jr., and Uchida, T., 1973, Diphtheria toxin, protein synthesis, and the cell, *Fed. Proc. Fed. Amer. Soc. Exp. Biol.* **32:**1508.

Glossmann, H., 1975, Adrenal cortex adenylate cyclase: Specific binding sites for 5'-guanylyl-imidodiphosphate in partially purified plasma membranes from bovine adrenal cortex, *Naunyn-Schmiedeberg's Arch. Pharmacol.* **289:**99.

Glossmann, H., and Gips, H., 1975, Bovine adrenal cortex adenylate cyclase: Properties of the particulate enzyme and effects of guanyl nucleotides, *Naunyn-Schmiedeberg's Arch. Pharmacol.* **289:**77.

Goldstein, A., Lowney, L. I., and Pal, B. K., 1971, Stereospecific and nonspecific interactions of the morphine congener levorphanol in subcellular fractions of mouse brain, *Proc. Nat. Acad. Sci. U.S.A.* **68:**1742.

Goldstein, G., and Schlesinger, D. H., 1975, Thymopoietin and myasthenia gravis: Neostigmine-responsive neuromuscular block produced in mice by a synthetic peptide fragment of thymopoietin, *Lancet* **2:**256.

Gullis, R., Traber, J., and Hamprecht, B., 1975, Morphine elevates levels of cyclic GMP in a neuroblastoma X glioma hybrid cell line, *Nature* **256:**57.

Guttler, R. B., Shaw, J. W., Otis, C., and Nicoloff, J. T., 1975, Epinephrine-induced alterations in urinary cyclic AMP in hyper- and hypothyroidism, *J. Clin. Endocrinol.* **41:**707.

Hanoune, J., Lacombe, M.-L., and Pecker, F., 1975, The epinephrine-sensitive adenylate cyclase of rat liver plasma membranes: Role of guanyl nucleotides, *J. Biol. Chem.* **250:**4569.

Hardman, J. G., Davis, J. W., and Sutherland, E. W., 1966, Measurement of guanosine 3',5'-monophosphate and other cyclic nucleotides, *J. Biol. Chem.* **241:**4812.

Heath, D. A., and Aurbach, G. D., 1975, Studies on the binding of ^{125}I-parathyroid hormone to renal cortical membranes, *in: Calcium-Regulating Hormones* (R. V. Talmage, M. Owen, and J. A. Parsons, eds.), pp. 159–162, Excerpta Medica, Amsterdam.

Hepp, K. D., Langley, J., von Funcke, H. J., Renner, R., and Kemmler, W., 1975, Increased insulin binding capacity of liver membranes from diabetic Chinese hamsters, *Nature* **258:**154.

Hewlett, E. L., Guerrant, R. J., Evans, D. J., Jr., and Greenough, W. B., III, 1974, Toxins of *Vibrio cholerae* and *Escherichia coli* stimulate adenyl cyclase in rat fat cells, *Nature* **249**:371.

Hinkle, P. M., and Tashjian, A. H., Jr., 1975, Degredation of thyrotropin-releasing hormone by the GH-3 strain of pituitary cells in culture, *Endocrinology* **97:** 324.

Hollenberg, M. D., and Cuatrecasas, P., 1975, Insulin and epidermal growth factor; human fibroblast receptors related to deoxyribonucleic acid synthesis and amino acid uptake, *J. Biol. Chem.* **250**:3845.

Hosey, M., and Tao, M., 1975, Effect of 5'-guanylylimidodiphosphate on prostaglandin- and fluoride-sensitive adenylate cyclase of rabbit red blood cells, *Biochem. Biophys. Res. Commun.* **64:**1263.

Huang, D., and Cuatrecasas, P., 1975, Insulin-induced reduction of membrane receptor concentrations in isolated fat cells and lymphocytes, *J. Biol. Chem.* **250:**8251.

Hughes, J., 1975, Isolation of an endogenous compound from the brain with pharmacological properties similar to morphine, *Brain Res.* **88:**295.

Hughes, J., Smith, T. W., Kosterlitz, H. W., Fothergill, L. A., Morgan, B. A., and Morris, H. R., 1975, Identification of two related pentapeptides from the brain with potent opiate agonist activity, *Nature* **258:**577.

Imbert, M., Chabardes, D., Montegut, M., Clique, A., and Morel, F., 1975, Vasopressin dependent adenylate cyclase in single segments of rabbit kidney tubule, *Pflügers Arch.* **357:**173.

Insel, P., Balakir, R., and Sacktor, B., 1975, Binding of cyclic AMP to renal brush border membranes, *J. Cyclic Nucleotide Res.* **1:**107.

Issekutz, T. B., 1975, Estimation of cyclic AMP turnover in normal and methyl-prednisolone-treated dogs: Effect of catecholamines, *Amer. J. Physiol.* **229:**291.

Jard, S., and Bockaert, J., 1975, Stimulus–response coupling in neurohypophysical peptide target cells, *Physiol. Rev.* **55:**489.

Jard, S., Roy, C., Barth, T., Rajerison, R., and Bockaert, J., 1975, Antidiuretic hormone-sensitive kidney adenylate cyclase, *Adv. Cyclic Nucleotide Res.* **5:**31.

Jarett, L., and Smith, R. M., 1975, Ultrastructural localization of insulin receptors on adipocytes, *Proc. Nat. Acad. Sci. U.S.A.* **72:**3526.

Kahn, C. R., and Roth, J., 1975, Cell membrane receptors for polypeptide hormones, *Amer. J. Clin. Pathol.* **63:**656.

Kakiuchi, S., Yamazaki, R., Teshima, Y., Uenishi, K., and Miyamoto, E., 1975, Ca^{2+}/Mg^{2+}-dependent cyclic nucleotide phosphodiesterase and its activator protein, *Adv. Cyclic Nucleotide Res.* **5:**163.

Kaminsky, N. I., Broadus, A. E., Hardman, J. G., Jones, D. J., Jr., Ball, J. H., Sutherland, E. W., and Liddle, G. W., 1970, Effects of parathyroid hormone on plasma and urinary adenosine 3',5'-monophosphate in man, *J. Clin. Invest.* **49:**2387.

Kern, P., Picard, J., Caron, M., and Veissiere, D., 1975, Decreased binding of insulin to liver plasma membrane receptors in hereditary diabetic mice, *Biochim. Biophys. Acta* **389:**281.

Kimberg, D. V., Field, M., Johnson, J., Henderson, A., and Gershaw, E., 1971,

Stimulation of intestinal mucosal adenyl cyclase by cholera enterotoxin and prostaglandins, *J. Clin. Invest.* **50:**1218.

Kinne, R., Shlatz, L. J., Kinne-Saffran, E., and Schwartz, I. L., 1975, Distribution of membrane-bound cyclic AMP–dependent protein kinase in plasma membranes of cells of the kidney cortex, *J. Membrane Biol.* **24:**145.

Klee, W. A., and Nirenberg, M., 1974, A neuroblastoma X glioma hybrid cell line with morphine receptors, *Proc. Nat. Acad. Sci. U.S.A.* **71:**3474.

Klee, W. A., Sharma, S. K., and Nirenberg, M., 1975, Opiate receptors as regulators of adenylate cyclase, *Life Sci.* **16:**1869.

Kono, T., 1969, Destruction of insulin effector system of adipose tissue cells by proteolytic enzymes, *J. Biol. Chem.* **244:**1772.

Kono, T., Robinson, F. W., and Safvef, J. A., 1975, Insulin-sensitive phosphodiesterase: Its localization, hormonal stimulation, and oxidative stabilization, *J. Biol. Chem.* **250:**7826.

Kriss, J. P., Pleshakov, V., and Chien, J. R., 1964, Isolation and identification of the long-acting thyroid stimulator and its relation to hyperthyroidism and circumscribed pretibial myxedema, *J. Clin. Endocrinol.* **24:**1005.

Kuchel, O., Hamet, P., Cuche, J. L., Tolis, G., Fraysse, J., and Genest, J., 1975, Urinary and plasma cyclic adenosine 3′,5′-monophosphate in patients with idiopathic edema, *J. Clin. Endocrinol.* **41:**282.

Lands, A. M., Arnold, A., McAuliff, J. P., Luduena, F. P., and Brown, T. G., Jr., 1967, Differentiation of receptor systems activated by sympathomimetic amines, *Nature* **214:**597.

Lee, C. Y., Stolman, S., Akera, T., and Brody, T. M., 1973, Saturable binding of [³H]-dihydromorphine to rat brain tissue *in vitro:* Characterization and effect of morphine pretreatment, *Pharmacologist* **15:**202 (Abstract No. 258).

Lefkowitz, R. J., 1975, Guanosine triphosphate binding sites in solubilized myocardium, *J. Biol. Chem.* **250:**1006.

Lefkowitz, R. J., and Caron, M. G., 1975, Characteristics of 5′-guanylyl-imidodiphosphate-activated adenylate cyclase, *J. Biol. Chem.* **250:**4418.

Lefkowitz, R. J., Mukherjee, C., Coverstone, M., and Caron, M. G., 1974, Stereospecific [³H](−)alprenolol binding sites, β-adrenergic receptors and adenylate cyclase, *Biochem. Biophys. Res. Commun.* **60:**703.

Lennon, V. A., Lindstrom, J. M., and Seybold, M. E., 1975, Experimental autoimmune myasthenia: A model of myasthenia gravis in rats and guinea pigs, *J. Exp. Med.* **141:**1365.

Levey, G. S., Fletcher, M. A., and Klein, I., 1975, Glucagon and adenylate cyclase: Binding studies and requirements for activation, *Adv. Cyclic Nucleotide Res.* **5:**53.

Levitzki, A., Atlas, D., and Steer, M. L., 1974, The binding characteristics and number of β-adrenergic receptors on the turkey erythrocyte, *Proc. Nat. Acad. Sci. U.S.A.* **71:**2773.

Liljenquist, J. E., Bomboy, J. D., Lewis, S. B., Sinclair-Smith, B. C., Felts, P. W., Lacy, W. W., Crofford, O. B., and Liddle, G. W., 1974, Effect of glucagon on net aplanchnic cyclic AMP production in normal and diabetic men, *J. Clin. Invest.* **53:**198.

Limbird, L. E., De Meyts, P., and Lefkowitz, R. J., 1975, β-Adrenergic receptors: Evidence for negative cooperativity, *Biochem. Biophys. Res. Commun.* **64:**1160.

Lin, T., Kopp, L. E., and Tucci, J. R., 1973, Urinary excretion of cyclic 3′,5′-adenosine monophosphate in hyperthyroidism, *J. Clin. Endocrinol.* **36:**1033.

Linarelli, L. G., 1972, Newborn urinary cyclic AMP and developmental renal responsiveness to parathyroid hormone, *Pediatrics* **50:**14.

Loten, E. G., and Sneyd, J. G. T., 1970, An effect of insulin on adipose-tissue adenosine 3′,5′-cyclic monophosphate phosphodiesterase, *Biochem. J.* **120:**187.

Lowney, L. I., Schultz, K., Lowery, P. J., and Goldstein, A., 1974, Partial purification of an opiate receptor from mouse brain, *Science* **183:**749.

Maguire, M. E., Wiklund, R. A., Anderson, H. J., and Gilman, A. G., 1976, Binding of [^{125}I]iodohydroxybenzylpindolol to putative β-adrenergic receptors of rat glioma cells and other cell clones, *J. Biol. Chem.* **251:**1221.

Mallette, L. E., Bilezikian, J. P., Heath, D. A., and Aurbach, G. D., 1974, Primary hyperparathyroidism: clinical and biochemical features, *Medicine* **53:**127.

Manley, S. W., Bourke, J. R., and Hawker, R. W., 1974, The thyrotropin receptor in guinea pig thyroid homogenate: Interaction with the long-acting thyroid stimulator, *J. Endocrinol.* **61:**437.

Marx, S. J., and Aurbach, G. D., 1975, Renal receptors for calcitonin: Coordinate occurrence with calcitonin-activated adenylate cyclase, *Endocrinology* **97:**448.

Marx, S. J., Woodard, C. J., and Aurbach, G. D., 1972, Calcitonin receptors of kidney and bone, *Science* **178:**999.

McKenzie, J. M., 1958, Delayed thyroid response to serum from thyrotoxic patients, *Endocrinology* **62:**865.

Meek, J. C., Jones, A. E., Lewis, U. J., and VanderLaan, W. P., 1964, Characterization of the long-acting thyroid stimulator of Graves' disease, *Proc. Nat. Acad. Sci. U.S.A.* **52:**342.

Megyesi, K., Kahn, C. R., Roth, J., Neville, D. M., Jr., Nissley, S. P., Humbel, R. E., and Froesch, E. R., 1975, The NSILA-s receptor in liver plasma membranes: Characterization and comparison with the insulin receptor, *J. Biol. Chem.* **250:**8990.

Mehdi, S. Q., and Nussey, S. S., 1975, A radio-ligand receptor assay for the long-acting thyroid stimulator: Inhibition by the long-acting thyroid stimulator of the binding of radioiodinated thyroid-stimulating hormone to human thyroid membranes, *Biochem. J.* **145:**105.

Mickey, J., Tate, R., and Lefkowitz, R. J., 1975, Subsensitivity of adenylate cyclase and decreased β-adrenergic receptor binding after chronic exposure to (−)isoproterenol *in vitro, J. Biol. Chem.* **250:**5727.

Morel, F., Chabardes, D., and Imbert, M., 1975, Target sites of antidiuretic hormone (ADH) and parathyroid hormone (PTH) along the segments of the nephron, *Adv. Nephrol.* **5:**283.

Mukherjee, C., Caron, M. G., Coverstone, M., and Lefkowitz, R. J., 1975a, Identification of adenylate cyclase–coupled β-adrenergic receptors in frog erythrocytes with (−)-[^{3}H]alprenolol, *J. Biol. Chem.* **250:**4869.

Mukherjee, C., Caron, M. G., and Lefkowitz, R. J., 1975b, Catecholamine-induced subsensitivity of adenylate cyclase associated with loss of β-adrenergic receptor binding sites, *Proc. Nat. Acad. Sci. U.S.A.* **72:**1945.

Murad, F., 1973, Clinical studies and application of cyclic nucleotides, *Adv. Cyclic Nucleotide Res.* **3:**355.

Murad, F., Moss, W. W., Johanson, A. J., and Selden, R. F., 1975, Urinary excretion of adenosine 3′,5′-monophosphate and guanosine 3′,5′-monophosphate in normal children and those with cystic fibrosis, *J. Clin. Endocrinol.* **40:**552.

Neelon, F. A., Drezner, M., Birch, B. M., and Lebovitz, H. E., 1973, Urinary cyclic adenosine monophosphate as an aid in the diagnosis of hyperparathyroidism, *Lancet* **1:**631.

Olefsky, J. M., and Reaven, G. M., 1975, Effects of age and obesity on insulin binding to isolated adipocytes, *Endocrinology* **96:**1486.

Orly, J., and Schramm, M., 1975, Fatty acids as modulators of membrane functions: Catecholamine-activated adenylate cyclase of the turkey erythrocyte, *Proc. Nat. Acad. Sci. U.S.A.* **72:**3433.

Pak, C. Y. C., Kaplan, R., Bone, H., Townsend, J., and Waters, O., 1975, A simple test for the diagnosis of absorptive, resorptive and renal hypercalciurias, *N. Engl. J. Med.* **292:**497.

Pasternak, G. W., Goodman, R., and Snyder, S. H., 1975, An endogenous morphine-like factor in mammalian brain, *Life Sci.* **16:**1765.

Patrick, J., and Lindstrom, J., 1973, Autoimmune response to acetylcholine receptor, *Science* **180:**871.

Patrick, J., Lindstrom, J., Culp, B., and McMillan, J., 1973, Studies on purified eel acetylcholine receptor and anti-acetylcholine receptor antibody, *Proc. Nat. Acad. Sci. USA* **70:**3334.

Pert, C. B., and Snyder, S. H., 1973, Opiate receptor: Demonstration in nervous tissue, *Science* **179:**1011.

Peytremann, A., Nicholson, W. E., Hardman, J. G., and Liddle, G. N., 1973, Effect of adrenocorticotropic hormone on extracellular adenosine 3′,5′-monophosphate in the hypophysectomized rat, *Endocrinology* **92:**1502.

Pfeuffer, T., and Helmreich, E. J. M., 1975, Activation of pigeon erythrocyte membrane adenylate cyclase by guanylnucleotide analogues and separation of a nucleotide binding protein, *J. Biol. Chem.* **250:**867.

Pittman, R. C., Khoo, J. C., and Steinberg, D., 1975, Cholesterol esterase in rat adipose tissue and its activation by cyclic adenosine 3′,5′-monophosphate-dependent protein kinase, *J. Biol. Chem.* **250:**4505.

Queener, S. F., Fleming, J. W., and Bell, N. H., 1975, Solubilization of calcitonin-responsive renal cortical adenylate cyclase, *J. Biol. Chem.* **250:**7586.

Robison, G. A., Butcher, R. W., and Sutherland, E. W., 1971, *Cyclic AMP,* Academic Press, New York, 531 pp.

Rodbell, M., Krans, H. M. J., Pohl, S. L., and Birnbaumer, L., 1971, The glucagon-sensitive adenyl cyclase system in plasma membranes of rat liver. IV. Effects of guanyl nucleotides on binding of ^{125}I-glucagon, *J. Biol. Chem.* **246:**1872.

Rodbell, M., Lin, M. C., Salomon, Y., Londos, C., Harwood, J. P., Martin, B. R., Rendell, M., and Berman, M., 1975, Role of adenine and guanine nucleotides in the activity and response of adenylate cyclase systems to hormones: Evidence for multisite transition states, *Adv. Cyclic Nucleotide Res.* **5**:3.

Romero, J. A., Zatz, M., Kebabian, J. W., and Axelrod, J., 1975, Circadian cycles in binding of ^{3}H-alprenolol to β-adrenergic receptor sites in rat pineal, *Nature* **258**:435.

Rosen, O. M., Erlichman, J., and Rubin, C. S., 1975, Molecular structure and characterization of bovine heart protein kinase, *Adv. Cyclic Nucleotide Res.* **5**:253.

Roth, J., Kahn, C. R., Lesniak, M. A., Gorden, P., De Meyts, P., Megyesi, K., Neville, D. M., Jr., Gavin, J. R., III, Soll, A. H., Freychet, P., Goldfine, I. D., Bar, R. S., and Archer, J. A., 1975, Receptors for insulin, NSILA-s, and growth hormone: Applications to disease states in man, *Recent Prog. Horm. Res.* **31**:95.

Rudolph, S. A., and Greengard, P., 1974, Regulation of protein phosphorylation and membrane permeability by β-adrenergic agents and cyclic adenosine 3′,5′-monophosphate in the avian erythrocyte, *J. Biol. Chem.* **249**:5684.

Salomon, Y., Lin, M. C., Londos, C., Rendell, M., and Rodbell, M., 1975, The hepatic adenylate cyclase system. I. Evidence for transition states and structural requirements for guanine nucleotide activation, *J. Biol. Chem.* **250**:4239.

Schramm, M., 1975, The catecholamine-responsive adenylate cyclase system and its modification by 5′-guanylylimidodiphosphate, *Adv. Cyclic Nucleotide Res.* **5**:105.

Schramm, M., and Rodbell, M., 1975, A persistent active state of the adenylate cyclase system produced by the combined actions of isoproterenol and guanylylimidodiphosphate in frog erythrocyte membranes, *J. Biol. Chem.* **250**:2232.

Schwartz, R. H., Bianco, A. R., Handwerger, B. S., and Kahn, C. R., 1975, Demonstration that monocytes rather than lymphocytes are the insulin-binding cells in preparations of human peripheral blood mononuclear leukocytes: Implications for studies of insulin-resistant states in man, *Proc. Nat. Acad. Sci. U.S.A.* **72**:474.

Scurry, M. T., and Pauk, G. L., 1974, Renal tubular localization of parathyroid hormone induced urinary cyclic adenosine 3′,5′-monophosphate, *Acta Endocrinol.* **77**:282.

Sebens, J. B., and Korf, J., 1975, Cyclic AMP in cerebrospinal fluid: Accumulation following probenecid and biogenic amines, *Exp. Neurol.* **46**:333.

Sharma, S. K., Klee, W. A., and Nirenberg, M., 1975a, Dual regulation of adenylate cyclase accounts for narcotic dependence and tolerance, *Proc. Nat. Acad. Sci. U.S.A.* **72**:3092.

Sharma, S. K., Nirenberg, M., and Klee, W. A., 1975b, Morphine receptors as regulators of adenylate cyclase activity, *Proc. Nat. Acad. Sci. U.S.A.* **72**:590.

Sharp, G. W. G., and Hynie, S., 1971, Stimulation of intestinal adenyl cyclase by cholera toxin, *Nature* **229**:266.

Schlatz, L. J., Schwartz, I. L., Kinne-Saffran, E., and Kinne, R., 1975, Distribution of parathyroid hormone–stimulated adenylate cyclase in plasma membranes of cells of the kidney cortex, *J. Membrane Biol.* **24**:131.

Simon, E. J., Hiller, J. M., and Edelman, I., 1973, Stereospecific binding of the potent narcotic analgesic [^{3}H]etorphine to rat-brain homogenate, *Proc. Nat. Acad. Sci. U.S.A.* **70:**1947.

Smith, B. R. and Hall, R., 1974, Thyroid-stimulating immunoglobulins in Graves' disease, *Lancet* **2:**427.

Soll, A. H., Kahn, C. R., and Neville, D. M., Jr., 1975a, Insulin binding to liver plasma membranes in the obese hyperglycemic (ob/ob) mouse: Demonstration of a decreased number of functionally normal receptors, *J. Biol. Chem.* **250:**4702.

Soll, A. H., Kahn, C. R., Neville, D. M., Jr., and Roth, J., 1975b, Insulin receptor deficiency in genetic and acquired obesity, *J. Clin. Invest.* **56:**769.

Spiegel, A. M., and Aurbach, G. D., 1974, Binding of 5'-guanylyl-imidodiphosphate to turkey erythrocyte membranes and effect on β-adrenergic-activated adenylate cyclase, *J. Biol. Chem.* **249:**7630.

Spiegel, A. M., Bilezikian, J. P., and Aurbach, G. D., 1975, Increased adrenergic receptor content in membranes of stress-induced erythrocytes, *Clin. Res.* **23:**390A (abstract).

Spiegel, A. M., Brown, E. M., Fedak, S. A., Woodard, C. J., and Aurbach, G. D., 1976, Holocatalytic state of adenylate cyclase in turkey erythrocyte membranes: Formation with guanylylimidodiphosphate plus isoproterenol without effect on affinity of β-receptor, *J. Cyclic Nucleotide Res.* **2:**47.

Stephenson, R. P., 1956, A modification of receptor theory, *Brit. J. Pharmacol.* **11:**379.

Strange, R. C., and Mjøs, O. D., 1975, The sources of plasma cyclic AMP: Studies in the rat using isoprenaline, nicotinic acid and glucagon, *Eur. J. Clin. Invest.* **5:**147.

Terenius, L., 1973, Stereospecific interaction between narcotic analgesics and a synaptic plasma membrane fraction of rat cerebral cortex, *Acta Pharmacol.* **32:**317.

Terenius, L., and Wahlström, A., 1975, Search for an endogenous ligand for the opiate receptor, *Acta Physiol. Scand.* **94:**74.

Teschemacher, H., Opheim, K. E., Cox, B. M., and Golstein, A., 1975, A peptide-like substance from pituitary that acts like morphine. 1. Isolation, *Life Sci.* **16:**1771.

Tomlinson, S., Hendy, G. N., and O'Riordan, J. L. H., 1976, A simplifed assessment of response to parathyroid hormone in hypoparathyroid patients, *Lancet* **1:**62.

Van Heyningen, S., and King, C. A., 1975, Subunit A from cholera toxin is an activator of adenylate cyclase in pigeon erythrocytes, *Biochem. J.* **146:**269.

Van Wyk, J. J., Underwood, L. E., Baseman, J. B., Hintz, R. L., Clemmons, D. R., and Marshall, R. N., 1975, Explorations of the insulin-like and growth-promoting properties of somatomedin by membrane receptor assays, *Adv. Metab. Disord.* **8:**127.

Wang, J. H., Teo, T. S., Ho, H. C., and Stevens, F. C., 1975, Bovine heart protein activator of cyclic nucleotide phosphodiesterase, *Adv. Cyclic Nucleotide Res.* **5:**179.

Wehmann, R. E., Blonde, L., and Steiner, A. L., 1974, Sources of cyclic nucleotides in plasma *J. Clin. Invest.* **53:**173.

Wilfong, R. F., and Neville, D. M., Jr., 1970, The isolation of a brush border membrane fraction from rat kidney, *J. Biol. Chem.* **245**:6106.

Williams, L. T., Snyderman, R., and Lefkowitz, R. J., 1976, Identification of β-adrenergic receptors in human lymphocytes by (−)[^{3}H]alprenolol binding, *J. Clin. Invest.* **57**:149.

Winand, R. J., and Kohn, L. D., 1974, Stimulation of adenylate cyclase activity in retro-orbital tissue membranes by thyrotropin and an exophthalmogenic factor derived from thyrotropin, *J. Biol. Chem.* **250**:6522.

Wolff, J., and Cook, G. H., 1975a, Choleragen stimulates steroidogenesis and adenylate cyclase in cells lacking functional hormone receptors, *Biochim. Biophys. Acta* **413**:283.

Wolff, J., and Cook, G. H., 1975b, Endotoxic lipopolysaccharides stimulate steroidogenesis and adenylate cyclase in adrenal tumor-cells, *Biochim. Biophys. Acta* **413**:291.

Yamashita, K. and Field, J. B., 1972, Effects of long-acting thyroid stimulator on thyrotropin stimulation of adenyl cyclase activity in thyroid plasma membranes, *J. Clin. Invest.* **51**:463.

Diabetes Mellitus

Stefan S. Fajans

2.1. Introduction

In this chapter, the author has attempted to review publications during the past year in the field of diabetes mellitus that have contributed to new points of view, that constitute progress in a particular area, or that expand significantly on previously reported information. To achieve appropriate perspective, work appearing in earlier years has been cited where necessary.

2.2. Heterogeneity in Etiology and Pathogenesis

There has been an accumulation of evidence suggesting that there is heterogeneity in the etiology and pathogenesis of diabetes. Hypergly-

---

STEFAN S. FAJANS • Department of Internal Medicine, Division of Endrocinology and Metabolism and the Metabolism Research Unit, The University of Michigan, Ann Arbor, Michigan 48109.

cemia and the chronic complications of diabetes (complications of pregnancy, cataracts, neuropathy, atherosclerosis, microangiopathy) are found in both the juvenile-onset, ketosis-prone, and the maturity-onset, or "ketosis-resistant," type of diabetes. These two types of diabetes have usually been thought to represent only a quantitative difference in the defect in insulin secretion or action. However, a growing body of evidence suggests the existence of heterogeneity of "idiopathic diabetes mellitus" in terms of inheritance, insulin responses to glucose in maturity-onset diabetes, and prevalence of vascular disease. Thus, it appears that "idiopathic" diabetes mellitus is not a single disease entity. In this respect, diabetes can be likened to hypertension and its vascular complications, hypertension being the result of a variety of pathogenetic mechanisms.

2.2.1. Heterogeneity of Heredity

There are multiple lines of evidence to indicate that there is heterogeneity of inheritance of "idiopathic" diabetes mellitus (as distinguished from secondary types of diabetes or carbohydrate intolerance associated with a variety of well-defined genetic syndromes).

2.2.1.1. Patterns of Inheritance

A difference in patterns of inheritance has been shown between the families of 26 propositi with the *maturity-onset* type of *diabetes* in *young* people (MODY; under 25 years of age at diagnosis) and families of 35 propositi with the classic *juvenile-onset* type of *diabetes* (JOD) (Tattersall and Fajans, 1975a). In the families of Mody: (1) 85% of propositi had a diabetic parent, (2) 46% of families showed direct vertical transmission of diabetes through three generations, (3) 53% of tested siblings had latent* diabetes, and (4) the diabetic phenotype in the families was consistent, most affected patients having a type of diabetes not requiring insulin. These findings are compatible with autosomal dominant inheritance of MODY, although they do not exclude multifactorial inheritance. In contrast, in the families of JOD, only 11% of propositi had a diabetic parent, and three-generation inheritance was found in only 6% of JOD families. Of 74 tested siblings, 8% had the JOD type of diabetes, and only 3% had

---

*A latent (or asymptomatic or chemical) diabetic is a patient who has no signs, symptoms, or complications referable to the disease (except for reactive hypoglycemia in some patients), but in whom a definite diagnosis of diabetes can be established by presently accepted laboratory procedures. This stage may be characterized by an occasional elevated fasting blood glucose level, but when present, it is of lesser severity than in overt diabetes. When the fasting blood glucose is below diagnostic levels, latent diabetes can be recognized by an abnormal glucose tolerance test.

latent diabetes. This difference not only provides evidence of genetic heterogeneity, but also further indicates that there is a need for careful definition of the phenotype of diabetes in populations in which the genetics of diabetes is to be analyzed.

In contrast to the high prevalence of the maturity-onset type of diabetes among the parents and grandparents of MODY-propositi (mean age 19 years at diagnosis), there is an equal prevalence of the adult-onset type of diabetes among ancestors of juvenile diabetics and nondiabetics (MacDonald, 1974). The families of 118 ketosis-prone, insulin-requiring diabetic children who were diagnosed before age 16, and the families of 118 nondiabetics with a family history of no individuals diagnosed as diabetic prior to age 30, were interviewed. The incidence of individuals diagnosed as diabetic after age 45 among 423 grandparents of the diabetic children (0.078) was not significantly different from that among 395 grandparents of the children in whose families there was no childhood diabetes (0.071). This finding is also interpreted as evidence that juvenile and adult-onset diabetes are under different genetic control.

The prevalence of diabetes and glucose intolerance among offspring of conjugal adult-onset type diabetic parents was found to be 45–60% (Tattersall and Fajans, 1975b; Radder and Terpstra, 1975). No data are available to ascertain the prevalence and type of diabetes among offspring of conjugal juvenile-onset type diabetic patients.

2.2.1.2. Histocompatibility Typing

A difference in the inheritance between the juvenile-onset and maturity-onset types of diabetes may be associated with a difference in the frequency of occurrence of certain histocompatibility types or HLA antigens (HLA-B8 or Bw15 or both) (Nerup et al., 1974; Cudworth and Woodrow, 1975), and a difference in the frequency with which viral or autoimmune processes, or both, may be involved. When 146 diabetics were HLA typed, HLA-B8 and Bw15 were significantly more frequent in the diabetics than in 967 controls (Nerup et al., 1974). The increase was found almost exclusively in insulin-dependent diabetics. These findings support the concept that insulin-dependent and insulin-independent diabetes are two different disease entities. Similar data supporting a positive association of acute-onset juvenile diabetes with HLA-B8 and Bw15 antigens were found among 100 diabetic patients (Cudworth and Woodrow, 1975). In addition, 4 families were described with 2 or more members with this type of diabetes, and in each family, affected individuals share a haplotype including HLA-B8 or Bw15. A further implication of these findings is the possibility that the HLA determinants themselves might be involved in promoting disease susceptibility. A more likely possibility, however, is that immune response genes at loci closely linked with HLA loci are involved. Genes in the HLA chromosomal region may impart increased susceptibility to beta cell damage by viral agents by influencing virus receptor sites or by failing to eliminate an infective virus that might destroy pancreatic beta cells, or they may play a role in an immune response leading to an autoimmune process.. The presence of cell-mediated immunity to pancreas antigens has been reported to be more frequent in patients with insulin-dependent than in patients with insulin-independent diabetes (Nerup et al., 1974; McCuish et al., 1974). These findings also support the concept that the two types of diabetes differ from each other, and have been cited to indicate that they are two different diseases in etiology and pathogenesis (Nerup et al., 1974).

2.2.1.3. Twin Studies

2.2.1.3a. Prevalence of Diabetes. Genetic heterogeneity has been found among sets of identical twins of which at least one had diabetes mellitus (Tattersall and Pyke, 1972). Concordance of diabetes among the pairs of identical twins was very high (92%) among those in whom the age of onset of diabetes in the index twin was 40 years or more (mostly maturity-onset type), while concordance was found with a frequency of only 53% in those in whom diabetes was diagnosed under 40 years of age in one twin (mostly juvenile-onset type). This finding suggests that there is a difference in genetic as well as environmental factors in the etiology and pathogenesis of diabetes between these two groups of identical twins.

2.2.1.3b. HLA Typing. Histocompatibility typing performed in 84 pairs of identical twins of whom at least one was diabetic (Nelson et al., 1975) has given further evidence for possible differences in a hereditary predisposition to diabetes. Twenty-two pairs of identical twins were maturity-onset diabetics; all were concordant, and they showed no disturbance of HLA frequencies. Of the remaining 62 pairs of juvenile-onset diabetics, 31 were discordant and 31 concordant. Frequency of the Bw15 antigen was equally increased in both the concordant and discordant pairs. That Bw15 is increased in the discordant pairs shows that there is a genetic predisposition to diabetes even in the nondiabetic twin. The HLA-B8 antigen was increased only in the concordant pairs. That HLA-B8 is not increased in the discordant pairs suggests that different alleles may underlie susceptibility in the two groups of twins. The increased frequency of HLA-B8 in the concordant twins and the normal frequency in the discordant twins provides some support for there being more than one allele.

2.2.1.4. Autoimmunity

Autoimmunity has been linked to insulin-dependent juvenile-onset type diabetes (Editorial, 1974). The evidence supporting such an association can be summarized as follows: (1) the clinical association of diabetes with other diseases that have acute immune features, including antibody-positive thyroid disorders (Hashimoto thyroiditis, primary hypothyroidism), Graves' disease, pernicious anemia, Addison's disease, and hypoparathyroidism, and the coexistence of diabetes with multiple autoimmune disorders; (2) the finding of increased incidence of organ-specific humoral antithyroid, gastric-parietal cell, and adrenal antibodies in diabetes; (3) the demonstration of insulitis in patients dying soon after the onset of diabetes, suggesting a cellular immune response; (4) demonstration by leukocyte migration inhibition tests of antipancreatic cell–mediated immunity to pancreatic antigens of animal and human pancreases in juvenile diabetes; and (5) detection by immunofluorescence of humoral islet cell antibodies in patients with diabetes associated with other autoimmune polyendocrine disease.

During 1975, more direct evidence has been presented suggesting that autoimmune beta cell damage occurs in most insulin-dependent diabetics. Circulating antibodies to live, tissue-cultured, human insulinoma cells were identified in 34 of 39 insulin-dependent diabetic patients by an indirect immunofluorescent technique (MacLaren *et al.*, 1975). The antibodies were not related to therapy with exogenous insulin. They were of the IgM and IgG classes. These findings, if confirmed, would also suggest that autoimmune mechanisms are important in the pathogenesis of most cases of insulin-requiring diabetes. In another study, antibodies reacting with human pancreatic islet cells were found by immunofluorescence in the serum of 51 of 105 children with diabetes mellitus of recent onset (Lendrum *et al.*, 1975). These antibodies were of the IgG class. These patients had no other evidence of autoimmune disease. Of 54 sera scored negative, 32 showed a faint fluorescence, compared with only 5 of 71 similar controls. It seems likely, therefore, that there may be autoimmune activity directed against islet cells of a substantial proportion, if not of a majority, of cases of childhood diabetes of recent onset. The age distribution and seasonal variation in onset that occur in juvenile diabetes suggested to the authors that autoimmune damage may be combined with a seasonal factor, e.g., viral.

2.2.2. Environmental Factors

Environmental factors superimposed on an inherited predisposition may be essential for the development of recognizable or clinical diabetes.

Heterogeneity of environmental factors that precipitate or cause the emergence of the disease may also exist. Recently, viruses have been implicated in the pathogenesis of the juvenile-onset type of diabetes, while nutritional factors have been thought for many decades to play a role in the pathogenesis of the maturity-onset type of diabetes.

2.2.2.1. Viral Factors—Multiple

Excellent reviews have summarized the epidemiological evidence that suggests a temporal association between viral infection and the onset of the juvenile-onset type of diabetes (Maugh, 1975a,b; Craighead, 1975a). A seasonal variation in the incidence of the juvenile-onset type of diabetes has been reported. The incidence varies with an autumn peak about October and a winter peak from December to March. This variation implies the presence of seasonal, environmental etiological factors, and virus infection seems a likely candidate.

The epidemiological studies of Gamble and Taylor have shown an interesting correlation between Coxsackie virus B_4 infection and the onset of diabetes mellitus in patients under 30 years of age. These investigators noted that insulin-dependent diabetic patients possessed higher titers of neutralizing antibodies against Coxsackie virus group B, type 4, than did selected control subjects. These differences were observed only when the disease was of relatively short duration, i.e., less than 3 months. The incidence of the juvenile-onset type of diabetes has also been said to parallel the incidence for mumps and mumps encephalitis, if allowance is made for a 4-year lag time (Sultz et al., 1975).

Other infective agents implicated have included hepatitis, congenital rubella, and other viruses. Although some of this evidence is contradictory and inconclusive, it is nonetheless likely that viruses play some role in the initiation of the juvenile-onset type of diabetes. If viruses are in fact involved in the pathogenesis of diabetes, it is likely that they can initiate pancreatic damage only in persons who are genetically predisposed to such damage. As reviewed above, the juvenile form of diabetes appears to be linked to histocompatibility antigens that may be associated with certain genes controlling immune responses. Thus, the failure to find an increased prevalence of diabetes in a population infected with Coxsackie B_4 (Dippe et al., 1975) does not rule out the potential importance of viruses in the pathogenesis of insulin-dependent diabetes in predisposed persons.

Diabetes could also result from many different series of infections producing cumulative pancreatic damage. Alternatively, one might expect an autoimmune process to be a self-feeding mechanism, and once it is triggered, the resulting tissue damage would sustain the process.

Although studies of virus-induced diabetes in animals provide circumstantial support for the virus theory in man, there is as yet little direct evidence for it.

Craighead has shown that a diabeteslike disease can be produced in certain strains of mice by the M variant of the encephalomyocarditis (EMC) virus (Craighead, 1975b). After inoculation, viremia is relatively transient, and is followed by the abrupt appearance of circulating neutralizing antibody in the serum. Virus can be recovered from the pancreas, heart, and brain for as long as 18 days after inoculation. Immunofluorescence studies of the pancreas have demonstrated viral antigens exclusively in the insular tissue. The severity of the diabetic syndrome is directly related to the amount of necrosis of beta cells. The most important factor in the development of diabetes in mice seems to be a genetic susceptibility to pancreatic damage resulting from the infection. Results of genetic studies showed that several strains of mice regularly develop hyperglycemia during the acute stages of infection, whereas other strains infrequently exhibit evidence of abnormal carbohydrate metabolism. Other investigators have shown that several strains of mice were resistant to the diabetogenic effects of EMC virus.

Further evidence has been presented that subjects who may have a genetic predisposition to JOD diabetes need not have an impaired or subnormal insulin response to glucose or a raised or supernormal insulin response as the basic or initial lesion. Among young nondiabetic monozygotic twins of JOD-type diabetic patients, a normal insulin secretory response to glucose has been found (Johansen et al., 1975). As reviewed earlier, discordance of diabetes in monozygotic twins has been found to be relatively high in those pairs when the index twin developed diabetes under the age of 40. This finding suggests that in these twins, diabetes evolves from a genetic predisposition only with the superimposition of a specific environmental factor such as a viral infection or development of autoimmunity, or both.

2.2.2.2. Nutritional Factors

In the maturity-onset type of diabetes, which represents a different type of genetic predisposition (no disturbance of HLA frequencies) from the juvenile-onset type of diabetes, other environmental factors such as overnutrition and resulting obesity (or pregnancy) may lead to hyperglycemia (Tattersall and Fajans, 1975b; Radder and Terpstra, 1975).

Insulin levels were determined prospectively in subjects before and after they developed the maturity-onset type of diabetes. Immunoreactive insulin levels were studied in 13 obese Pima Indians who initially had glucose tolerance tests within normal limits, but when followed longitudinally became unequivocally diabetic (Savage *et al.*, 1975b). The insulin and glucose values for the group that became diabetic, but that were studied prior to the development of diabetes, were not different from the insulin and glucose values of a matched control group. There were no differences between the values of these two groups in the fasting state or at 1/2, 1, or 2 hr after the oral administration of glucose. This study indicates that these "prediabetics"* who developed the maturity-onset type of diabetes also secreted neither excess nor deficient insulin prior to the development of diabetes.

2.2.3. Insulin Secretion

2.2.3.1. Heterogeneity of Insulin Responses to Glucose in the Maturity-Onset Type of Diabetes

In addition to evidence that there are differences in genetic and environmental factors between insulin-dependent and insulin-independent diabetes, there is also evidence for heterogeneity of insulin responses in asymptomatic diabetes. From cross-sectional studies, it has been suggested that the magnitude of the insulin response to glucose depends on the severity of carbohydrate intolerance, mild carbohydrate intolerance being associated with supernormal 2-hr insulin levels and more severe carbohydrate intolerance being associated with low insulin levels (Savage *et al.*, 1975a). However, other investigators have found, in groups of patients with comparable glucose intolerance, either an impaired initial and subnormal insulin secretory response (hypoinsulinemia) (Fujita *et al.*, 1975) or a supernormal insulin response (hyperinsulinemia) (Ginsberg *et al.*, 1974) to a glycemic stimulus, suggesting insulin resistance.

In a longitudinal prospective study, most of the latent diabetic patients had a significantly delayed and subnormal increment in plasma insulin in response to glucose, but the magnitude of the individual responses to glucose encompassed a wide spectrum (Fajans *et al.*, 1974a,b). At one extreme, greatly decreased insulin responses appear to be the determinant, at least in part, of abnormal carbohydrate tolerance. On follow-up with therapy, the insulin responses were greater, and glucose levels were lower. At the other extreme were the patients with glucose intolerance, who had insulin responses that were supernormal. On follow-up with therapy, their insulin responses decreased toward or to normal, and carbohydrate tolerance improved. These results suggest that in these patients, hyperinsulinemia is secondary or compensatory to the factors that cause glucose intolerance. Progression to insulin-requiring diabetes

---

*By definition, these are true "prediabetics"; i.e., they progress from the nondiabetic to the diabetic state.

(some to the ketosis-prone type) occurred only in patients who had insulin responses that were subnormal or lower than the mean response of the control subjects. Such an insulin response appears to be a more reliable prognostic indicator of decompensation to insulin-requiring diabetes than the degree of abnormality of carbohydrate intolerance or the fasting level of glucose at presentation. None of these patients with supernormal insulin responses progressed to fasting hyperglycemia or insulin-requiring diabetes. Between the two extremes, there was a continuum of insulin responses. One interpretation of these data would be that the variation in insulin responses represents a gradation in pancreatic reserve from severe (absolute insulinopenia) to mild (absolute hyperinsulinemia, but relative hypoinsulinemia in terms of compensation for carbohydrate intolerance). Another interpretation would favor a heterogeneity of insulin responses to glucose in nonobese patients with latent diabetes (Fajans et al., 1974a), a concept that is supported by the difference in insulin responses with improvement of carbohydrate intolerance. Such a concept would support the view that so-called idiopathic diabetes includes more than one disorder associated with hyperglycemia.

2.2.3.2. Insulin Resistance

2.2.3.2a. In Vivo. When hyperinsulinemia is found in diabetes, it appears to be secondary to insulin resistance. Resistance to insulin-mediated glucose uptake has been demonstrated in nonobese patients with the maturity-onset type of diabetes. This resistance had been reported previously in patients with chemical diabetes. The same authors (Ginsberg et al., 1975) concluded that insulin resistance exists in adult-onset diabetes with fasting hyperglycemia. Insulin resistance was assessed again by administering constant infusions of epinephrine, propranolol, glucose, and exogenous insulin. This study protocol is based on the assumptions that endogenous insulin secretion is suppressed by epinephrine and propranolol (by α-adrenergic stimulation), and that hepatic glucose output is suppressed by the infusion of glucose and insulin. The rationale of this method is to measure the ability of similar plasma levels of insulin to induce glucose uptake. Similar steady-state plasma insulin levels were achieved in all subjects of this study. The mean steady-state glucose level of the 14 diabetic patients was 350 mg/dl; that of 12 normal subjects was 121 mg/dl. Additional studies indicated that a difference in initial plasma glucose levels could not account for the different glucose responses of the two groups to the basic infusion. There was no insulin resistance in patients with hyperglycemia due to chronic pancreatitis. The data reported with this experimental design do not exclude the possibility that healthy and diabetic patients have different counterregulatory responses to the pharmacological mixture administered, rather than different degrees of resistance to insulin in the basal state.

2.2.3.2b. In Vitro—Receptor-Binding Studies. A defect in insulin-binding to target cells due to a decrease in the number of available insulin-receptor sites (as demonstrated by the use of circulating monocytes) has been evoked to explain the hyperinsulinemia of insulin-resistant diabetic subjects (Olefsky and Reaven, 1974).

Patients with a unique and rare form of diabetes associated with extreme insulin resistance and acanthosis nigricans have markedly reduced insulin-binding to specific receptors on their circulating monocytes (Flier *et al.*, 1975). When normal insulin receptors were exposed to serum or immunoglobulin fractions from 3 of these patients *in vitro*, the specific binding defect was reproduced. A serum factor, most probably an antibody from these patients, alters the insulin receptor and impairs subsequent binding of insulin. This factor recreates *in vitro* the defect in insulin-binding observed with these patients' own cells, and accounts reasonably for the extreme resistance to the effect of insulin. The binding of insulin to the insulin receptor in four well-characterized systems— circulating human monocytes, cultured human lymphocytes, highly purified plasma membranes of rat liver, and fresh avian erythrocytes—was used. It is likely that the serum factor that inhibits insulin-binding to its receptors is an immunoglobulin. The inhibitory effect is not due to antiinsulin antibodies. The antibody might occupy the receptor site directly, or bind to the cell on or near the insulin receptor, producing steric hindrance of insulin-binding. The antibody might also interact with a membrane component distant from the receptor, inducing a change in the membrane that subsequently alters the insulin-receptor interaction (Flier *et al.*, 1975).

Indeed, it has been postulated that this type of diabetes may be an example of an "antireceptor disease" (Carnegie and MacKay, 1975). Possibly this may apply to other types of diabetes when more sensitive methods for measurement of receptor-binding become available.

2.2.3.3. Glucose Receptors—D-Glucose Anomers

Glucose anomers have been used to characterize further the events that can be coupled with the induction of insulin secretion. In 1974, several investigators demonstrated that the α-D-glucose anomer is a more potent stimulator of insulin release than the β-anomer (Niki *et al.*, 1974; Grodsky *et al.*, 1974). This finding suggested that the plasma membrane of the beta cell contains specific receptors to glucose, and that the induction of stimulation of insulin release is due to the occupation of an anomer-specific recognition site of glucose on the cell membrane of the beta cell. In addition, the α-anomer of glucose is a more effective stimulus for enhanced release of [^{32}P] orthophosphate ("phosphate flush"—one of the earliest indices of islet excitation) than is the β-anomer (Pierce and Freinkel, 1975). The efficacy of α- and β-D-glucose in causing insulin release and in suppressing glucagon release from the isolated perfused rat pancreas was tested further (Matchinsky et al., 1975). In order to allow simultaneous assessment of the glucose effect on both alpha and beta cells, the pancreas was continually perfused with a physiological amino acid mixture that provokes glucagon secretion and also stimulates the beta cells, provided glucose is present. Under these conditions, the α-anomer of D-glucose proved significantly more potent than the β-anomer in inducing insulin release and in inhibiting glucagon secretion. These data lend support to the concept that the alpha cells as well as the beta cells contain direct glucoreceptors controlling glucagon and insulin secretion, and that certain properties of these receptors are alike in both types of cells. The pancreatic beta cells appear to recognize the α-anomer of D-glucose in controlling insulin secretion at a step before membrane transport, since the β-anomer is transported and phosphorylated more effectively than the α-anomer (Idahl et al., 1975). The possibility that a stimulation of a pathway of glucose utilization that is anomer-sensitive but does not entail initial phosphorylation (Pierce and Freinkel, 1975) has not been tested.

On the basis of their own previous work and that of other investigators supporting the concept of a cell membrane glucoreceptor, Niki and Niki (1975) have suggested a hypothesis for diabetes as a generalized disorder of glucoreceptors, including disturbances in insulin and glucagon release. Although this is an interesting concept, further work is necessary to substantiate whether even one form of diabetes mellitus is due to a generalized disorder of glucose receptors.

2.2.4. Glucagon Secretion—Somatostatin

Glucagon secretion in diabetes mellitus and the effect of somatostatin on hormonal release will not be reviewed in this chapter, since they are discussed extensively in Chapter 3.

2.3. Measurement of Insulin Secretory Products

Measurements of insulin secretory products in the peripheral circulation have been utilized to understand abnormalities of insulin secretion in pathological states, and have been applied as aids in diagnosis. Small amounts of proinsulin, the single-chain precursor of insulin, have been found in normal plasma (usually 10–15%, and less than 22% of total immunoreactive insulin). Insulin and connecting-peptide (C-peptide), generated from cleavage of proinsulin, are secreted in equimolar concentrations (Horwitz *et al.*, 1975b). Measurements of proinsulin, free insulin, and C-peptide have provided additional or alternative means of measuring beta cell secretion, and have proved useful in the study of islet cell function in certain diabetic patients and in patients with islet cell tumors. The absolute basal concentration of proinsulin and the percentage of basal proinsulin may be increased in some diabetic patients. This has been demonstrated in some middle-aged or older diabetic patients with fasting hyperglycemia and hypoinsulinemic responses to administered glucose (Gorden *et al.*, 1974), as well as in 4 of 9 pregnant diabetic patients with mild fasting hyperglycemia and hypoinsulinemia (Phelps *et al.*, 1975). These data suggest that diseases that affect the beta cell's ability to store and secrete insulin, or prevent the secretory granule from undergoing full maturation because of continuous stimulation to insulin secretion, will be associated with an increased extrusion of immature granules containing a high percentage of proinsulin. In patients with fasting hypoglycemia, elevated levels of proinsulin point to a diagnosis of hyperinsulinism due to islet cell tumor, in the absence of renal insufficiency.

In insulin-treated diabetic patients in whom plasma levels of insulin cannot be estimated because of the presence of antibodies to exogenous insulin, free insulin can be measured after extraction of serum with polyethylene glycol (Nakagawa *et al.*, 1973). In such patients, direct measurement of C-peptide by radioimmunoassay after administration of glucose allows estimation of residual insulin secretory reserve (Block *et al.*, 1973). Serum C-peptide immunoreactivity increased during the remission phase (honeymoon period) of the diabetic state, suggesting that improvement in carbohydrate tolerance was due to increased beta cell secretory activity. In patients with hypoglycemia and hyperinsulinism, determination of C-peptide can indicate whether insulin in the circulation is of endogenous origin or due to surreptitious insulin administration (Couropmitree *et al.*, 1975; Sandler *et al.*, 1975). In healthy subjects, suppression of beta cell secretion by prolonged insulin-induced hypoglycemia can be ascertained by measuring the concentration of circulating C-peptide (Horwitz *el al.*, 1975a). Failure of suppression of C-peptide, indicating autonomous insulin-secreting tissue, may facilitate a diagnosis of insulinoma.

2.4. Acute Complications

2.4.1. Ketoacidosis

Some long-held concepts regarding the treatment of diabetic ketoacidosis have been questioned recently, and others, previously largely ignored, have been found valid and have been reemphasized.

2.4.1.1. Low-Dose Insulin Treatment

Diabetic ketoacidotic coma is an acute medical emergency. Prompt and effective fluid and electrolyte therapy, administration of insulin, and close monitoring of the patient are essential to successful treatment. For years, it has been generally accepted that diabetic ketoacidosis is associated with acute insulin resistance and a requirement for large doses of insulin, although there has been no agreement on what constitutes a rational "insulin program." Several reports appearing in 1974 have emphasized that small doses of insulin (hourly intramuscular injections of 10 U regular insulin, or, preferably continuous infusion of insulin at low dosages, - 2.4–10 U/hr) are equally effective and safe, and a simple form of treatment (Page et al., 1974; Kidson et al., 1974; Semple et al., 1974). It has been stated that this procedure allows for a standard initial protocol for insulin administration, with less subsequent hypoglycemia or hypokalemia. In a recent comparative prospective study (Soler et al., 1975), 36 patients with severe diabetic ketoacidosis were treated with small doses of insulin, the first 18 by the intramuscular route (10 U every hour), and the remainder by continuous intravenous infusion (8 U/hr). These patients were compared with 25 ketoacidotic patients who were treated with large intravenous boluses of insulin (100 U every 2–3 hr). With the intramuscular administration, the fall in blood sugar was significantly slower (9 hr) than with either the continuous infusion or the intravenous bolus of insulin (5.5–6 hr). Absorption of intramuscular insulin may be delayed in the hypotensive patient. With several exceptions, the smaller doses of insulin were as effective in controlling the hyperglycemia as the large bolus of insulin injected intravenously every 2–3 hr.

In patients treated without bicarbonate, when small doses of insulin were given intramuscularly or by continuous infusion, the acidosis was corrected (HCO_3 >20 mmole/liter) in 14–15 hr, as compared to a mean of 11½ hr with a large intravenous bolus. This difference was not significant. The intravenous-bolus regimen corrected both the blood sugar and the acidosis in shorter periods than intramuscular insulin. The time lag between the correction of blood sugar and correction of acidosis varied from 5 hr in patients given intramuscular insulin to 6 hr for the intravenous-bolus regimen, and 9 hr for the continuous infusion of insulin. In severe cases, acidosis may have important cardiovascular and cerebral effects. The authors commented on the danger that the acidosis may remain unaffected despite a quick response of the hyperglycemia. This problem is more prominent among patients with low initial blood sugars (<500 mg/dl) and severe acidosis, a group constituting a third of all ketoacidotic patients in the authors' experience.

In a majority of patients with moderately severe diabetic ketoacidosis, the mode of administration of insulin appears to be of limited significance,

and small doses, although effective in most cases, are not clearly superior
to conventional treatment with larger doses. The possibility of larger
insulin requirements in a few severely ketoacidotic, comatose patients
should be recognized and anticipated. Individualization of insulin administration superimposed on any of a number of conventional regimens
appears most important in the successful management of any given
patient with severe ketoacidosis.

Potassium requirements during treatment were identical (30–40
mmole/liter fluid infused) and independent of the insulin regimen (Soler
et al., 1975). However, small doses of insulin led to poor retention of
potassium. Independent of the insulin regimen, potassium retention was
considerable when large amounts of bicarbonate (> 250 mmole) were
used.

2.4.1.2. Bicarbonate Therapy

The use of bicarbonate in concentrations above that contained in
extracellular fluid remains controversial. In a series of patients with
moderate to severe diabetic ketoacidosis and impaired levels of consciousness who were treated with 180–300 mEq sodium bicarbonate in addition
to saline and insulin, the patients did not have deterioration or improvement in clinical status, as compared to a group of patients treated without
bicarbonate (Assal *et al.*, 1974). In general, bicarbonate replacement
therapy in concentrations above those found in extracellular fluid is to be
avoided, because by correcting arterial pH more rapidly, there is a shift of
the oxygen disassociation curve to the left, causing increased oxygen
affinity and the danger of tissue hypoxia (see below). Supplemental
bicarbonate therapy in pharmacological concentrations and amounts is
indicated primarily in patients with severe metabolic acidosis (pH <7.0),
which itself impairs already compromised circulatory and ventilatory
function.

2.4.1.3. 2,3-Diphosphoglycerate and Phosphate Therapy

In diabetic ketoacidosis, particularly during recovery, there is an
abnormality in the oxygen transport system of red blood cells. In the
1940's, it was recognized that there is a striking decrease in the content of
the 2,3-diphosphoglycerate (2,3-DPG) in the red blood cells, and it has
been realized in recent years that this decrease causes increased oxygen
affinity and decreased delivery of oxygen to the tissues by the microcirculation. 2,3-Diphosphoglycerate is formed as an intermediary product of
glycolysis in the red cells, and this fraction is decreased in acidosis due to
the inhibitory effect of increased hydrogen ion concentration and of

dehydration on enzymes involved in its resynthesis (Ditzel and Standl, 1975a). In diabetic ketoacidosis, there is also a significant depletion of the phosphorus stores in the body, as shown by the immediate response of plasma and urinary phosphorus to insulin. With insulin treatment, there occurs a precipitous fall in both plasma and urinary phosphorus levels, and the plasma phosphate level may remain subnormal for as long as a week. Since inorganic phosphate (Pi) is known to act as a cofactor in the glycolysis of the red cells by stimulating enzymatic formation of 2,3-DPG, the concentration of Pi may be a determining factor for the rate of resynthesis of red cell 2,3-DPG and the normalization of the affinity of hemoglobin for oxygen. On the other hand, when 2,3-DPG has been depleted, acidosis shifts the oxygen disassociation curve to the right, causing a reduction in the oxygen affinity of hemoglobin. This is a mechanism by which more oxygen is delivered to tissues by the microcirculation at a given partial pressure of oxygen. With correction of acidosis, at a time when 2,3-DPG is still depleted, the oxygen affinity of hemoglobin is increased, and oxygenation of tissues is decreased. Resynthesis of 2,3-DPG is a slow event, and it may take up to 1 week for the 2,3-DPG to return to approximately normal levels. It is closely related to serum phosphate levels when the phosphate has fallen to very low levels following treatment with insulin and fluids. The decrease of oxygen disassociation at low 2,3-DPG concentrations during ketoacidosis and after correction of acidosis was shown to be preventable by higher inorganic phosphate concentrations (Ditzel and Standl, 1975b). This is a strong indication for adding phosphate early to intravenous replacement regimens in ketoacidosis, as first recommended in 1948 (Franks et al., 1948). Potassium can be administered as phosphate salts. In view of the disordered erythrocyte oxygen transport system, it is conceivable that hypoxic tissue injury might occur during recovery from diabetic ketoacidosis. There is a marked reduction in cerebral utilization of oxygen that occurs despite generally augmented cerebral blood flow.

2.4.2. Alcoholic Ketoacidosis

Alcoholic ketoacidosis is being recognized more frequently (Fulop and Hoberman, 1975). It is easily distinguished from diabetic ketoacidosis and lactic acidosis. It is encountered in chronic alcoholics who have starved for several days while maintaining some caloric intake by drinking alcohol. Patients present with hyperpnea, ketonemia, ketonuria, mild acidosis, and high levels of free fatty acids, cortisol, and growth hormone. Most patients are not diabetic; there is mild or no hyperglycemia or glycosuria. The condition is easily treated with infusion of glucose and saline. The precise mechanism by which ingestion of alcohol induces augmented ketonemia is unknown.

2.4.3. Lactic Acidosis

Lactic acidosis can be induced by therapy with phenformin in diabetic patients in the presence of even mild renal insufficiency (Assan *et al.*, 1975). The role of renal failure in the accumulation of phenformin was suggested by the frequency of lactic acidosis when phenformin therapy was associated with renal failure. Higher concentrations of phenformin were found in plasmas from lactic-acidotic patients than in plasmas from phenformin-treated patients without lactic acidosis. Phenformin should not be given to patients with serum creatinine of 1.5 mg/dl or above. Disappearance of the drug accumulated in plasma can be accelerated by dialysis or furosemide-induced diuresis, or both. The usefulness of insulin therapy has been stressed: insulin can decrease peripheral lactate release. Inhibition of lipolysis prevents additional acidosis.

2.5. Long-Term Complications

New data have been published that increase our understanding of the pathogenesis of some of the long-term complications associated with the diabetic state, and indicate that insulin deficiency and hyperglycemia may evoke specific complications.

2.5.1. Diabetic Neuropathy

Further experimental evidence is accumulating that diabetic peripheral neuropathy is secondary to insulin insufficiency and possibly hyperglycemia. In addition to abnormalities secondary to activation of the sorbitol pathway in Schwann cells, nerve free myoinositol, a component of membrane phospholipid, is depleted in acute streptozotocin-diabetic rats (Greene *et al.*, 1975). In these rats, the development of impaired sciatic motor nerve conduction velocity (MNCV) was examined. Decreased MNCV developed by the fourteenth day after streptozotocin administration, but only in rats that became hyperglycemic. Insulin treatment, begun on day 3, failed to prevent MNCV and depletion of nerve free myoinositol in diabetic rats in which improved or normal weight gain and a decreased degree of hyperglycemia were induced. However, insulin treatment prevented the development of impaired MNCV and depletion of nerve myoinositol in a group of diabetic rats in which plasma glucose concentration was never found to exceed the upper limits of normal of 160 mg/dl during days 6–14, and in which the mean of the average plasma glucose concentration for each animal during the same period was 75 mg/dl. In diabetic rats, the decrease in nerve free myoinositol and the development of impaired MNCV was largely or totally prevented by supplementing the diet with 1% myoinositol, despite persistent hyperglycemia and elevated nerve sorbitol and fructose concentrations. These studies suggest that insulin deficiency and possibly hyperglycemia are primary features in the development of impaired MNCV in acute experimental diabetes. However, the development of impaired MNCV appears to be related in some manner to a derangement in the regulation of nerve free myoinositol, which appears to be subject to modification by increases in plasma myoinositol concentration over a critical range (Greene *et al.*, 1975). Feeding a diet supplemented with 3% free myoinositol had a deleterious effect, in that these diabetic rats exhibited significantly depressed mean sciatic MNCV (and elevated plasma levels of myoinositol), compared to rats supplemented with 1% myoinositol.

Other experiments suggest that insulin plays a role in myelin synthesis or maintenance, and that insulin-deficient states may be associated with impairment of this function (Spritz *et al.*, 1975a). In insulin-deficient rabbits, the incorporation of isotopic precursors into myelin components, both lipid and protein, is decreased. Because myelin is an extension of the plasma membrane of the Schwann cell, it can be concluded from these studies that the Schwann cell is insulin-sensitive. Further, in nondiabetic animals, insulin *in vitro* stimulates the incorporation of leucine into myelin proteins. In experimentally diabetic rabbits, there is a progressive decrease in myelin content of sciatic nerve with aging, and this occurs earlier and is greater than the decrease with aging found in control animals (Spritz *et al.*, 1975b).

2.5.2. Accelerated Aging

It had been postulated previously that one of the basic tissue abnormalities that characterizes the human diabetic state and its complications is accelerated aging or senescence (Vracko and Benditt, 1974). It may be on a genetic basis, and it may be exacerbated by hyperglycemia. This accelerated senescence of tissue may be manifested by a decreased replication rate of beta cells of the pancreatic islets in response to injury, an accelerated rate of cell death in basal lamina, or a decreased replication rate of cultured fibroblasts from diabetic patients (Goldstein *et al.*, 1975), and it may be responsible for the increased incidence of senile cataracts and osteoporosis and the accelerated atherosclerosis found in diabetic patients. The width of muscle capillary basement membrane increases with age in healthy subjects, and this thickening is accelerated in diabetes (Kilo *et al.*, 1972).

The chronological ages of human subjects were determined experimentally by enzymatic digestion of diaphragm tendon collagen samples

(Hamlin *et al.*, 1975). Determined age closely matched actual age for 14 subjects dying with a variety of major diseases. However, 3 juvenile diabetics did not fit this pattern; their experimentally determined ages were 51–65 years greater than their actual ages. These findings support the possibility of relationships among diabetes mellitus, changes in connective tissue, and accelerated aging.

2.5.3. Diabetic Microangiopathy

2.5.3.1. Basement Membrane Thickening

Controversy continues in regard to the relation of microangiopathy to insulin insufficiency and hyperglycemia in the diabetic syndrome, although experimental evidence strongly favors such a relationship. Since muscle capillary basement membrane thickening (BMT) was present in only 40% of diabetic patients below the age of 20, the Siperstein group (Raskin *et al.*, 1975) now agree, contrary to their former suggestion, that basement membrane hypertrophy does not represent the primary lesion of the diabetic syndrome. Since BMT is not present in 60% of children with diabetes, they also concur with previous conclusions of others that hyperglycemia must precede the appearance of microangiopathy. These investigators still conclude that microangiopathy is not the result of hyperglycemia, but probably represents an independent lesion, since BMT is unrelated to the "duration of diabetes," and since in 30% of children, BMT was found at the time of "onset of hyperglycemia." However, they equate the "onset of hyperglycemia" with, or date the "duration of hyperglycemia" from, the onset of symptomatology. It has been shown repeatedly, however, that postprandial or fasting hyperglycemia can precede symptoms or diagnosis by months or years in all age groups (Fajans *et al.*, 1974a,b).

The thickness of capillary basement membrane of femoral muscle was examined in normal and spontaneously diabetic monkeys (Howard, 1975). The thickness correlated significantly with the degree and severity of diabetes; greater thickness was associated with decreased glucose tolerance, decreased serum insulin, and increased fasting plasma glucose. Average basement membrane thickness and minimum basement membrane thickness were increased to the same extent.

Another study demonstrated an apparent relationship between the thickness of basal laminae of muscle capillaries and the presence of clinical retinopathy (Yodaiken *et al.*, 1975). The focal and segmental nature of the basal laminar thickening was confirmed. There was a clear-cut difference between the capillaries of patients with and those of patients without retinopathy.

2.5.3.2. Diabetic Glomerulosclerosis

2.5.3.2a. Human. The onset and progression of diabetic glomeru-losclerosis (DGS) were evaluated in a prospective study based on serial renal biopsies in 23 diabetic patients (Takazakura *et al.,* 1975). The authors concluded that the type of diabetes (juvenile-onset type vs. maturity-onset type) was more closely related to the development and progression of DGS than was the control of blood glucose to the progres-sion of DGS. If this closer relationship in fact obtains, it would be further evidence for heterogeneity (in terms of the degree of susceptibility of vascular tissue to metabolic insult) between the two types of diabetes. However, the authors did not exclude the significance of an elevated blood glucose as a cause of DGS. In none of the juvenile and intermedi-ate types of diabetes was it possible to maintain good control. Most showed moderate progression of DGS. Of 11 adult-onset type diabetics maintained under good control, 6 showed no progression of renal lesions during the follow-up period. Poor control was associated with progression of renal lesions even in cases of adult-type diabetes. The authors thought that "strict" control may prevent the development and progression of DGS in such patients. Even though the evidence that good control may modify DGS is only suggestive, it would seem desirable to attempt to keep blood glucose as near physiological limits as feasible. The authors did not find a correlation between duration of diabetes and progression of DGS.

On the other hand, a correlation between duration of diabetes and the renal lesion of diabetes was found in another study (Klein *et al.,* 1975). A marked increase was found in the collagen content of the glomerulus of the diabetic over that of the nondiabetic, which correlated with the duration of the disease and with the pathologist's estimate of the glomeru-lar lesion in the stained kidney section. Diabetic glomeruli were larger and had a greater hydroxyproline content per glomerulus than nondiabetic glomeruli. There was a high correlation between the hydroxyproline content and the histological determination of the extent of the renal lesion. Glomeruli from diabetics of longest duration showed the greatest increases in mass and hydroxyproline values.

One report questions the relationship between glucose intolerance and DGS (Nash *et al.,* 1975). Four patients had renal abnormalities suggestive of diffuse DGS. Early intercapillary nodule formation was seen in 2 of the 4 patients. Other pathological findings suggestive of diabetic nephropathy included efferent arteriolosclerosis and linear immunoflu-orescence without electron-dense deposits or inflamation. Sketetal muscle capillary basement membrane was demonstrated to be significantly thick-ened. Although the authors stated that these patients had no evidence of carbohydrate intolerance by standard clinical techniques, they commented that in 2 patients, glucose values during the glucose tolerance test were abnormally high. In the discussion, they also commented that intermittent carbohydrate intolerance may have existed for years and could be directly responsible for the microangiopathy, and that the severity of glucose intolerance may periodically be mild enough to escape detection by standard clinical studies. Spontaneous progression and regression of carbohydrate intolerance have been demonstrated even in young people with diabetes mellitus.

2.5.3.2b. Experimental. Induction of diabetes by streptozotocin in Lewis rats results in the development of progressive glomerular lesions (Mauer *et al.*, 1975). These lesions are characterized by thickening of the glomerular mesangium and increased mesangial matrix material with deposition of large quantities of immunoglobulins (IgG and IgM) and complement (C3) by immunofluorescent microscopy. Successful pancreatic transplantation resulting in normal glucose and insulin levels was followed within 2–3 weeks by rapid regression of these lesions. Transplantation of kidneys from diabetic rats to normal recipients also resulted in arrest or reversal of the lesion within 2 months. Kidneys transplanted from normal donors into diabetic rats developed the renal lesions. Although the lesions seen in these diabetic rats differ from human DGS, they develop in a milieu of insulin insufficiency and hyperglycemia, and they regress in a normal environment. One need not expect the tissues from different species to react to injury in the same fashion. In addition, although differing from the lesions in rats, deposition of immunoglobulins in glomerular basement membrane as a result of nonimmunological mechanisms has been found in human DGS as well (Westberg and Michael, 1973).

2.5.3.3. Diabetic Retinopathy and Intravascular Factors

It has been suggested that intravascular factors may play a role in the pathogenesis of microangiopathy. Abnormalities in platelet aggregation and fibrinolytic activity may be involved in capillary closure, which is one of the earliest manifestations of diabetic retinopathy. Increased sensitivity to platelet aggregation has been demonstrated *in vitro* in response to adenosine diphosphate, epinephrine, and collagen in diabetic patients (Sagel *et al.*, 1975), particularly in patients with severe and overt disease and with severe retinopathy (Bensoussan *et al.*, 1975). The major abnormality is seen during the second phase of platelet aggregation, probably because of release of intracellular platelet material such as prostaglandins or prostaglandin precursors. Inhibition of prostaglandin synthesis by a competitive inhibitor of the labile aggregation-stimulating substance inhibits platelet aggregation in diabetic subjects (Colwell *et al.*, 1975). Platelet aggregation was reversed by aspiring, tolbutamide, and glucose as well (Sagel *et al.*, 1975). Abnormal platelet aggregation has also been reported in patients with diabetic peripheral neuropathy with evidence of microvascular thrombosis (O'Malley *et al.*, 1975). Thus, metabolic and vascular factors in the pathogenesis of diabetic neuropathy need not be mutually exclusive. Abnormalities in the fibrinolytic system have also been found in patients with retinopathy (Almer *et al.*, 1975). In a study of 135 randomly selected diabetic patients, those with long-standing (10 years or more) diabetes who had not developed retinopathy had a much higher and almost normal fibrinolytic response to venous occlusion, and also a higher spontaneous fibrinolytic activity, than those who had developed retinopathy. There were other differences as well. Serum fibrinogen and α-macroglobulin concentrations were greater among patients with retinopathy.

2.5.4. Evidence for Heterogeneity

Variations in occurrence of significant vascular disease in diabetes also suggests that we are dealing with a syndrome that includes entities in which different pathogenetic factors (genetic, environmental) are at play. Among a group of patients with the classic juvenile-onset, ketoacidosis-prone type of diabetes of more than 30 years' duration and with continuous hyperglycemia ("poorly controlled"), 20% did not have clinically significant retinopathy or nephropathy (Knowles, 1971). As reported from at least six clinics in five different countries, among insulin-requiring ketosis-prone patients who have survived diabetes for 20–40 years or more, clinical evidence of microvascular disease, atherosclerosis, or neuropathy has been found in only 20–40% (Oakley *et al.*, 1974). In a further report, 73 patients with juvenile diabetes mellitus of 40 years' or more duration were studied retrospectively (Paz-Guevara *et al.*, 1975). No diabetic retinal changes were demonstrable on funduscopic examination in about 1/4 of the patients. Further findings were that 59% were free of renal involvement and were normotensive, 79% had no coronary artery disease, and 60% had no evidence of peripheral vascular disease. Thus, the juvenile-onset type of diabetes can be compatible with long survival and minor complications. As implied in section 2.5.3.2a, there may be genetic differences in the vulnerability of vascular tissue to the environmental metabolic abnormalities accompanying the diabetic state, such as hyperglycemia, hyperlipidemia, disordered amino acid metabolism, and other disturbances in metabolism or hormonal release.

2.5.5. Changes in Hemoglobin Components

2.5.5.1. Changes in Concentration of Hemoglobin A1$_c$

Abnormalities in the oxygen-carrying capacity of blood and in oxygenation of tissues are found not only in diabetic ketoacidosis, but also in the uncontrolled diabetic state. Hemoglobin A1$_c$, a "fast" hemoglobin (F-Hb), is a minor hemoglobin component, and is increased to more than twice its normal level in diabetics, accounting for more than 10% of total erythrocyte hemoglobin (Trivelli et al., 1971; Paulsen, 1973). The altered hemoglobin molecule is a glycoprotein with a hexose attached to the terminal nitrogen of both β-peptide chains of the globulin. It binds 2,3-DPG much less firmly than does normal adult hemoglobin, thereby increasing the affinity of the hemoglobin molecule for oxygen. This increase in affinity for oxygen reduces its ability to yield its oxygen to tissues. The F-Hb is elevated 4–5-fold in gestational and insulin-dependent diabetic patients (Gandhi and Bleicher, 1975); elevated F-Hb may impair fetal oxygenation. The increase in concentration of this glycohemoglobin, another example of increased glycoproteins in diabetes, is dependent on the disordered carbohydrate metabolism, and is not an independent component or genetic marker of the diabetic syndrome (Tattersall et al., 1975). Incubation of normal red blood cells in buffers with a high glucose concentration in vitro causes an increase in F-Hb (Gandhi and Bleicher, 1975). In diabetic patients, the material that accumulates in human glomerulus and in capillary basement membrane of muscle is also a glycoprotein.

2.5.5.2. Changes in Concentration of 2,3-DPG

In newly discovered and poorly controlled diabetic patients, the erythrocyte 2,3-DPG concentration has been found to be low even in the absence of ketosis (Ditzel and Standl, 1975a). The amount of 2,3-DPG reduction is sufficient to reduce significantly the availability of oxygen at the venous end of the capillary bed in tissues. This reduction may have clinical significance, as the effect of oxygen lack is increased by the increased oxygen requirement of the diabetic retina and by the decreased blood supply of tissues affected by vascular insufficiency. The 2,3-DPG concentration has been shown to vary much more in diabetic patients than in normal subjects (Ditzel and Standl, 1975a). It may be increased in ambulatory nonacidotic patients, and may represent a compensatory mechanism. Kanter et al. (1975) determined the red cell 2,3-DPG levels among diabetic patients with and without vascular complications. Nonacidotic diabetic patients with vascular complications had significantly elevated levels of 2,3-DPG. The elevation of the 2,3-DPG level may be a reflection of red blood cell compensation for tissue hypoxia in a diabetic patient with progressive vascular insufficiency.

References

Almer, L. O., Pandolfi, M., and Nilsson, I. M., 1975, Diabetic retinopathy and fibrinolytic system, *Diabetes* **24:**529.

Assal, J. P., Aoki, T. T., Manzano, F. M., and Kozak, G. P., 1974, Metabolic effects of sodium bicarbonate in management of diabetic ketoacidosis, *Diabetes* **23:**405.

Assan, R., Heuclin, C., Girard, J. R., LeMaire, F., and Attali, J. R., 1975, Phenformin-induced lactic acidosis in diabetic patients, *Diabetes* **24:**791.

Bensoussan, D., Levy-Toledano, S., Passa, P., Caen, J., and Canivet, J., 1975, Platelet hyperaggregation and increased plasma level of Von Willebrande factor in diabetics with retinopathy, *Diabetologia* **11:**307.

Block, M. B., Rosenfield, R. L., Mako, M. E., Steiner, D. F., and Rubenstein, A. H., 1973, Sequential changes in beta-cell function in insulin-treated diabetic patients assessed by C-peptide immunoreactivity, *N. Engl. J. Med.* **288:**1144.

Carnegie, P. R., and Mackay, I. R., 1975, Vulnerability of cell-surface receptors to autoimmune reactions, *Lancet* **2:**684.

Colwell, J. A., Chambers, A., and Laimins, M., 1975, Inhibition of labile aggregation-stimulating substance (LASS) and platelet aggregation in diabetes mellitus, *Diabetes* **24:**684.

Couropmitree, C., Freinkel, N., Nagel, T. C., Horwitz, D. L., Metzger, B., Rubenstein, A. H., and Hahnel, R., 1975, Plasma C-peptide and diagnosis of factitious hyperinsulinism. Study of an insulin-dependent diabetic patient with "spontaneous" hypoglycemia, *Ann. Intern. Med.* **82:**201.

Craighead, J. E., 1975a, The role of viruses in the pathogenesis of pancreatic disease and diabetes mellitus, *Prog. Med. Virol.* **19:**161.

Craighead, J. E., 1975b, Animal model of human disease: Diabetes mellitus (juvenile- and maturity-onset types), *Amer. J. Pathol.* **78:**537.

Cudworth, A. G., and Woodrow, J. C., 1975, HL-A system and diabetes mellitus, *Diabetes* **24:**345.

Dippe, S. E., Miller, M., Bennett, P. H., Maynard, J. E., and Berquist, K. R., 1975, Lack of causal association between coxsackie B_4 virus infection and diabetes, *Lancet* **1:**1314.

Ditzel, J., and Standl, E., 1975a, The problem of tissue oxygenation in diabetes mellitus. II. Evidence of disordered oxygen release from the erythrocytes of diabetics in various conditions of metabolic control, *in: Diabetic Mircoangiopathy* (August Krogh Memorial Symposium, *Acta Med. Scand. Supple.* 578, J. Ditzel and J. E. Poulsen, eds.), p. 59.

Ditzel, J., and Standl, E., 1975b, The oxygen transport system of red blood cells during diabetic ketoacidosis and recovery, *Diabetologia* **11:**255.

Editorial, 1974, Autoimmune diabetes mellitus, *Lancet* **2:**1549.

Fajans, S. S., Floyd, J. C., Jr., Taylor, C. I., and Pek, S., 1974a, Heterogeneity of insulin responses in latent diabetes, *Trans. Assoc. Amer. Physicians* **87**:83.

Fajans, S. S., Taylor, C. I., Floyd, J. C., Jr., and Conn, J. W., 1974b, Some aspects of the natural history of diabetes mellitus, *Proceedings of the 8th Congress of the International Diabetes Federation,* Excerpta Medica International Congress Series No. 312, p. 329.

Flier, J. S., Kahn, C. R., Roth, J., and Bar, R. S., 1975, Antibodies that impair insulin receptor binding in an unusual diabetic syndrome with severe insulin resistance, *Science* **190**:63.

Franks, M., Berris, R. F., Kaplan, N. O., and Myers, G. B., 1948, Metabolic studies in diabetic acidosis II. The effect of the administration of sodium phosphate, *Arch. Intern. Med.* **81**:42.

Fujita, Y., Herron, A. L., and Seltzer, H. S., 1975, Confirmation of impaired early insulin response to glycemic stimulus in nonobese mild diabetics, *Diabetes* **24**:17.

Fulop, M., and Hoberman, H. D., 1975, Alcoholic ketosis, *Diabetes* **24**:785.

Gandhi, V. S., and Bleicher, S. J., 1975, "Fast" hemoglobin, diabetes and pregnancy, *Diabetes* **24**:(Supple. 2):415.

Ginsberg, H., Olefsky, J. M., and Reaven, G. M., 1974, Further evidence that insulin resistance exists in patients with chemical diabetes, *Diabetes* **23**:674.

Ginsberg, H., Kimmerling, G., Olefsky, J. M., and Reaven, G. M., 1975, Demonstration of insulin resistance in untreated adult onset diabetic subjects with fasting hyperglycemia, *J. Clin. Invest.* **55**:454.

Goldstein, S., Niewiarowski, S., and Singal, D. P., 1975, Pathological implications of cell aging *in vitro, Fed. Amer. Soc. Exp. Biol. Proc.* **34**:56.

Gorden, P., Hendricks, C. M., and Roth, J., 1974, Circulating proinsulin-like component in man: Increased proportion in hypoinsulinemic states, *Diabetologia* **10**:469.

Greene, D. A., DeJesus, P. V., Jr., and Winegrad, A. I., 1975, Effects of insulin and dietary myoinositol on impaired peripheral motor nerve conduction velocity in acute streptozotocin diabetes, *J. Clin. Invest.* **55**:1326.

Grodsky, G. M., Fanska, R., West, L., and Manning, M., 1974, Anomeric specificity of glucose-stimulated insulin release: Evidence for a glucoreceptor?, *Science* **186**:536.

Hamlin, C. R., Kohn, R. R., and Luschin, J. H., 1975, Apparent accelerated aging of human collagen in diabetes mellitus, *Diabetes* **24**:902.

Horwitz, D. L., Rubenstein, A. H., Reynolds, C., Molnar, G. D., and Yanaihara, N., 1975a, Prolonged suppression of insulin release by insulin-induced hypoglycemia: Demonstration by C-peptide assay, *Horm. Metab. Res.* **7**:449.

Horwitz, D. L., Starr, J. I., Mako, M. E., Blackard, W. G., and Rubenstein, A. H., 1975b, Proinsulin, insulin, and C-peptide concentrations in human portal and peripheral blood, *J. Clin. Invest.* **55**:1278.

Howard, C. F., 1975, Basement membrane thickness in muscle capillaries of normal and spontaneously diabetic *Macaca nigra, Diabetes* **24**:201.

Idahl, L-Å., Sehlin, J., and Taljedal, I-B., 1975, Metabolic and insulin-releasing activities of D-glucose anomers, *Nature* **254**:75.

Johansen, K., Soeldner, J. S., Gleason, R. E., Gottlieb, M. S., Park, B. N., Kaufmann, R. L., and Tan, M. H., 1975, Serum insulin and growth hormone response patterns in monozygotic twin siblings of patients with juvenile-onset diabetes, *N. Engl. J. Med.* **293:**57.

Kanter, Y., Bessman, S. P., and Bessman, A. N., 1975, Red cell 2,3-diphosphoglycerate levels among diabetic patients with and without vascular complications, *Diabetes* **24:**724.

Kidson, W., Casey, J., Kraegen, E., and Lazarus, L., 1974, Treatment of severe diabetes mellitus by insulin infusion, *Br. Med. J.* **2:**691.

Kilo, C., Vogler, N., and Williamson, J. R., 1972, Muscle capillary basement membrane changes related to aging and to diabetes mellitus, *Diabetes* **21:**881.

Klein, L., Butcher, D. L., Sudilovsky, O., Kikkawa, R., and Miller, M., 1975, Quantification of collagen in renal glomeruli isolated from human nondiabetic and diabetic kidneys, *Diabetes* **24:**1057.

Knowles, H., 1971, Long-term juvenile diabetes treated with unmeasured diet, *Trans. Assoc. Amer. Physicians* **84:**95.

Lendrum, R., Walker, G., and Gamble, D. R., 1975, Islet-cell antibodies in juvenile diabetes mellitus of recent onset, *Lancet* **1:**880.

MacCuish, A. C., Jordan, J., Campbell, C. J., Duncan, L. J. P., and Irvine, W. J., 1974, Cell-mediated immunity to human pancreas in diabetes mellitus, *Diabetes* **23:**693.

MacDonald, M. J., 1974, Equal incidence of adult-onset diabetes among ancestors of juvenile diabetics and nondiabetics, *Diabetologia* **10:**767.

MacLaren, N. K., Huang, S. -W., and Fogh, J., 1975, Antibody to cultured human insulinoma cells in insulin-dependent diabetes, *Lancet* **1:**997.

Matschinsky, F. M., Pagliara, A. S., Hover, B. A., Haymond, M. W., and Stillings, S. N., 1975, Differential effects of α- and β-D-glucose on insulin and glucagon secretion from the isolated perfused rat pancreas, *Diabetes* **24:**369.

Mauer, S. M., Steffes, M. W., Sutherland, D. E. R., Najarian, J. S., Michael, A. F., and Brown, D. M., 1975, Studies of the rate of regression of the glomerular lesions in diabetic rats treated with pancreatic islet transplantation, *Diabetes* **24:**280.

Maugh, T. H., 1975a, Diabetes: Epidemiology suggests a viral connection, *Science* **188:**347.

Maugh, T. H., 1975b, Diabetes (II): Model systems indicate viruses a cause, *Science* **188:**436.

Nakagawa, S., Nakayama, H., Sasaki, T., Yoshino, K., Yu, Y. Y., Shinozaki, K., Aoki, S., and Mashimo, K., 1973, A simple method for the determination of serum free insulin levels in insulin-treated patients, *Diabetes* **22:**590.

Nash, D. A., Rogers, P. W., Langlinais, P. C., and Bunn, S. M., 1975, Diabetic glomerulosclerosis without glucose intolerance, *Amer. J. Med.* **59:**191.

Nelson, P. G., Pyke, D. A., Cudworth, A. G., Woodrow, J. C., and Batchelor, J. R., 1975, Histocompatibility antigens in diabetic identical twins, *Lancet* **2:**193.

Nerup, J., Platz, P., Andersen, O. O., Christy, M., Lyngsøe, J., Poulsen, J. E., Ryder, L. P., Thomsen, M., Nielson, L. S., and Svejgaard, A., 1974, HL-A antigens and diabetes mellitus, *Lancet* **2:**864.

Niki, A., and Niki, H., 1975, Is diabetes mellitus a disorder of the glucoreceptor?, *Lancet* **2:**658.

Niki, A., Niki, H., Miwi, I., and Okuda, J., 1974, Insulin secretion by anomers of D-glucose, *Science* **186**:150.
Oakley, W. G., Pyke, D. A., Tattersall, R. B., and Watkins, P. J., 1974, Long-term diabetes. A clinical study of 92 patients after 40 years, *Q. J. Med.* **43**:145.
Olefsky, J. M., and Reaven, G. M., 1974, Decreased insulin binding to lymphocytes from diabetic subjects, *J. Clin. Invest.* **54**:1323.
O'Malley, B. C., Timperley, W. R., Ward, J. D., Porter, N. R., and Preston, F. E., 1975, Platelet abnormalities in diabetic peripheral neuropathy, *Lancet* **2**:1274.
Page, M. McB., Alberti, K. G. M. M., Greenwood, R., Gumaa, K. A., Hockaday, T. D. R., Lowy, C., Nabarro, J. D. N., Pyke, D. A., Sönksen, P. H., Watkins, P. J., and West, T. E. T., 1974, Treatment of diabetic coma with continuous low-dose infusion of insulin, *Br. Med. J.* **2**:687.
Paulsen, E. P., 1973, Hemoglobin A1$_c$ in childhood diabetes, *Metabolism* **22**:269.
Paz-Guevara, A. T., Hsu, T. -H., and White, P., 1975, Juvenile diabetes mellitus after forty years, *Diabetes* **24**:559.
Phelps, R. L., Bergenstal, R., Freinkel, N., Rubenstein, A. H., Metzger, B. E., and Mako, M., 1975, Carbohydrate metabolism in pregnancy: XIII. Relationships between plasma insulin and proinsulin during late pregnancy in normal and diabetic subjects, *J. Clin. Endocrinol. Metab.* **41**:1085.
Pierce, M., and Freinkel, N., 1975, Anomeric specificity for the rapid transient efflux of phosphate ions from pancreatic islets during secretory stimulation with glucose, *Biochem. Biophys. Res. Commun.* **63**:870.
Radder, J. K., and Terpstra, J., 1975, The incidence of diabetes mellitus in the offspring of diabetic couples. Investigation based on the oral glucose tolerance test, *Diabetologia* **11**:135.
Raskin, P., Marks, J. F., Burns, H., Jr., Plumer, M. E., and Siperstein, M. D., 1975, Capillary basement membrane width in diabetic children, *Amer. J. Med.* **58**:365.
Sagel, J., Colwell, J. A., Crook, L., and Laimins, M., 1975, Increased platelet aggregation in early diabetes mellitus, *Ann. Intern. Med.* **82**:733.
Sandler, R., Horwitz, D. L., Rubenstein, A. H., and Kuzuya, H., 1975, Hypoglycemia and endogenous hyperinsulism complicating diabetes mellitus: Application of the C-peptide assay to diagnosis and therapy, *Amer. J. Med.* **59**:730.
Savage, P. J., Dippe, S. E., Bennett, P. H., Gorden, P., Roth, J., Rushforth, N. B., and Miller, M., 1975a, Hyperinsulinemia and hypoinsulinemia. Insulin responses to oral carbohydrate over a wide spectrum of glucose tolerance, *Diabetes* **24**:362.
Savage, P. J., Gorden, P., Bennett, P. H., and Miller, M., 1975b, Insulin responses to oral carbohydrate in true prediabetics and matched controls, *Lancet* **1**:300.
Semple, P. F., White, C., and Manderson, W. G., 1974, Continuous intravenous infusion of small doses of insulin in treatment of diabetic ketoacidosis, *Br. Med. J.* **2**:694.
Soler, N. G., Wright, A. D., FitzGerald, M. G., and Malins, J. M., 1975, Comparative study of different insulin regimens in management of diabetic ketoacidosis, *Lancet* **2**:1221.

Spritz, N., Singh, H., and Marinan, B., 1975a, Metabolism of peripheral nerve myelin in experimental diabetes, *J. Clin. Invest.* **55:**1049.

Spritz, N., Singh, H., and Marinan, B., 1975b, Decrease in myelin content of rabbit sciatic nerve with aging and diabetes, *Diabetes* **24:**680.

Sultz, H. A., Hart, B. A., Zielenzny, M., and Schlesinger, E. R., 1975, Is mumps virus an etiologic factor in juvenile diabetes mellitus? *J. Ped.* **86:**654.

Takazakura, E., Nakamoto, Y., Hayakawa, H., Kawai, K., Muramoto, S., Yoshida, K., Shimizu, M., Shinoda, A., and Takeuchi, J., 1975, Onset and progression of diabetic glomerulosclerosis. A prospective study based on serial renal biopsies, *Diabetes* **24:**1.

Tattersall, R. B., and Fajans, S. S., 1975a, A difference between the inheritance of classical juvenile-onset and maturity-onset type diabetes of young people, *Diabetes* **24:**44.

Tattersal, R. B., and Fajans, S. S., 1975b, Prevalence of diabetes and glucose intolerance in 199 offspring of thirty-seven conjugal diabetic parents, *Diabetes* **24:**452.

Tattersall, R. B., and Pyke, D. A., 1972, Diabetes in identical twins, *Lancet* **2:**1120.

Tattersall, R. B., Pyke, D. A., Ranney, H. M., and Bruckheimer, S. M., 1975, Hemoglobin components in diabetes mellitus: Studies in identical twins, *N. Engl. J. Med.* **293:**1171.

Trivelli, L. A., Ranney, H. M., and Lai, H. T., 1971, Hemoglobin components in patients with diabetes mellitus, *N. Eng. J. Med.* **284:**353.

Vracko, R., and Benditt, E. P., 1974, Manifestations of diabetes mellitus—Their possible relationships to an underlying cell defect, *Amer. J. Pathol.* **75:**204.

Westberg, N. G., and Michael, A. F., 1973, Human glomerular basement membrane: chemical composition in diabetes mellitus, *Acta. Med. Scand.* **194:** 39.

Yodaiken, R. E., Menefee, M., Seftel, H. C., Kew, M. C., and McClaren, M. J., 1975, Capillaries of South African diabetics, IV. Relation to retinopathy, *Diabetes* **24:**286.

Glucagon

Roger H. Unger

3.1. Immunoreactive Glucagon in Tissues and Plasma

3.1.1. Primary Structure of Glucagon

True glucagon, i.e., the 3485 mol. wt. biologically active immunoreactive polypeptide present in pancreas, appears to have the same amino acid sequence in all the mammalian species thus far studied—pork (Bromer (*et al.*, 1957), beef (Bromer *et al.*, 1971), man (Thomsen *et al.*, 1972), rat (Sundby and Markussen, 1971), and rabbit (Sundby and Markussen, 1972)—suggesting the possible importance of these primary structural features. The primary sequences of avian glucagons differ (Markussen *et al.*, 1972; Sundby *et al.*, 1972; Pollock and Kimmel, 1975), and these differences appear to influence their immunological properties (Markussen *et al.*, 1972).

ROGER H. UNGER • University of Texas Southwestern Medical School and Veterans Administration Hospital, Dallas, Texas 75216.

3.1.2. Biosynthesis

Study of the biosynthesis of glucagon is still in its infancy. The pulse-chase experiments of Noe and Bauer (1971) and Noe *et al.*, (1975) suggest that a precursor or intermediate of glucagon biosynthesis with a molecular weight of about 9000 may exist both in anglerfish and in man. This material may be the same as the so-called "large glucagon immunoreactivity" ("LGI") of pancreatic extracts, a material found to be devoid of glycogenolytic activity when perfused in a rat liver (Rigopoulou *et al.*, 1970). Tryptic digestion of proglucagon gives rise to an immunoreactive derivative slightly smaller in molecular size than glucagon, and lacking glycogenolytic activity (Rigopoulou *et al.*, 1970).

Tager and Steiner (1973) have identified the primary structure of a 37-amino-acid fragment of proglucagon containing the 29-amino-acid primary structure of bovine glucagon; the remaining 8 residues were at the C-terminus. Trakatellis *et al.* (1975) have reported that anglerfish proglucagon is a 78-amino-acid single-chain polypeptide from which glucagon is liberated by tryptic cleavage, the conversion occurring very rapidly within 3–10 min at a 1:500–1:1000 molar ratio of enzyme to substrate, making it a far more sensitive polypeptide than glucagon, and very similar to proinsulin with respect to its conversion to active hormone.

3.1.3. Plasma Immunoreactive Glucagon

The studies of Valverde *et al.* (1974, 1975) make it clear that immunoreactive glucagon (IRG) fractions other than true glucagon are present in plasma. Four fractions have thus far been identified (Fig. 1). These fractions include a glucagon-sized immunoreactive fraction, presumed to be true glucagon; a quantitatively small immunoreactive substance with a molecular weight less than that of true glucagon, presumed to be a derivative of glucagon; an immunoreactive fraction in the 9000 mol. wt. zone thought to be proglucagon; and a globulin-sized immunoreactive substance identified independently by several groups and referred to as *interfering factor* (Weir *et al.*, 1973), *big plasma glucagon* (*BPG*) (Valverde *et al.*, 1974), or *macro-IRG* (Valverde *et al.*, 1975). Its biological activity remains to be determined. It appears, however, that maneuvers that suppress or increase plasma IRG do so largely by suppressing or increasing the amount of true glucagon in the plasma, with only modest changes in proglucagon (Valverde *et al.*, 1975). With prolonged stimulation, proglucagon may also be increased (Valverde *et al.*, 1975). Clearly, interpretation of IRG determinations must be made cautiously, with full knowledge of their heterogeneity. However, there is at present no evidence to suggest

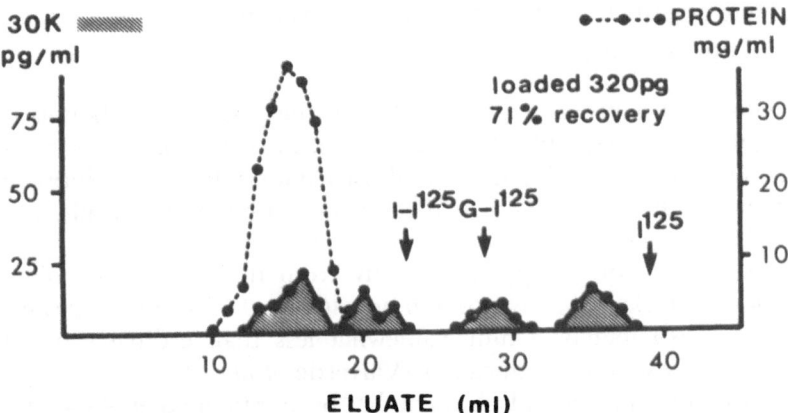

Fig. 1. Chromatographic pattern on Biogel P-10 of 4 ml basal plasma from a normal dog. The shaded area represents glucagon immunoreactivity; the broken line, the protein content of the eluate. The arrows indicate the elution volumes of the markers (insulin-I^{125}: $I\text{-}I^{125}$; glucagon-I^{125}: $G\text{-}I^{125}$; iodide^{125}: I^{125}). (Reprinted with permission of Valverde *et al.* (1975) and *Metabolism.*)

that the published conclusions of physiological or clinical studies in man or animals, normal or diabetic, based on measurements of total plasma IRG, are qualitatively invalidated by the recent recognition of the heterogeneity of the IRG elements.

In order to simplify an already complex nomenclature, it is suggested that the term *plasma glucagon* be restricted to the glucagon-sized polypeptide, and that all four immunoreactive moieties be referred to collectively as *IRG*, i.e., *immunoreactive glucagon.* The globulin-sized immunoreactive fraction can be referred to as *big* or *macro-IRG* or BPG. The 9000 mol. wt. IRG can be referred to as IRG^{9000}, and the tiny and quantitatively unimportant low-molecular-weight fraction can be referred to as IRG^{2000}.

3.1.4. Tissue Immunoreactive Glucagon

Extracts of glucagon-containing tissues such as the pancreas and the fundus of the canine stomach have also been shown to contain four immunoreactive components, including true biologically active glucagon, biologically inactive small IRG^{2000} and IRG^{9000}, and substantial quantities of a large IRG component estimated to have a molecular weight of approximately 65,000, and having biological activity comparable to glucagon (Srikant *et al.*, 1976). Its relationship to the much larger BPG of plasma, if any, is obscure, as is the whole question of the significance of plasma BPG. Interestingly, Ensinck (1974, personal communication) has discovered an otherwise healthy family with high IRG levels that may be the result of increased BPG.

3.2. Glucagon Metabolism—Clearance and Degradation

Glucagon is presumed to circulate in the plasma in unbound form, although it is conceivable that the big plasma IRG represents a carrier protein to which several IRG molecules are bound. Plasma is glucagonolytic, particularly in man and in the rat, but just how much glucagon is degraded within the circulation is uncertain.

True glucagon disappears rapidly from the circulation. When its secretion is blocked by somatostatin, its estimated half-time of disappearance is approximately 3 min, somewhat less than estimates based on injections of exogenous glucagon (Valverde *et al.*, 1975). In the portal blood, the concentration of glucagon has been estimated at 300–5000 pg/ml (Blackard *et al.*, 1974; Felig *et al.*, 1974), compatible with the estimate of Rodbell *et al.* (1971) of physiological binding of glucagon to hepatic receptors (K_m of 4.5×10^{-9}). Blackard *et al.* (1974) report a basal concentration of 160 pg/ml in the portal blood at a time when peripheral venous glucagon averaged 100 pg/ml, but during stimulation by arginine, portal glucagon rose to above 1000 pg/ml before a change in peripheral plasma levels was observed. Felig *et al.* (1974) have obtained similar results, reporting a portal–peripheral vein glucagon gradient of 1.3. In normal human subjects, Dencker *et al.* (1975) have observed that portal vein glucagon may rise after an ordinary meal without a measurable change in the peripheral plasma levels, indicating that small changes in glucagon secretion may not be reflected by measurable changes in the peripheral plasma.

Removal of glucagon from the plasma may, in part, involve its degradation within the liver at a site considered to be separate from the glucagon receptor. Kakiuchi and Tomazawa (1964) report a glucagon-degrading enzyme system that they have purified from hepatic glutathione–insulin–transhydrogenase. Duckworth and Kitabchi (1974) have observed an "insulin–glucagon specific protease" in muscle, but as of the present, this has not been reported in liver. Assan (1972) considers that 0.5 mg/day of glucagon is excreted in the bile, and that biliary excretion may be a physiological route of glucagon removal.

However, the kidneys appear to be the major site of glucagon removal (Lefebvre and Luyckx, 1975). The disappearance curve of intravenously injected crystalline glucagon is markedly prolonged in severe renal failure following bilateral nephrectomy, as is the hyperglycemic effect of the hormone. The hyperglucagonemia of renal insufficiency (Bilbrey *et al.*, 1974) is believed to result in large part from the decreased removal of glucagon. Ligation of the renal vessels in dogs is accompanied by a prompt increase in plasma glucagon, which can be entirely attributed to reduced clearance by the kidney (Lefebvre and Luyckx, 1976). Recent work suggests that proglucagon is disproportionately increased in patients with chronic renal insufficiency (Kuku *et al.*, 1976), raising the possibility that impaired conversion of proglucagon to glucagon may contribute to the high IRG levels of renal failure patients.

3.3. Actions of Glucagon on the Liver

3.3.1. Glucagon and Hepatic Glucose Production

The glycogenolytic action of glucagon is a noncontroversial effect of the hormone, and is easily demonstrated *in vivo* as well as *in vitro*, using the isolated perfused rat liver. By contrast, the gluconeogenic actions of glucagon, readily demonstrable in the isolated liver preparation, have been difficult to show in intact animals. Difficulties in demonstrating the gluconeogenic activity of glucagon *in vivo* may, in large part, be due to the potent antigluconeogenic effect of insulin, the secretion of which increases whenever exogenous glucagon is infused, thus masking the gluconeogenic actions of the hormone. However, the gluconeogenic action of glucagon is readily demonstrated *in vivo* when the concentrations of insulin are low relative to those of glucagon. Brockman and Bergman (1975) measured net hepatic uptakes of alanine, glutamate, and glutamine before and during intraportal glucagon infusions in insulin-treated alloxan-diabetic sheep, in which plasma insulin levels were maintained at a constant level during the infusion of glucagon. The net hepatic uptake of alanine and glutamine increased significantly, and conversion of alanine to glucose almost doubled.

Moreover, it now appears that demonstration of the gluconeogenic effects of glucagon may require more than simple studies of splanchnic substrate balance. Chiasson *et al.* (1975) have studied gluconeogenesis from alanine in normal postabsorptive human subjects, examining both *hepatic uptake* of alanine and *intrahepatic shunting* of extracted alanine into gluconeogenic pathways. They found that while glucagon given by constant infusion at a rate of 15–50 ng/kg per min had no effect on splanchnic extraction of alanine, net splanchnic glucose production from labeled alanine doubled during the glucagon infusion. Thus, in normal man, a glucagon effect on gluconeogenesis from alanine was exerted primarily within the liver by shunting of extracted alanine toward new glucose formation *without* a demonstrable increase in hepatic alanine extraction.

3.3.2. Glucagon and Ketogenesis

Teleologically, the concept of glucagon as a regulator of the production of calories for the brain demands that in time of diminished exogenous caloric availability or increased caloric requirements, it produce an alternative fuel to glucose so as to avoid serious depletion of protein stores. Ketones constitute the alternative fuel, and glucagon may well be essential for the ketogenesis of starvation. The reduced insulin levels that accompany starvation result in increased lipolysis and increased delivery of free fatty acids to the liver, thus providing the substrate required for enhanced ketogenesis. However, McGarry *et al.* (1975a,b) have proposed that unless glucagon is present to convert the liver to a "ketogenic mode," the increased availability of substrate will not increase ketogenesis. They suggest that glycogen depletion and an increase in intrahepatic carnitine are prerequisites for the increased ketogenic capacity of the liver that glucagon appears to generate (McGarry *et al.*, 1975a). Schade and Eaton (1975a,b) have reported studies in man suggesting that glucagon is involved in the ketonemic response in insulin-deficient diabetics. Further evidence of glucagon's involvement in ketogenesis in man is obtained from the studies of Gerich *et al.* (1975a) and of Alberti *et al.* (1975), in which juvenile diabetics withdrawn from insulin treatment failed to develop the usual rise in ketonemia when glucagon secretion was suppressed by somatostatin. Thus, a powerful array of evidence points to a role of glucagon in ketone production, both in health and in disease. The physiological importance of ketonemia for protein conservation is further emphasized by the studies of Sherwin *et al.* (1975), which suggest that in addition to its caloric contribution to the brain, the hyperketonemia of prolonged fasting may reduce the availability of circulating alanine, and thus further curtail protein catabolism in normal man.

3.4. Physiological Roles of Glucagon and Insulin in Fuel Homeostasis—The Concept of a Bihormonal Unit

The concept of an A-cell–B-cell bihormonal unit has its roots in classic studies by Park and Exton (1972) and Mackrell and Sokal (1969), in which the net biological antagonism of insulin and glucagon to hepatic glucose metabolism was established *in vitro*. The concept assigns to the islets of Langerhans the role of regulator of metabolic traffic throughout the body, with glucoregulation taking precedence over regulation of other fuels because of the glucose dependence of the CNS under normal circumstances. Of all the key fuels, only glucose is kept within an extremely narrow concentration range despite wide variations in its flux, indicating that in normal persons glucose efflux and influx rates are never very far apart. Only by means of a "push–pull" system is it possible

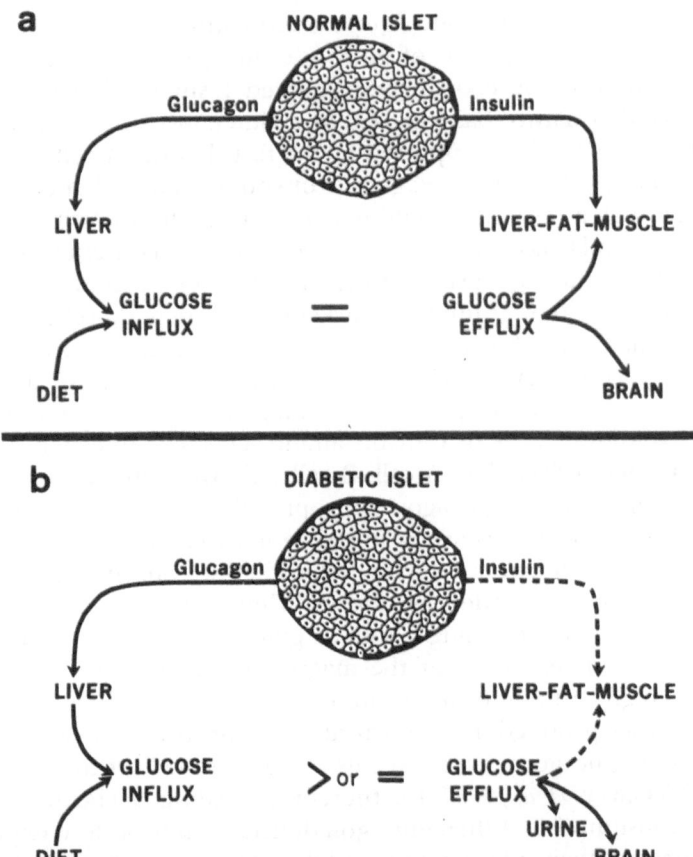

Fig. 2. (a) Bihormonal hypothesis for normal glucoregulation, in which influx from endogenous sources alone in the fasting state, and from exogenous sources during meals, is almost always equal to glucose efflux, which is presumably constant in the glucose-independent tissues such as the brain, but which is varied by change in insulin secretion in the major insulin-sensitive tissues—liver, fat, and muscle. In starvation, glucose efflux is reduced by lowering of insulin levels, and glucose influx is maintained at an equal rate by the appropriate level of glucagon. During increased fuel need, the greater efflux of glucose is met by a rise in glucagon to maintain a comparable level of glucose influx. During an influx of dietary glucose, glucose efflux is proportionately increased to avoid hyperglycemia. (b) In diabetes, glucose influx, even in the fasting state, may, at least periodically, exceed glucose efflux, which is reduced by the absence of insulin. The presence of glucagon maintains an inappropriately high rate of glucose production, inasmuch as hyperglycemia fails to stimulate insulin or suppress glucagon and thereby fails to raise glucose efflux or reduce glucose influx to a level that would tend to correct hyperglycemia. Insulin administration will increase glucose efflux and perhaps reduce glucose influx to a modest degree, but glucagon suppression will more effectively reduce hepatic glucose production.

to limit concentration changes of a substance traveling through a space at greatly changing flux rates. The "push–pull" system is believed to consist of glucagon, regulator of endogenous glucose influx into the extracellular space, and insulin, regulator of glucose efflux from that space (Fig. 2a), operating in properly coordinated coupled fashion. The physiological importance that nature has assigned to maintenance of a normal glucose concentration is further supported by the fact that the A-cells and B-cells respond to physiological secretagogues or suppressants other than glucose only when such a response would not result in undesirable hypoglycemia or hyperglycemia, i.e., violate the narrow glucose concentration range. For example, during carbohydrate deprivation, insulin secretion in response to protein or arginine is markedly obtunded, thereby preventing hypoglycemia, and favoring repletion of glycogen stores through increased gluconeogenesis. Conversely, during carbohydrate abundance, glucagon secretion in response to aminogenic stimulation is reduced, thereby avoiding a waste of valuable amino acids for unneeded gluconeo-genesis (Unger, 1971). The A-cell–B-cell unit, by changing the secretory mixture of insulin and glucagon appropriately, can bring about changes in glucose flux as wide as are required to meet changing needs for fuel, while restricting changes in extracellular glucose concentration to within the narrow limits regarded as normal. Glucagon functions to prevent hypoglycemia by maintaining a rate of glucose production equal to glu-cose utilization irrespective of the magnitude of net glucose utilization. When the high cost of gluconeogenesis in terms of protein loss makes this means of fuel production impractical, as in protracted fasting, the low insulin–high glucagon mixture seems to convert the liver into a ketogenic organ (McGarry *et al.*, 1975b), thereby providing a cheaper fuel for cerebral consumption. When glucagon deficiency is produced experimen-tally in normal man, plasma glucose falls, evidence of its contribution to maintenance of normoglycemia. Insulin, of course, prevents hypergly-cemia irrespective of the rate of glucose influx by somehow increasing glucose entry into insulin-sensitive tissues and promoting incorporation of glucose into glycogen and fat. When the insulin–glucagon mixture is high, as it normally is during the influx of exogenous nutrients, the incorporation of these nutrients into macromolecules will be rapid, and the hyperglycemia relatively modest and transient. When exogenous fuels are not available—i.e., in starvation, or when fuel needs increase, as during exercise, or both—a secretory mixture low in insulin and high in glucagon will result in the retrieval of energy-yielding components of the macromolecules glycogen, triglycerides, and proteins (Unger, 1976).

This bihormonal concept provides an attractive explanation for the precise regulation of extracellular concentrations of nutrients when their rates of entry and exit from the extracellular space may suddenly change so markedly. It suggests, too, that malfunction of this precisely titrated bihormonal unit will result in disorders of nutrient metabolism, such as diabetes mellitus and certain hypoglycemic states, all of which are characterized by a disparity between the rate of glucose influx and that of glucose efflux, as the result of which extracellular glucose concentration moves beyond its normally narrow range.

3.5. Proposed Mechanisms of Glucagon Action

3.5.1. Glucagon and Its Receptors

The actions of glucagon on its target cells involve its interaction with glucagon receptors in the cell membranes. In the case of its major target organ, the liver, this interaction is believed by Lin *et al.* (1975) to involve the hydrophilic amino acid residues at the C-terminal region of the glucagon molecule, but it is the amino-terminal histidyl residue that plays an important role in the expression of hormone action, contributing to the recognition of the hormone by the receptor.

3.5.2. Mechanism of Adenylate Cyclase Activation

The elegant studies of Rodbell and colleagues (Rodbell *et al.*, 1974, 1975; Solomon *et al.*, 1975) have greatly advanced our understanding of the molecular events leading to the activation by glucagon of the enzyme adenylate cyclase, thus generating the cAMP that mediates the glycogenolytic response of liver cells to glucagon. They propose a model in which guanine nucleotide induces the formation of an intermediate transition state of the enzyme without an increase in adenylate cyclase activity over the basal state, but one in which slow isomerization to a high activity state of the enzyme is occurring. They suggest that glucagon acts by accelerating the rate of isomerization. Using a variety of glucagon derivatives to determine structure–function relationships of the hormone, they conclude that the hydrophilic residues of the terminus of the carboxy region of glucagon are involved in the process of recognition of the glucagon receptor, but do not participate in the sequence of events that leads to activation of the adenylate cyclase (Solomon *et al.*, 1975).

In fat cells, in which glucagon has a lipolytic effect also believed to be mediated by an increase in cAMP, Cuatrecasas *et al.* (1975) have also studied the enzyme activation process by analogues of GTP, and they suggest that GTP, after binding, may activate the enzyme by forming a labile pyrophosphoryl enzyme intermediate, and that hormone receptors may function to increase the rate of formation, and thus concentration, of the active enzyme.

The mechanism by which gluconeogenesis is enhanced by glucagon is unknown. Recent studies indicate that glucagon-induced gluconeogenesis is accompanied by a rise in the cytosolic and mitochondrial state of reduction of the NAD system and a fall in the ATP:ADP ratio, effects abolished by insulin. It would appear that pyruvate carboxylation is an important site of glucagon interaction with the gluconeogenic pathway (Parrilla *et al.*, 1975; Garrison and Haynes, 1975).

3.6. Control of Glucagon Secretion

3.6.1. Glucose

The physiological importance of glucose as a fuel is reflected by the fact that the arterial glucose level dominates the secretory responses of the islet cells in an obligatory fashion. Glucose abundance is the single most potent physiological suppressor of glucagon, while glucose lack is its single most potent stimulus. The reverse is true for insulin secretion, which is obtunded by glucose lack and enhanced by glucose abundance (Unger, 1971).

The mechanism by which glucose blocks the secretion of glucagon is unknown. The concept of a specific A-cell glucoreceptor is supported by the fact that the α-anomer of glucose is more potent than the β-anomer in suppressing glucagon secretion, as it is in stimulating insulin secretion (Matschinsky *et al.*, 1975). This suggests that a stereospecific site, perhaps on the A-cell membrane, recognizes the molecular structure of α-D-glucose, and that this interaction, rather than the metabolism of glucose, evokes the A-cell response to glucose.

3.6.2. Amino Acids

Amino acids, particularly arginine, alanine, and several others (Rocha *et al.*, 1972), are powerful stimuli of pancreatic glucagon secretion. Ingested protein hydrolysates or protein are well recognized as a major glucagon-stimulating factor. Aminogenic release of glucagon is believed to prevent hypoglycemia secondary to aminogenic insulin secretion (Unger *et al.*, 1969). Its secretion during a protein meal is probably augmented by the release of gut hormones such as pancreozymin (Unger *et al.*, 1967) and GIP (Rabinovitch and Dupré, 1974), which serve an anticipatory and enhancing function with respect to directing an appropriate insular response (Unger and Eisentraut, 1969).

3.6.3. Free Fatty Acids

Free fatty acids (FFA), ketones, and glycerol may to a varying degree influence the response of the A-cell. However, the physiological importance of the suppressive action on the A-cell of high levels of FFA

(Madison *et al.,* 1968) is open to question, since it is precisely in those states in which FFA are elevated—e.g., starvation, exercise, stress, hypogly- cemia, and insulin deficiency—that glucagon secretion is maximal. Per- haps the influence of concomitant stimulating factors on the A-cell is so overpowering that the modest suppressive effect of high FFA levels in the plasma is masked; indeed, the high glucagon–low insulin state may well be the major cause of the increased lipolysis. Similarly, the importance of the suppressive effect of ketones on glucagon secretion demonstrated *in vitro* (Edwards and Taylor, 1970) is difficult to establish *in vivo,* because glucagon levels are almost always high when ketone production is increased, and, as discussed previously, these high levels may be essential in ketogenesis.

3.6.4. Cyclic 3′,5′-Adenosine Monophosphate

The role of cAMP in glucagon secretion is controversial. Weir *et al.* (1975) report stimulation of glucagon secretion by the isolated perfused rat pancreas with increasing concentrations of cAMP, in agreement with several other groups (Iversen and Rodriquez, 1970; Rosselin *et al.,* 1973; Braaten *et al.,* 1974). Yet inhibitory effects of dibutyrl cAMP on glucagon release were reported by Toyota *et al.* (1975), and in monolayer cultures by Wollheim *et al.* (1973).

3.6.5. Hormones

Gut hormones such as gastrin (Unger *et al.,* 1967), pancreozymin– cholecystokinin (Unger *et al.,* 1967; Frame *et al.,* 1975), and gastric inhibitory peptide (Rabinovitch and Dupré, 1974) have all been identified as glucagon secretagogues, and are candidate hormones for a role in an enteroinsular axis involving the A-cells.

Catecholamines are considered to stimulate glucagon secretion via a β-adrenergic mechanism (Iversen, 1973a).

3.6.6. Sympathetic Nerves

The sympathetic nervous system is considered to stimulate glucagon via a β-adrenergic mechanism that can be blocked by propranolol (Marliss *et al.,* 1973). The increase in glucagon secretion that occurs in exercise and stress is thought to be mediated by this system. During exercise, glucose suppresses glucagon secretion and stimulated insulin (Böttger *et al.,* 1972). During severe stress, however, glucagon cannot be suppressed by a rise in glycemia, nor is insulin stimulated; the lack of insulin may contrib- ute to the lack of A-cell suppression. In fact, stress hyperglycemia coexists with and is attributed to the hyperglucagonemia coupled with hypoinsulinemia (Unger, 1976). Hyperglucagonemia has been reported in experimentally induced hemorrhagic shock in dogs, and was largely blocked by propranolol, but not by phentolamine (Lindsey et al., 1975). Järhult (1975) conducted more elegant experiments in cats, and observed that hemorrhagic hypotension of 50 mm Hg was accompanied by a rapid rise in arterial plasma glucose, which was the consequence of increased hepatic glucose production. Neither bilateral adrenalectomy nor sectioning of the hepatic sympathetic nerves eliminated this response, although the latter procedure somewhat reduced it; however, sectioning of the splanchnic nerves in adrenalectomized cats virtually abolished both the hyperglycemia and the glucagon rise. He suggests that the sympathoadrenal system may influence glucose output from the liver by three different mechanisms: (1) release of catecholamines from the adrenal glands; (2) direct sympathetic nerve influence on the liver; and (3) release of glucagon from the pancreas. Kaneto et al. (1975) have reported that stimulation of the left splanchnic nerve causes a rapid increase in both glucose and glucagon.

3.6.7. Exercise

Exercise raises plasma glucagon levels (Böttger et al., 1972), and is thought to contribute to the augmentation of hepatic glucose production that occurs under such circumstances. In man, Nilsson et al. (1975) observed little increase in glucagon with workloads up to 900 kpm/min for consecutive 5-min periods, circumstances in which catecholamine levels rose. It seems likely that longer periods of strenuous exercise are required to increase peripheral vein glucagon levels in man. Galbo et al. (1975) observed only a 35% increase in glucagon concentrations after graded exercise, but a 300% rise during prolonged exercise, while insulin levels dropped. There was a significant correlation between glucagon and the norepinephrine and epinephrine levels during prolonged exercise, but with epinephrine only during graded exercise. The authors have concluded that increments of catecholamines may explain increased glucagon secretion during graded exercise, but they do not completely explain the rise in glucagon during prolonged exercise.

3.6.8. Severe Stress

At the clinical level, hyperglucagonemia has been observed in acute trauma patients (Lindsey et al., 1974; Meguid et al., 1973) and during surgery (Russell et al., 1975), and in patients with thermal injury (Wilmore et al., 1974; Orton et al., 1975), infection (Rocha et al., 1973), and cardiogenic shock (Willerson et al., 1974).

3.6.9. Acetylcholine

The cholinergic system is now believed to influence A-cell secretion. Acetylcholine has been found to stimulate both glucagon and insulin when perfused in the isolated dog pancreas (Iversen, 1973b). Moreover, atropine has been found to modify the response of glucagon to the ingestion of food (Dobbs and Unger, unpublished data).

3.6.10. Calcium

The importance of calcium in glucagon secretion has only recently received attention. Leclercq-Meyer *et al.* (1975) report that in the absence of calcium the rate of glucagon release by the isolated perfused rat pancreas is *positively*, rather than negatively, related to glucose concentration in the perfusing medium. This paradoxical behavior of the A-cell is reminiscent of that in diabetes. It appears that in contrast to many other secretory processes, the secretion of glucagon, or at least its release, can take place in the absence of calcium.

3.6.11. Somatostatin

The discovery, purification, and synthesis of the 14-amino-acid polypeptide somatostatin by Guillemin's group (Brazeau *et al.*, 1973) has been a major landmark in the history of glucagon research. Its unique ability to suppress glucagon secretion (Koerker *et al.*, 1973), as well as secretion of insulin, growth hormone, and thyrotropin, has provided researchers with a means of assessing for the first time the true importance of glucagon's contribution to glucoregulation and ketogenesis in man and animals.

The mechanism by which somatostatin blocks both basal and stimulated glucagon secretion is uncertain, but studies in the perfused rat pancreas suggest that it has a direct effect on the islets (Iversen, 1974; Gerich *et al.*, 1975d).

3.7. Studies of Glucagon Physiology Using Somatostatin

The availability of glucagon-suppressing agent has generated a large body of work in which glucagon's role in glucoregulation has been defined. That somatostatin causes a lowering of the plasma glucose concentration (Alberti *et al.*, 1973) while suppressing insulin prompted studies of its effect on glucagon, which was also found suppressed (Koerker *et al.*, 1974; Mortimer *et al.*, 1974). This finding suggested that glucagon-controlled basal glucose production exceeded insulin-controlled basal glucose utilization—or that in the absence of both hormones, basal glucose production was less than glucose utilization by insulin-independent tissues. It strongly supported the concept of a bihormonal system for control of glycemia and glucose flux.

The magnitude of glucagon's contribution relative to that of insulin in the regulation of glucose homeostasis has been explored by Liljenquist and his colleagues at Vanderbilt. They have provided quantitative information concerning the relative importance of insulin and glucagon in the "fine tuning" of hepatic glucose production (Jennings *et al.*, 1975) by exploiting the ability of somatostatin to block the secretion of both insulin and glucagon, and then varying the plasma concentrations of each hormone by various infusions of exogenous hormones so as to examine independently the effects of each. Their findings suggest that glucagon is responsible for approximately half of hepatic glucose production in the normal basal state, and that this contribution cannot be inhibited by insulin, the major effect of which is on glucose utilization. However, when, in the absence of both endogenous insulin and glucagon, hepatic glucose production is stimulated by an infusion of exogenous glucagon, exogenous insulin can reduce this increase.

The interplay of the two hormones would thus seem to be important in determining the net hepatic response. As is well known, insulin governs glucose efflux from the extracellular space into insulin-sensitive tissues, and glucagon, as long suspected but never before so clearly shown, controls glucose influx into the extracellular space, thus preventing hypoglycemia. Gerich *et al.* (1975b) have in effect confirmed and extended in man earlier studies by Koerker *et al.* (1974) in baboons by demonstrating that glucagon suppression by somatostatin lowers glucose, which again supports the role of glucagon in preventing hypoglycemia. Chideckel *et al.* (1975), studying baboons fasted overnight, found that despite the somatostatin-induced decrease in plasma insulin levels, a decrease in hepatic glucose production attributed to glucagon suppression occurred. This agrees with the earlier study of Sakurai *et al.* (1974), which interpreted similar experiments in dogs in this manner.

These findings fit well with other studies supporting the concept of the molar insulin–glucagon ratio (Unger, 1971) as a determinant of glucose flux rates and of glucose concentration.

3.8. Microanatomical Organization of the Islets of Langerhans

3.8.1. Functional Subdivisions of the Islets and the Role of the Insular D-Cell

Knowledge of the relationship of the pancreatic A-cells to the other islet cells has been advanced through the application, primarily by Orci's group, of powerful morphological technology. Immunofluorescent studies (Fig. 3) disclose that in man and in the rat, the A-cells are largely situated in the outer rim of the islet, and constitute approximately 25% of the total islet cell population (Orci and Unger, 1975; Orci *et al.*, 1976). The insulin-containing B-cells make up more than 60% of the islet cell population, and occupy the central area of the islet unit in these species. Approximately 10% of the cells are D-cells (Orci *et al.*, 1976), and have been shown by immunocytochemical techniques (Pelletier *et al.*, 1975; Orci *et al.*, 1975a) to contain the immunoreactive somatostatinlike material first observed in the islets by histocytochemical techniques (Luft *et al.*, 1974; Dubois, 1975) and by direct assay in extracts of pancreas (Arimura *et al.*, 1975). While the functional role of insular somatostatinlike immunoreactivity remains to be elucidated, as does the role of stomatostatin in the gastrointestinal tissues, it has been hypothesized on purely inferential grounds that the outer tricellular rim of the islets, composed of A- and D-cells and the outer layers of the B-cells, may form an extremely responsive "insular cortex," from which rapid bursts of hormones can be released and instantly stopped, thus avoiding the risk of hormonal "overshoots" and providing for precise bihormonal secretion (Orci and Unger, 1975). This hypothesis is based entirely on the fact that the D-cells, which are presumed to contain the powerful suppressor of both insulin and glucagon secretion (Koerker *et al.*, 1974; Alberti *et al.*, 1973; Mortimer *et al.*, 1974; Sakurai *et al.*, 1974), are located between the A- and B-cells. [It is noteworthy that this tricellular rim of the islet is said to have the most extensive relationships with vascular and neural elements (Fujita, 1976).] Because most A-cells are located adjacent to D-cells, while most B-cells are not (Orci and Unger, 1975), it has been proposed that any inhibitory action on hormone release would influence glucagon secretion more than insulin. Compatible with this concept is the fact that D-cell hyperplasia is observed in circumstances in which A-cells are increased in number or in activity, such as diabetes and glucagon-secreting tumors (Orci *et al.*, 1976), as if in a compensatory effort to reduce the hyperglucagonemia.

3.8.2. Ultrastructural Features of Islet Cells

3.8.2.1. Exocytosis

At the ultrastructural level, the application of conventional electron-microscopic techniques and freeze–fracture methodology by Orci and his co-workers has greatly advanced our understanding of A-cell function. It has been demonstrated, for example, that glucagon is secreted at least in part through the process of exocytosis (Orci *et al.*, 1970), as was established earlier for the B-cell (Lacy, 1970).

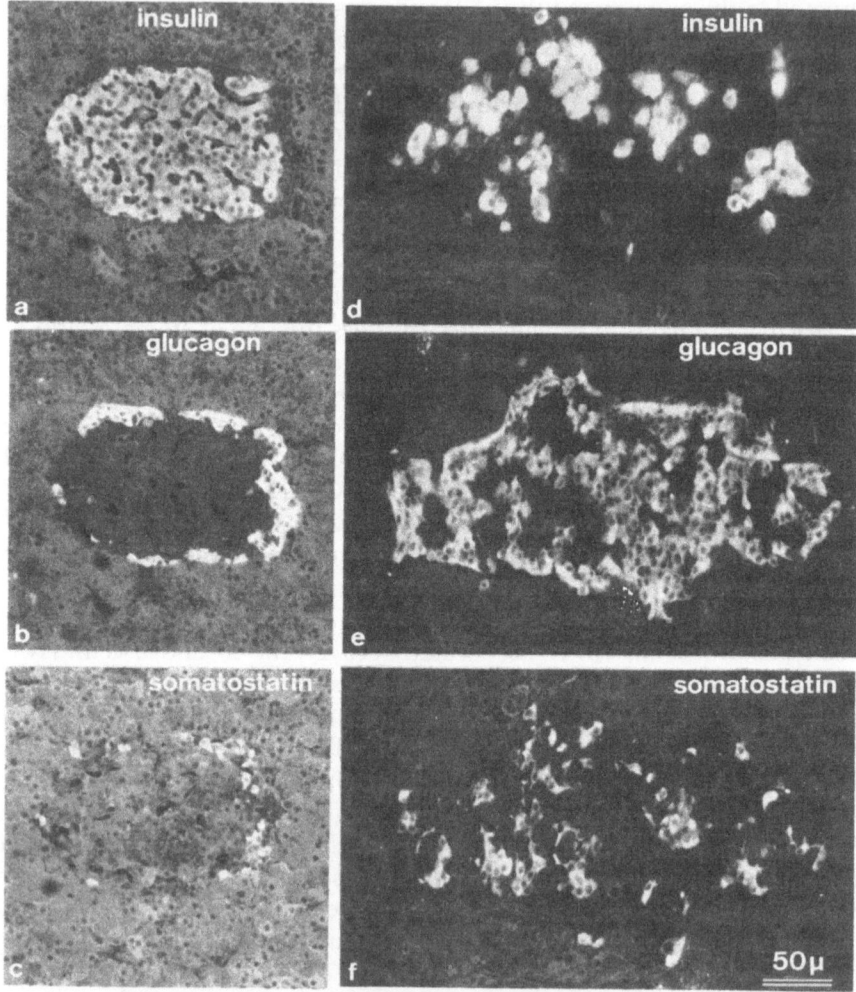

Fig. 3. (a–c) Distribution of B-, A-, and D-cells in serial sections of an islet from a normal rat, as determined by the indirect immunofluorescent technique against insulin (a), glucagon (b), and somatostatin (c). Both glucagon-fluorescent cells and somatostatin-fluorescent cells are located at the periphery of the islet, forming the so-called "mantle islet" surrounding the centrally located B-cells. (d–f) Distribution of B-, A-, and D-cells on serial sections of an islet from a 16 months' streptozotocin-diabetic rat, as determined by the indirect immunofluorescent technique, against insulin (d), glucagon (e), and somatostatin (f). Most of the fluorescent cells are glucagon- and somatostatin-containing cells, which are now seen both at the periphery and in the inner part of the islet. × 200 (reduced 20% for reproduction). (Reprinted with permission of *C. R. Acad. Sci. Paris.*)

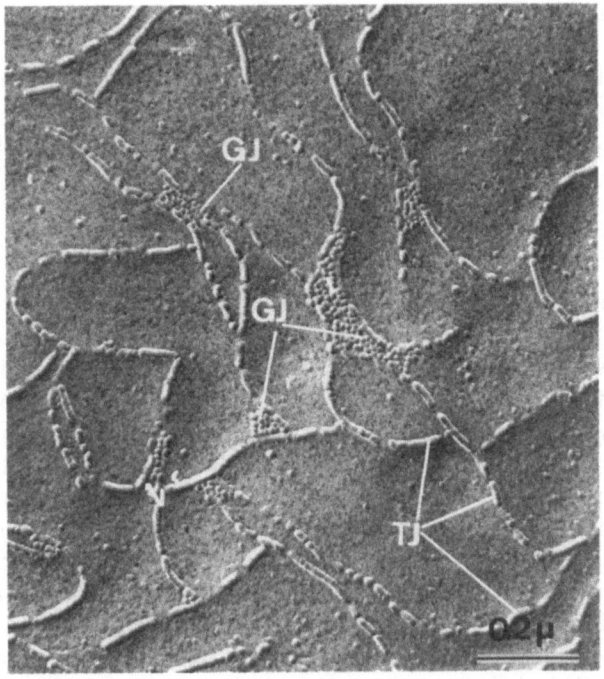

Fig. 4. High magnification of a freeze-fractured human islet cell membrane, showing the characteristic network of fibrils of the tight junction (TJ). In addition, localized domains in the network contain patches of closely packed globular subunits representing gap junctions (GJ). × 65,000. (Reprinted with permission of *J. Clin. Endocrinol. Metab.*)

3.8.2.2. Tight Junctions

Both conventional and freeze-fracture techniques have established in all species examined, including man, the presence within the islets of junctional complexes, providing morphological evidence of intercellular communication between A-cells and A-cells, B-cells and B-cells, and, interestingly, between A-cells and B-cells (Orci *et al.*, 1973; Orci *et al.*, 1975b,c). Junctional complexes consist of tight and gap junctions. Tight junctions are networks of anastomizing ridges representing a fusion of the outer leaflets of the plasma membrane's adjacent cells, which divide the intercellular space into compartments (Fig. 4). While their function is unknown, it has been suggested that they may serve to direct the flow of the various secretory products within the intercellular space so that secretory products intended for release into the circulation, such as insulin and glucagon, are channelled toward the effluent capillaries, rather than diffusing throughout the intercellular space; in the case of glucagon, uncontrolled diffusion through the intercellular spaces of the islets might stimulate inappropriate release of insulin. On the other hand, the tight junctions would channel secretory products that exert their effects primarily within the islet, as may be the case with somatostatin, toward their receptors on their nearby target cells, and prevent entry into the circulation, as a result of which unintended actions on distant target tissues might be elicited.

3.8.2.3. Gap Junctions

The function of the gap junctions of the islets of Langerhans is also unknown, but in other tissues, they are believed to constitute low-resistance pathways through which electrical and metabolic coupling of adjacent cells may occur (Staehelin, 1974). They can be viewed as channels through which molecules of less than 500 mol. wt. may traverse from one cell to another without entering the intercellular space. The A-cell–B-cell unit is the only known example of anatomically linked endocrine cells with different polypeptide products (Orci *et al.*, 1975c), a fact exploited in the argument that the A- and B-cells constitute a single functional unit secreting biologically antagonistic hormones in carefully titrated fashion (Unger and Orci, 1975). It may be relevant to this functional role of the gap junctions that when the isolated rat pancreas is perfused with a calcium-free solution, an experimental maneuver considered to disrupt junctional complexes, the normal suppressive effect of glucose on glucagon secretion is lost (Leclercq-Meyer *et al.* 1975). Perhaps normal A-cell–B-cell relationships and responses to external influences require cell-to-cell contacts.

3.9. Extrapancreatic Glucagon

3.9.1. Morphological and Biochemical Studies

Evidence in recent years strongly suggests that the pancreas is not the sole source of immunologically and biologically active glucagon. Sutherland and DeDuve (1948) first observed the hyperglycemic effect in extracts of canine gastric fundus and duodenum. Subsequently, Ferner (1953) suggested the presence of extrapancreatic A-cells. The demonstration by Vranic *et al.* (1974), Matsuyama and Foa (1975), and Mashiter *et al.* (1975) of residual glucagonemia in insulin-deprived dogs following total pancreatectomy led to a revival of interest in this possibility. The application of morphological techniques, as well as biochemical methods, has confirmed the existence of glucagon-containing cells in the upper gastrointestinal tract of dogs (Dobbs *et al.*, 1975; Sasaki *et al.*, 1975b; Baetens *et al.*, 1976a; Larsson *et al.*, 1975). Sasaki *et al.* (1975b) have found in

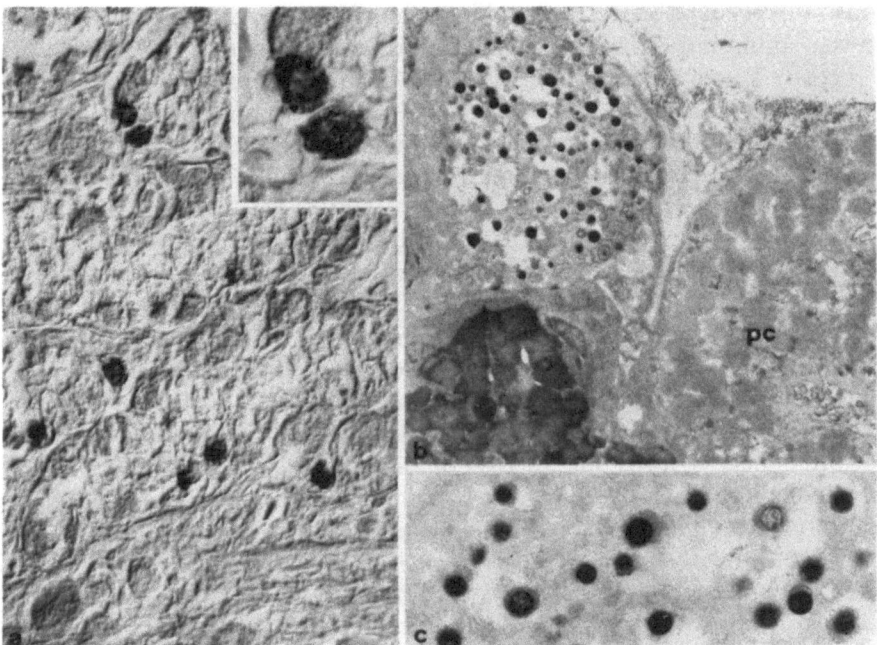

Fig. 5. Dog oxyntic mucosa. (a) Immunoperoxidase staining with antiglucagon serum (15K) of paraffin-embedded material, revealing several positive cells in the gastric glands. ×500. The inset shows two of these cells at higher magnification (×1300). (Reduced 24% for reproduction.) (b) Thin section of a gastric gland, treated by the immunoperoxidase technique for antiglucagon serum, showing an endocrine cell with positively stained granules (A-cell). (pc) Parietal cell. ×6000 (reduced 24% for reproduction). (c) Aspect of the peroxidase-stained granules at higher magnification. Note the presence of dense reaction product in the core and in the halo of the secretory granules. ×17600 (reduced 24% for reproduction). (Reprinted with permission of *C. R. Acad. Sci. Paris.*)

extracts of porcine duodenum a material that could not be distinguished by its immunological, physicochemical, or biological properties from pancreatic glucagon. Immunohistological and immunocytochemical techniques have demonstrated an abundance of glucagon-containing cells in the gastric fundus and corpus of the dog (Larsson *et al.*, 1975; Baetens *et al.*, 1976b). Not only do the secretory granules seem indistinguishable from those of pancreatic A-cells at the ultrastructural level, but immunoperoxidase methods reveal localization of specific antiglucagon serum to the secretory granules, as in the pancreatic A-cells (Baetens *et al.*, 1976a) (Fig. 5). These extrapancreatic A-cells are morphologically and immunocytochemically different from the glucagonlike immunoreactivity (GLI)–containing cells, which are abundant in the postduodenal small bowel (Orci *et al.*, 1968; Polak *et al.*, 1971).

In man, extrapancreatic A-cells have been far more difficult to demonstrate, perhaps because of problems in obtaining well-preserved human tissue. Immunoperoxidase positive cells were observed by Muñoz et al. (cited by Unger, 1976) in only 1 of 8 human subjects dying accidentally and autopsied within 4 hr of death. However, biopsies of the human duodenum have revealed cells containing granules ultrastructurally indistinguishable from the granules of pancreatic A-cells (Sasagawa et al., 1973; Baetens et al., cited by Unger, 1976). That glucagon has been measured with highly specific 30K antiserum in the plasma of a totally depancreatized patient, and was increased further by the infusion of arginine, strongly suggests an extrapancreatic source of glucagon (Palmer et al., 1976). It has recently been proposed that the salivary glands may also contain IRG and A-cells, thus providing an additional source of non-pancreatic glucagon secretion (Lawrence et al., 1975). Extracts of the canine fundus contain the same four IRG fractions observed in extracts of the pancreas, including an IRG of approximately 65,000 daltons, and the biological activity and isoelectric point of each fraction resemble those of the corresponding pancreatic IRG fraction. Until each fraction has been purified, however, their identities remain uncertain.

The glucagon extracted from porcine duodenum and from the canine fundus appears to be immunometrically similar to pancreatic glucagon and quite different from GLI of the postduodenal gut, with respect not only to its molecular size and charge, but also to its glycogenolytic activity, as estimated in the isolated perfused rat liver. Moreover, it is as active as glucagon in displacing [^{125}I] glucagon from binding sites, and in activating adenylate cyclase in isolated rat liver membranes (Sasaki et al., 1975b) (Table I).

3.9.2. Gastric Glucagon Secretion

Whereas extrapancreatic gastric glucagon appears to be secreted only in modest quantities in normal dogs, in the insulin-deprived state, whether induced by alloxanization or by total pancreatectomy, direct catheterization of the venous effluent of the gastric fundus of dogs has revealed increased production of IRG, both in the basal state and in reponse to intragastric or intravenously administered arginine solutions (Muñoz et al., 1975). Administration of insulin abolishes fundic glucagon secretion. Somatostatin also suppresses it (Sakurai et al., 1975), and thereby reduces the rise in hyperglycemia that otherwise follows the discontinuation of insulin in a totally depancreatized dog.

Lawrence et al. (1975) have reported an IRG in the salivary glands of rats, rabbits, dogs, and man that appears to be synthesized within the glands. On column chromatography, the IRG appears to be larger than

Table I. Comparison of Gastrointestinal Glucagon, GLI, and Pancreatic Glucagon

Properties	Pancreatic glucagon	GI glucagon	GLI
Mol.wt.	3485	3500	2900
Isoelectric point	6.2	6.2	>10
Ratio 78J/30K	1.0	0.9	61
Glycogenolytic activity:			
% of 10 μg glucagon	100	100	50
70% of maximum adenylate cyclase stimulation	10^{-8} M	10^{-8} M	10^{-7} M
Affinity for rat liver membranes	4×10^{-9}	3×10^{-9}	5×10^{-8}

true glucagon, and is converted by trypsin incubation to a smaller IRG. The authors conclude that it has biological activity, and that it is stimulated by low glucose concentrations and suppressed by high glucose concentrations. Immunoperoxidase studies suggest that the material is localized in the basal portion of the ductular cells. It remains to be determined whether extrapancreatic glucagon, which appears to play an important role in the pathogenesis of the diabetes of totally depancreatized dogs, is also of significance in other forms of insulin deficiency.

3.10. Diabetes Mellitus

3.10.1. A-Cell Function in Human Diabetes

In poorly controlled human diabetes, absolute hyperglucagonemia is present whether the metabolic picture is one of ketoacidosis or nonketotic hyperglycemia (Unger, 1976). The hyperglucagonemia present under such circumstances may be in part the result of diminished glucagon clearance by hypoperfused kidneys, as well as hypersecretion, and it recedes with conventional treatment as volume deficit is corrected and insulin is provided (Unger *et al.*, 1970). In the calorically balanced diabetic state, hyperglycemic diabetics exhibit fasting glucagon levels that are within the range of normoglycemic nondiabetics, in whom a similar level of hyperglycemia would lower glucagon by at least 50%. Consequently, hyperglucagonemia is present in the relative sense. Moreover, human diabetics of all types fail to respond with an appropriate reduction in plasma glucagon to further increase in hyperglycemia induced by carbohydrate feeding (Müller *et al.*, 1970). Finally, human diabetics, whether of the adult or juvenile type, exhibit a hyperresponsiveness to aminogenic stimulation, whether by an intravenous infusion or arginine or alanine or a protein meal (Unger *et al.*, 1970; Müller *et al.*, 1970).

3.10.2. The Bihormonal Abnormality Hypothesis

That hyperglucagonemia, at least in the relative sense, has been identified in every form of overt diabetes (Müller *et al.*, 1971), including total pancreatectomy (Vranic *et al.*, 1974; Matsuyama and Foa, 1975; Mashiter *et al.*, 1975), has led to the hypothesis that many of the metabolic manifestations of diabetes hitherto attributed to insulin lack are, in fact, the results of concomitant relative or absolute hyperglucagonemia, and that glucagon is essential for the full-blown diabetic syndrome (Unger and Orci, 1975). The ability to lower or to prevent severe endogenous hyperglycemia by suppressing either or both pancreatic and extrapancreatic glucagon with somatostatin (Sakurai *et al.*, 1974, 1975; Dobbs *et al.*, 1975; Gerich *et al.*, 1975a) has provided a means of testing this view, and the results support it. According to this hypothesis, which is schematized in Fig. 2b, the principal consequence of lack of insulin is underutilization of glucose by insulin-dependent tissues such as the liver, fat, and muscle; although insulin lack by itself will cause modest augmentation in hepatic glucose production even in the absence of glucagon, in the fasted state this lack will generate only modest endogenous hyperglycemia of approximately 160 mg/100 ml or less (Gerich *et al.*, 1975c; Sakurai *et al.*, 1975). However, the presence of glucagon when insulin is lacking will raise hepatic glucose production far more, and markedly enhance the disparity between production and utilization of glucose. This generates the severe *endogenous* hyperglycemia encountered in uncontrolled diabetes. [The bihormonal abnormality hypothesis may also apply to the pathogenesis of diabetic ketoacidosis (McGarry *et al.*, 1975a,b), as was discussed in Section 3.3.2.]

The validity of the bihormonal hypothesis is supported by the work of Sakurai *et al.* (1975) showing that in the absence of both insulin and glucagon, i.e., when glucagon is suppressed by somatostatin in the insulin-deprived severely diabetic animal, hyperglycemia recedes. They attribute the decline in hyperglycemia in the absence of insulin to a reduction in hepatic glucose production to below the rate of glucose utilization by insulin-dependent tissues of the CNS (Fig. 6). In man, as shown in Fig. 7, sudden insulin withdrawal during the infusion of somatostatin prevents the rise in glucagon, hyperglycemia, and hyperketonemia that would otherwise have occurred (Gerich *et al.*, 1975a). Proponents of the bihormonal abnormality hypothesis maintain that the uncontrolled diabetic state is, by definition, a state in which endogenous glucose production

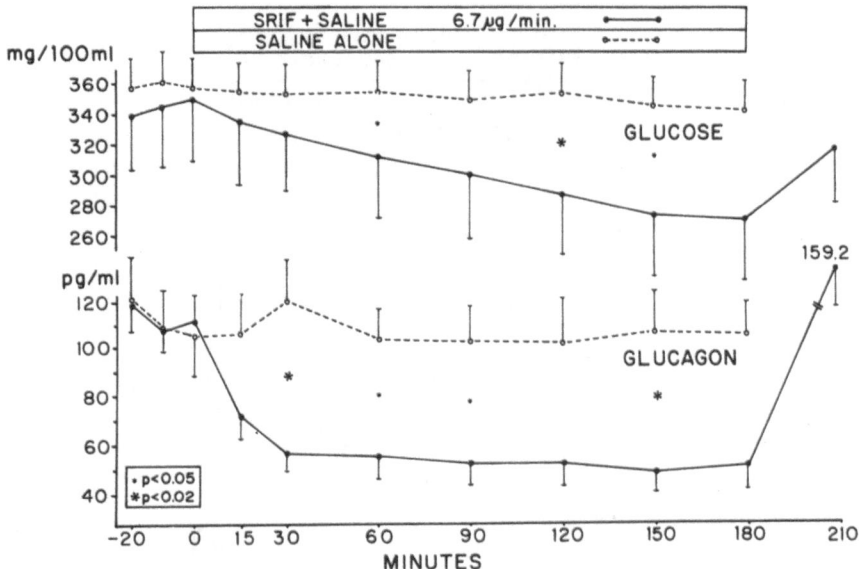

Fig. 6. Suppression of hyperglucagonemia by means of somatostatin infusion, causing a gradual decline in plasma glucose, in insulin-deprived alloxan-diabetic dogs. This suppression is attributed to a decrease in the rate of hepatic glucose production to below the rate of glucose utilization by insulin-independent tissues such as the brain. When the glucagon blockade is terminated and hyperglucagonemia returns, plasma glucose rises promptly. (Reprinted with permission of *Metabolism*.)

exceeds glucagon utilization, and that such a state is not easily produced unless glucagon is present in amounts that are high relative to the concomitant insulin level. They argue that while there may be circumstances in which glycogenolytic hormones other than glucagon bring about hyperproduction of glucose, in the ordinary insulin-deficient diabetic, glucagon is the usual cause of severe hyperglycemia of endogenous origin.

3.10.3. Evidence Against the Bihormonal Abnormality Hypothesis

While there is much to support the bihormonal abnormality hypothesis, it has not gone unchallenged. Sherwin *et al.* (1976) reported that in 2 juvenile-type diabetics receiving their usual dose of insulin, the continuous intravenous infusion of glucagon for 2 days failed to cause a clear-cut increase in hyperglycemia. They also found no increase in hyperglycemia in insulin-independent diabetics of the maturity-onset type, nor impairment in glucose tolerance in nondiabetics. Only in severe insulin deprivation did exogenous glucagon cause an obvious rise in glycemia. On the

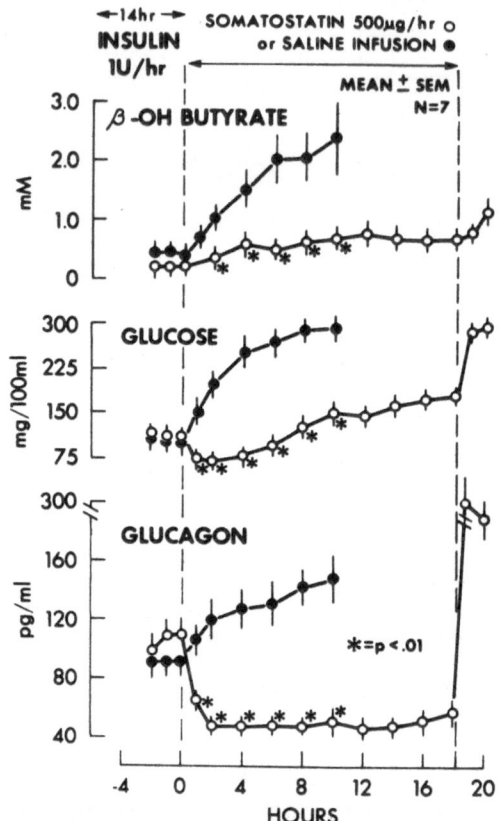

Fig. 7. Effect of glucagon blockade by somatostatin on glucose, β-hydroxybutyrate, and glucagon levels of juvenile diabetic patients following discontinuation of a constant infusion of insulin. (Reprinted with permission of *N. Engl. J. Med.,* courtesy of Dr. John E. Gerich.)

basis of these findings, they argue that the diabetogenic effects of glucagon are, at most, modest in the presence of insulin, whereas in the fully insulin-deprived state, the hyperglycemic effects of glucagon are striking.

However, it can be argued that in their studies, insulin must have been high relative to glucagon whenever glucagon appeared to be without effect. The 2 juvenile diabetic patients whom they studied were receiving long-acting insulin, and because their glucose levels dropped precipitously at various times during the glucagon infusion, the insulin effect must have been high relative to glucagon action—high enough to raise glucose utilization above glucose production, and thus lower plasma glucose. [The bihormonal hypothesis stresses that when insulin is high (molar insulin:glucagon ratio greater than 1.0) relative to glucagon, glucose utilization may exceed glucose production, and glycemia will decline (see Fig.

2).] Indeed, Raskin and Unger (1976a) administered glucagon subcutaneously to 5 juvenile diabetics receiving 28–50 U regular insulin administered 4 times/day, and, maintaining a low insulin:glucagon ratio, observed significant deterioration of glycemic control and a highly significant increase in glycosuria. This indicates that glucagon *can* increase hyperglycemia and glycosuria in the presence of insulin.

However, the concept of glucagon's essentiality in the pathogenesis of diabetes mellitus requires that it be present not only in the common forms of human diabetes, but also in the totally depancreatized human diabetic. Demonstration of extrapancreatic glucagon in man has been far more difficult than in the dog. Indeed, Barnes and Bloom (1976) have challenged the importance of glucagon's role in diabetes on the basis of their inability to measure with a highly sensitive glucagon assay any circulation glucagon in the plasma of 5 totally depancreatized diabetic patients. It can be argued, however, that the absence of circulating glucagon was the consequence of the insulin received on the previous day, and that, as in the dog (Mashiter *et al.*, 1975; Dobbs *et al.*, 1975), insulin effectively prevented extrapancreatic glucagon release. Furthermore, the fasting hyperglycemia in the absence of measurable glucagon in the plasma could have been the result of the meal ingested the evening before, rather than of endogenously produced hyperglycemia. In this regard, it is noteworthy that Palmer *et al.* (1976) have described a totally depancreatized patient in whom glucagon was present in the fasting state and increased further during the infusion of arginine, suggesting the presence of extrapancreatic glucagon; in contrast to the aglucagonemic patients of Barnes and Bloom, this patient exhibited a rise in plasma glucose similar to that of juvenile diabetics during the arginine-induced hyperglucagonemia (Unger *et al.*, 1970). (There are other methodologic variations in the glucagon assay used that may explain the results of Barnes and Bloom.)

3.10.4. Mechanism of Diabetic Hyperglucagonemia in Man

If glucagon is active in the insulin-treated juvenile type diabetic and the insulin-secreting adult-type diabetic, then the etiology of the A-cell dysfunction is important from the practical therapeutic standpoint, since correcting the dysfunction might improve the glucoregulation. Is it merely the consequence of insulin lack, is it an independent defect not secondary to insulin, or is it a combination of both? An abundance of evidence now suggests that the A-cell is an insulin-dependent cell, and that in the absence of insulin, it is incapable, at least in the intact animal, of either sensing or responding to hyperglycemia, or of both (Müller *et al.*, 1971). The restitution of insulin corrects this defect promptly in the experimentally insulin-deprived animal preparation. It is also clear that

the normal suppression of glucagon produced by the ingestion of carbohydrate involves a rise in *both* glucose and insulin; hyperglycemia in the
absence of a rise in insulin does not cause the suppression of glucagon,
and, in fact, may cause a paradoxical hyperglucagonemia (Buchanan and
McCarroll, 1972). Similarly, the exaggeration in aminogenic glucagon
secretion that characterizes the human diabetic can be produced experimentally by insulin deficiency. It is therefore well established that all
manifestations of A-cell dysfunction thus far reported in human diabetes
can be duplicated by the experimental induction of insulin deficiency by
any means—destruction of the B-cells with streptozotocin or alloxan,
neutralization of insulin by insulin antibody, or blockade of insulin secretion with mannoheptulose (Müller *et al.*, 1971). It would hardly be
expected that in man, whether nondiabetic or diabetic, the A-cell would
be "immune" from these effects of insulin lack. The question can then be
asked: Is the human diabetic A-cell as responsive to insulin repletion as
the A-cell of experimentally induced diabetes? Here the evidence is less
clear. An earlier claim of reduced A-cell responsiveness to insulin in adult-
type diabetics (Unger *et al.*, 1972) has recently been modified (Raskin *et
al.*, 1975). They report that in both juvenile- and adult-type diabetics, the
infusion of insulin at a rate that raises plasma insulin levels to between 30
and 50 μU/ml causes a significant reduction in circulating plasma glucagon, clearly indicating the ability of the human diabetic A-cell to respond
to insulin. Nevertheless, when compared to the response of nondiabetics
given glucose plus insulin in an attempt to simulate both the hyperglycemia and the insulin levels of the diabetic group, the glucagon levels of
the nondiabetics declined to levels significantly below those of the diabetics. Their study suggests that the diabetic A-cell requires higher than
normal levels of hyperglycemia or hyperinsulinemia or both in order to
reduce glucagon secretion to the level of hyperglycemic nondiabetics. In a
relative sense, then, the diabetic A-cell seems less responsive than normal
to the circulating insulin-glucose concentration.

The same conclusion might be reached on the basis of more chronic
studies in which both juvenile- and adult-type diabetics were subjected,
under the conditions of a clinical research center, to several days of
intensive treatment with mixtures of long- and short-acting insulins in an
effort to normalize glycemia (Raskin and Unger, 1976b). Even though
both glucose and insulin levels were well above the nondiabetic range, the
levels of glucagon at the time of optimal control were reduced only to
within the nondiabetic range; one can therefore argue that normal glucagon levels in the normal range were inappropriately high, relative to
insulin or glucose levels or both, and that in nondiabetics, glucagon
secretion would have been less under the same circumstances. In some of
the diabetic patients, absolute hyperglucagonemia persisted despite more

than 200 U insulin/day. However, further proof of the existence of an A-cell defect independent of insulin lack will be required.

If the administration of insulin could restore A-cell function to normal, a search for a glucagon suppressant as a possible therapeutic agent in the management of diabetes would be unnecessary. On the other hand, if insulin cannot completely restore A-cell function and glucose production to a level that is normal relative to the glycemia, the possible therapeutic value of glucagon suppression can be considered. The wide swings in plasma glucagon that characterize certain diabetic patients (Fig. 8) would be expected to contribute to the erratic glycemia. Evidence that glucagon suppression can abolish such changes in plasma glucagon has been provided by the studies of Gerich *et al.* (1975c) in man and Sakurai *et al.* (1974) in dogs; in both studies, postprandial hyperglucagonemia and hyperglycemia were prevented. Moreover, the studies of Pfeiffer's group (Meissner *et al.*, 1975), using the artificial pancreas, suggest that the infusion of somatostatin reduces the total insulin dose required to maintain euglycemia to approximately ⅓ of the level required when insulin alone is infused. Perhaps somatostatin reduces glycemia via mechanisms other than glucagon suppression alone; it may, for example, lower the rate of nutrient absorption. However, in view of the poor results obtained by present pharmacological management of diabetic glycemia, the value of efforts to control the hectic glucagon secretion in diabetes would seem to warrant scrutiny.

3.11. A-Cell Function in Prediabetes

That A-cells and B-cells originate from a common anlage has encouraged other efforts to document evidence of an A-cell defect not attributable to insulin deficiency. Day and Tattersall (1975) report abnormal A-cell responses in concordant, but not in discordant, nondiabetic identical twins of diabetics. While Kirk *et al.* (1975) have found nonsuppressibility of plasma glucagon by hyperglycemia in first-degree relatives of diabetic patients, Aronoff *et al.* (1976) were unable to identify an abnormality in the glucagon response to arginine in the nondiabetic offspring of conjugal diabetic Pima Indians as compared to matched controls. In gestational chemical diabetics, Daniel *et al.* (1974) observed impaired glucagon suppression during glucose tolerance tests conducted 5–8 weeks postpartum; during weeks 30–40 of gestation, however, when glucose and insulin levels were higher, glucagon suppression was normal. This finding could signify a decreased sensitivity of the diabetic A-cell to glucose, which was corrected by the impaired glucose tolerance and higher levels of insulin that characterized these diabetics' pregnancies.

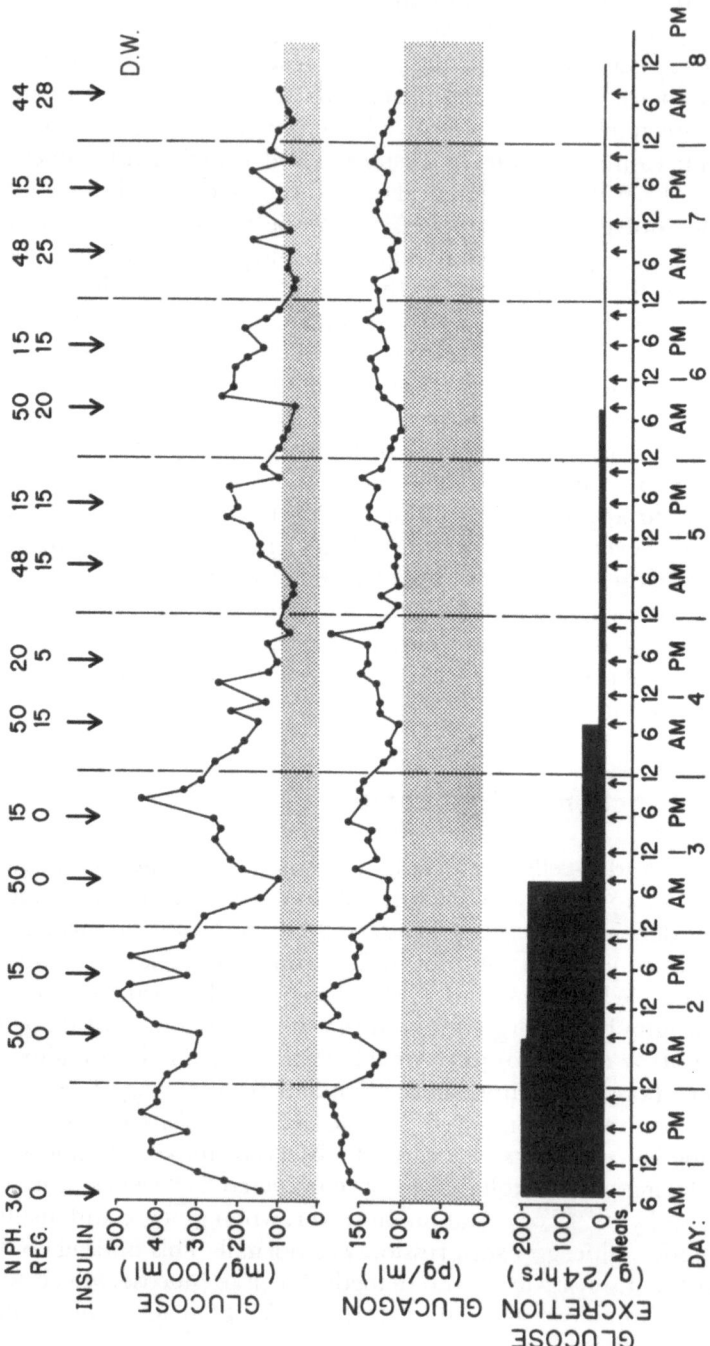

Fig. 8. Pattern of plasma glucagon and glucose observed at 2-hr intervals for several days in a juvenile-type diabetic during improving blood glucose control through increasing doses of insulin. Arrows at the top indicate the time of subcutaneous administration of insulin. Arrows at the bottom indicate mealtimes. Note the failure to abolish daytime rises in glucagon, despite an overall reduction of basal and daytime glucagon levels.

3.12. Catabolic Diseases

In severe illnesses with a negative nitrogen balance and prominent weight loss, the relative concentration of glucagon to insulin is increased. Insulin levels are low and are relatively unresponsive to stimulation, whereas glucagon is normal or increased. It has been suggested that the reduced molar ratio of insulin to glucagon may mediate the catabolic state (Unger, 1971) within a framework determined by other influential hormones such as cortisol. High levels of cortisol are reported to increase hepatic sensitivity to glucagon (Park and Exton, 1972), and to increase the sensitivity of the A-cell response to hyperaminoacidemia (Marco *et al.*, 1973; Wise *et al.*, 1973). One can envision increased mobilization of amino acids from tissues from which, because of the high cortisol and low insulin levels, release of gluconeogenic amino acids into the circulation may be increased; in the presence of a relatively high plasma glucagon, the conversion of amino acids into glucose, with loss of nitrogen as urea, would be inappropriately high. Thus, at a time when increased protein and DNA synthesis are needed to replace injured tissue and produce immunoglobulins, amino acids are wastefully preempted for unnecessary gluconeogenesis. Liver cells fill with lysosomes (Amherdt *et al.*, 1974), and DNA synthesis, at least in the liver, may be inhibited (Leffert *el al.*, 1975). Brief periods of increased catabolism may be essential for situations such as early in starvation and in acute stress, but when the regeneration of injured tissue is vital, this catabolic bihormonal mixture may be undesirable. It is noteworthy that by elevating the ratio of insulin to glucagon— whether by stimulating insulin with glucose as a supplement to amino acids (Dudrick *et al.*, 1970), or, if this fails to increase insulin, by giving exogenous insulin (Hinton *et al.*, 1971)—the negative nitrogen balance may be corrected to the benefit of the patient. The hepatotropic effects of insulin may be of clinical importance in many such disorders (Starzl *et al.*, 1975).

3.13. Glucagonoma

The first probable glucagonoma case was reported by Gössner and Korting (1960), but the first proven patient with this disorder was described by McGavran *et al.* in 1966. Since then, additional cases have been added to the literature. Mallinson *et al.* (1974) have attempted to characterize the glucagonoma syndrome. In 8 of their 9 patients, all postmenopausal females, they observed "necrolytic migratory erythema" and stomatitis associated with weight loss. In most of the patients, diabetes was diagnosed. Patients with the highest glucagon levels exhibited the most prominent weight loss. Glucagon levels ranged from 850 to 3500 pg/ml. In McGavran's case, however, plasma levels of glucagon as high as 50,000 pg/ml were observed, but despite this level, the diabetes was mild. The most striking abnormality in the patients was extensive replacement of the liver by metastases, with an inappropriately benign and protracted course for metastatic disease of the liver. In this syndrome, diabetes may be absent despite the hyperglucagonemia until underlying beta cell function is compromised by replacement of pancreas by tumor, as in the case of Yoshinaga *et al.* (1966). Glucagonoma patients reportedly exhibit marked increase in both the true glucagon and the proglucagon fractions of their plasma IRG (Valverde *et al.*, 1976).

References

Alberti, K. G. M. M., Christensen, N. J., Christensen, S. E., Hansen, A. P., Iversen, J., Lundbaek, K., Seyer-Hansen, K., and Orskov, H., 1973, Inhibition of insulin secretion by somatostatin, *Lancet* **2:**1299.

Alberti, K. G. M. M., Christensen, N. J., Iversen, J., and Orskov, H., 1975, Role of glucagon and other hormones in development of diabetic ketoacidosis, *Lancet* **1:**1307.

Amherdt, M., Harris, V., Renold, A. E., Orci, L., and Unger, R. H., 1974, Hepatic autophagy in uncontrolled experimental diabetes and its relationships to insulin and glucagon, *J. Clin. Invest.* **54:**188.

Arimura, A., Sato, H., Dupont, A., Nishi, N., and Schally, A. V., 1975, Somatostatin: Abundance of immunoreactive hormone in rat stomach and pancreas, *Science* **189:**1007.

Aronoff, S., Bennett, P. H., Rushforth, M. B., Miller, M., and Unger, R. H., 1976, Glucagon response to arginine infusion in "prediabetic" Pima Indians, *Diabetes* (in press).

Assan, R., 1972, *In vivo* metabolism of glucagon, *in: Glucagon: Molecular Physiology, Clinical and Therapeutic Implications* (P. J. Lefebvre and R. H. Unger, eds.), pp. 47–59, Pergamon Press, Oxford.

Baetens, D., Rufener, C., Srikant, B. C., Dobbs, R. E., Unger, R. H., and Orci, L., 1976a, Identification of glucagon-producing cells (A-cells) in dog gastric mucosa, *J. Cell Biol.* **69:**455.

Baetens, D., Rufener, C., Unger, R. H., Renold, A. E., and Orci, L., 1976b, Identification par immunocytochimie de la cellule secretant le glucagon dans la muqueuse gastrique, *C. R. Acad. Sci. Paris* **282:**195.

Barnes, A. J., and Bloom, S. R., 1976, Pancreatectomised man: A model for diabetes without glucagon, *Lancet* **1:**219.

Bilbrey, G. L., Faloona, G. R., White, M. C., and Knochel, J. P., 1974, Hyperglucagonemia of renal failure, *J. Clin. Invest.* **53:**841.

Blackard, W. G., Nelson N. C., and Andrews, S. S., 1974, Portal and peripheral vein immunoreactive glucagon concentrations after arginine or glucose infusions, *Diabetes* **23**:199.

Böttger, I., Schlein, E., Faloona, G. R., Knochel, J. P., and Unger, R. H., 1972, The effect of exercise on glucagon secretion, *J. Clin. Endocrinol. Metab.* **35**:117.

Braaten, J. T., Shenk, A., Lee, M. J., McGuigan, J. E., and Mintz, D. H., 1974, Cyclic nucleotide–mediated secretion of glucagon and gastrin in monolayer culture of rat pancreas, *J. Clin. Invest.* **53**:10A.

Brazeau, P., Vale, W., Burgus, R., Ling, N., Butcher, M., Rivier, J., and Guillemin, R., 1973, Hypothalamic polypeptide that inhibits the secretion of immunoreactive pituitary growth hormone, *Science* **179**:77.

Brockman, R. P., and Bergman, E. N., 1975, Effect of glucagon on plasma alanine and glutamine metabolism and hepatic gluconeogenesis in sheep, *Amer. J. Physiol.* **228**:1627.

Bromer, W. W., Sinn, L. G., and Behrens, O. K., 1957, The amino acid sequence of glucagon. V. Location of amide groups, acid degradation studies, and summary of sequential evidence, *J. Amer. Chem. Soc.* **79**:2807.

Bromer, W. W., Boucher, M. E., and Koffenberger, J. E., Jr., 1971, Amino acid sequence of bovine glucagon, *J. Biol. Chem.* **246**:2822.

Buchanan, K. D., and McCarroll, A. M., 1972, Abnormalities of glucagon metabolism in untreated diabetes mellitus, *Lancet* **2**:1394.

Chiasson, J. L., Liljenquist, J. E., Sinclair-Smith, B. C., and Lacy, W. W., 1975, Gluconeogenesis from alanine in normal postabsorptive man. Intrahepatic stimulatory effect of glucagon, *Diabetes* **24**:574.

Chideckel, E. W., Palmer, J., Koerker, D. J., Ensinck, J., Davidson, M. B., and Goodner, C. J., 1975, Somatostatin blockade of acute and chronic stimuli of the endocrine pancreas and the consequences of this blockade on glucose homeostasis, *J. Clin. Invest.* **55**:754.

Cuatrecasas, P., Jacobs, S., and Bennett, V., 1975, Activation of adenylate cyclase by phosphoramidate and phosphonate analogs of GTP: Possible role of covalent enzyme–substrate intermediates in the mechanism of hormonal activation, *Proc. Nat. Acad. Sci. U.S.A.* **72**:1739.

Daniel, R. R., Metzger, B. E., Freinkel, N., Faloona, G. R., Unger, R. H., and Nitzan, M., 1974, Carbohydrate metabolism in pregnancy. XI. Response of plasma glucagon to overnight fast and oral glucose during normal pregnancy and in gestational diabetes, *Diabetes* **23**:771.

Day, J. L., and Tattersall, R. B., 1975, Glucagon secretion in unaffected monozygotic twins of juvenile diabetics, *Metabolism* **24**:145.

Dencker, H., Hedner, P., Holst, J., and Tranberg, K. G., 1975, Pancreatic glucagon response to an ordinary meal, *Scand. J. Gastroenterol.* **10**:471.

Dobbs, R., Sakurai, H., Sasaki, H., Faloona, G., Valverde, I., Baetens, D., Orci, L., and Unger, R., 1975, Glucagon: Role in the hyperglycemia of diabetes mellitus, *Science* **187**:544.

Dubois, M. P., 1975, Immunoreactive somatostatin is present in discrete cells of the endocrine pancreas, *Proc. Nat. Acad. Sci. U.S.A.* **72**:1340.

Duckworth, W. C., and Kitabchi, A. E., 1974, Insulin and glucagon degradation by the same enzyme, *Diabetes* **23**:536.

Dudrick, S. J., Long, J. M., Steiger, E., and Rhoads, J. E., 1970, Intravenous hyperalimentation, *Med. Clin. North Amer.* **54:**577.

Edwards, J. C., Howell, S. L., and Taylor, K. W., 1970, Radioimmunoassay of glucagon release from isolated guinea-pig islets of Langerhans incubated *in vitro, Biochem. Biophys. Acta* **215:**297.

Felig, P., Gusberg, R., Hendler, R., Gump, F. E., and Kinney, J. M., 1974, Concentrations of glucagon and the insulin: glucagon ratio in the portal and peripheral circulation (38386), *Proc. Soc. Exp. Biol. Med.* **147:**88.

Ferner, H., 1953, The A- and B-cells of the pancreatic islets as sources of the antagonistic hormones glucagon and insulin. The shift of the AB-relation in diabetes mellitus, *Amer. J. Dig. Dis.* **20:**301.

Frame, C. M., Davidson, M. B., and Sturdevant, R. A. L., 1975, Effects of the octapeptide of cholecystokinin on insulin and glucagon secretion in the dog, *Endocrinology* **97:**549.

Fujita, T., 1976, *The 1975 International Symposium of the GEP Endocrine System,* Elsevier Scientific Publishing, Kyoto, Japan (in press).

Galbo, H., Holst, J. J., and Christensen, N. J., 1975, Glucagon and plasma catecholamine responses to graded and prolonged exercise in man, *J. Appl. Physiol.* **38:**70.

Garrison, J. C., and Haynes, R. C., Jr., 1975, The hormonal control of gluconeo-genesis by regulation of mitochondrial pyruvate carboxylation in isolated rat liver cells, *J. Biol. Chem.* **250:**2769.

Gerich, J. E., Lorenzi, M., Bier, D. M., Schneider, V., Tsalikian, E., Karam, J. H., and Forsham, P. H., 1975a, Prevention of human diabetic ketoacidosis by somatostatin. Evidence for an essential role of glucagon, *N. Engl. J. Med.* **292:**985.

Gerich, J. E., Lorenzi, M., Hane, S., Gustafson, G., Guillemin, R., and Forsham, P. H., 1975b, Evidence for a physiologic role of pancreatic glucagon in human glucose homeostasis: Studies with somatostatin, *Metabolism* **24:**175.

Gerich, J. E., Lorenzi, M., Karam, J. H., Schneider, V., and Forsham, P. H., 1975c, Abnormal pancreatic glucagon secretion and postprandial hyperglycemia in diabetes mellitus, *J. Amer. Med. Assoc.* **234:**159.

Gerich, J. E., Lovinger, R., and Grodsky, G. M., 1975d, Inhibition by somatostatin of glucagon and insulin release from the perfused rat pancreas in response to arginine, isoproterenol and theophylline: Evidence for a preferential effect on glucagon secretion, *Endocrinology* **96:**749.

Gössner, W., and Korting, G. W., 1960, Metastasierendes Inselzellkarzinom von A-Zelltyp bei einem Fall von Pemphigus foliaceus mit Diabetes renalis, *Dtsch. Med. Wochenschr.* **85:**434.

Hinton, P., Allison, S. P., Littlejohn, S., and Lloyd, J., 1971, Insulin and glucose to reduce catabolic response to injury in burned patients, *Lancet* **1:**767.

Iversen, J., 1973a, Adrenergic receptors in the secretion of glucagon and insulin from the isolated perfused canine pancreas, *J. Clin. Invest.* **52:**2102.

Iversen, J., 1973b, Effect of acetyl choline on the secretion of glucagon and in-sulin from the isolated perfused canine pancreas, *Diabetes* **22:**381.

Iversen, J., 1974, Inhibition of pancreatic glucagon release by somatostatin: *In vitro*, *Scand. J. Clin. Lab. Invest.* **33**:125.

Iversen, J., 1970, *Program of the Seventh Congress of the International Diabetes Federation*, International Congress Series 209:46 (F. J. G. Ebling, I. Henderson, and R. Assan, eds.), Excerpta Medica, Amsterdam.

Järhult, J., 1975, Role of the symphato–adrenal system in hemorrhagic hyperglycemia, *Acta Physiol. Scand.* **93**:25.

Jennings, A. S., Cherrington, A. D., Chiasson, J. L., Liljenquist, J. E., and Lacy, W. W., 1975, The fine regulation of basal hepatic glucose production, *Clin. Res.* **23**:323A.

Kakiuchi, S., and Tomizawa, H. H., 1964, Properties of a glucagon-degrading enzyme of beef liver, *J. Biol. Chem.* **239**:2160.

Kaneto, A., Kajinuma, H., and Kosaka, K., 1975, Effect of splanchnic nerve stimulation on glucagon and insulin output in the dog, *Endocrinology* **96**:143.

Kirk, R. D., Dunn, P. J., Smith, J. R., Beaven, D. W., and Donald, R. A., 1975, Abnormal pancreatic alpha-cell function in first-degree relatives of known diabetics, *J. Clin. Endocrinol. Metab.* **40**:913.

Koerker, D. J., Ruch, W., Chideckel, E., Palmer, J., Goodner, C. J., Ensinck, J., and Gale, C. C., 1974, Somatostatin: Hypothalamic inhibitor of the endocrine pancreas, *Science* **184**:482.

Kuku, S. F., Zeidler, A., Emmanouel, D. S., Katz, A. I., Levin, N. W., Tello, A., and Rubenstein, A. H., 1976. Heterogeneity of circulating glucagon in renal failure and diabetic hyperglycemic syndromes, *Clin. Res.* **23**:536A.

Lacy, P. E., 1970, Beta-cell secretion—function from the standpoint of pathologist (Banting Memorial Lecture), *Diabetes* **19**:895.

Larsson, L. I., Holst, J., Håkanson, R., and Sundler, F., 1975, Distribution and properties of glucagon immunoreactivity in the digestive tract of various mammals: An immunohistochemical and immunochemical study, *Histochemistry* **44**:281.

Lawrence, A. M., Kirsteins, L., Hojvat, S., Rubin, L., and Paloyan, V., 1975, Salivary gland glucagon: A potent extrapancreatic hyperglycemic factor, *Clin. Res.* **23**:536A.

Leclercq-Meyer, V., Rebolledo, O., Marchano, J., and Malaisse, W., 1975, Glucagon release: Paradoxical stimulation by glucose during calcium deprivation, *Science* **189**:897.

Lefebvre, P. J., and Luyckx, A. S., 1975, Effect of acute kidney exclusion by ligation of renal arteries on peripheral plasma glucagon levels and pancreatic glucagon production in the anesthetized dog, *Metabolism* **24**:1169.

Lefebvre, P. J., and Luyckx, A. S., 1976, Plasma glucagon after kidney exclusion: Experiments in somatostatin-infused and in eviscerated dogs, *Metabolism* **25**:761.

Leffert, H., Alexander, N. M., Faloona, G. R., Rubalcava, B., Steiner, A., and Unger, R. H., 1975, Specific endocrine and hormonal receptor changes associated with liver regeneration in adult rats, *Proc. Nat. Acad. Sci. U.S.A.* **72**:4033.

Lin, M. C., Wright, D. E., Hruby, V. J., and Rodbell, M., 1975, Structure–function relationships in glucagon: Properties of highly purified DES-HIS-l-, mon-oiodo-, and (DES-ASN-28, THR-29) (homoserine lactone-27)-glucagon, *Bio-chemistry* **14**:1559.

Lindsey, C. A., Santeusanio, F., Braaten, J., Faloona, G. R., and Unger, R. H., 1974, Pancreatic alpha cell function in trauma, *J. Amer. Med. Assoc.* **227**:757.

Lindsey, C. A., Faloona, G. R., and Unger, R. H., 1975, Plasma glucagon levels during rapid exsanguination with and without adrenergic blockade, *Diabetes* **24**:313.

Luft, R., Efendic, S., Hökfelt, T., Johansson, O., and Arimura, A., 1974, Immu-nohistochemical evidence for the localization of somatostatin-like immuno-reactivity in a cell population of the pancreatic islets, *Med. Biol.* **52**:428.

Mackrell, D. J., and Sokal, J. E., 1969, Antagonism between the effects of insulin and glucagon on the isolated liver, *Diabetes* **18**:724.

Madison, L. L., Seyffert, W. A., Jr., Unger R. H., and Barker, B., 1968, Effect of plasma free fatty acids on plasma glucagon and serum insulin concentrations, *Metabolism* **17**:301.

Mallison, C. N., Bloom, S. R., Warin, A. P., Salmon, P. R., and Cox, B., 1974, A glucagonoma syndrome, *Lancet* **2**:1.

Marco, J., Calle, C., Román, D., Díaz-Fierros, M., Villanueva, M. L., and Valverde, I., 1973, Hyperglucagonism induced by glucocorticoid treatment in man, *N. Engl. J. Med.* **288**:128.

Markussen, J., Frandsen, E., Heding, L. G., and Sundby, F., 1972, Turkey glu-cagon: Crystallization, amino acid composition, and immunology, *Horm. Metab. Res.* **4**:360.

Marliss, E. B., Girardier, L., Seydoux, J., Wollheim, C. B., Kanazawa, Y., Orci, L., Renold, A. E., and Porte, D., Jr., 1973, Glucagon release induced by pan-creatic nerve stimulation in the dog, *J. Clin. Invest.* **52**:1246.

Mashiter, K., Harding, P. E., Chou, M., Mashiter, G. D., Stout, J., Diamond, D., and Field, J. B., 1975, Persistent pancreatic glucagon but not insulin response to arginine in pancreatectomized dogs, *Endocrinology* **96**:678.

Matschinsky, F. M., Pagliara, A. S., Hover, B. A., Haymond, M. W., and Stillings, S. N., 1975, Differential effects of α- and β-D-glucose on insulin and gluca-gon secretion from the isolated perfused rat pancreas, *Diabetes* **24**:369.

Matsuyama, T., and Foá, P. P., 1975, Plasma glucose, insulin, pancreatic and entero-glucagon levels in normal and depancreatized dogs (38288), *Proc. Soc. Exp. Biol. Med.* **147**:97.

McGarry, J. D., Robles-Valdes, C., and Foster, D. W., 1975a, Role of carnitine in hepatic ketogenesis, *Proc. Nat. Acad. Sci. U.S.A.* **72**:4385.

McGarry, J. D., Wright, P. H., and Foster, D. W., 1975b, Hormonal control of ketogenesis: Rapid activation of hepatic ketogenic capacity in fed rats by anti-insulin serum and glucagon, *J. Clin. Invest.* **55**:1202.

McGavran, M. H., Unger, R. H., Recant, L., Polk, H. C., Kilo, C., and Levin, M. E., 1966, A glucagon-secreting alpha cell carcinoma of the pancreas, *N. Engl. J. Med.* **274**:1408.

Meguid, M. M., Brennan, M. F., Aoki, T. T., Müller, W. A., Ball, M. R., and Moor, F. D., 1973, The role of insulin and glucagon in acute trauma, *Surg. Forum* **24**:97.

Meissner, C., Thum, C., Beischer, W., Winkler, G. Schröder, K. E., and Pfeiffer, E. F., 1975, Antidiabetic action of somatostatin—assessed by the artificial pancreas, *Diabetes* **24**:988.

Mortimer, C. H., Turnbridge, W. M. G., Carr, D., Yeomans, L., Lind, T., Coy, D. H., Bloom, S. R., Kastin, A., Mallinson, C. N., Besser, G. M., Schally, A. V., and Hall, R., 1974, Effects of growth hormone release–inhibiting hormone on circulating glucagon, insulin, and growth hormone in normal, diabetic, acromegalic, and hypopituitary patients, *Lancet* **1**:697.

Müller, W. A., Faloona, G. R., Unger, R. H., and Aguilar-Parada, E., 1970, Abnormal alpha cell function in diabetes. Response to carbohydrate and protein ingestion, *N. Engl. J. Med.* **283**:109.

Müller, W. A., Faloona, G. R., and Unger, R. H., 1971, The effect of experimental insulin deficiency on glucagon secretion, *J. Clin. Invest.* **50**:1992.

Muñoz, L., Blazquez, E., and Unger, R., 1975, Gastric A-cell function in normal and diabetic dogs, *Diabetes* **24**:411(Suppl. 2).

Nilsson, K. O., Heding, L. G., and Hokfelt, B., 1975, The influence of short term submaximal work on the plasma concentrations of catecholamines, pancreatic glucagon, and growth hormone in man, *Acta Endocrinol. KBH* **79**:286.

Noe, B. D., and Bauer, G. E., 1971, Evidence for glucagon biosynthesis involving a protein intermediate in islets of the anglerfish *(Lophius americanus)*, *Endocrinology* **89**:642.

Noe, B. D., Bauer, G. E., Steffes, M. W., Sutherland, D. E. R., and Najarian, J. S., 1975, Glucagon biosynthesis in human pancreatic islets: Preliminary evidence for a biosynthetic intermediate, *Horm. Metab. Res.* **7**:314.

Orci, L., and Unger, R. H., 1975, Functional subdivision of islets of Langerhans and possible role of D-cells, *Lancet* **2**:1243.

Orci, L., Pictet, R., Forssmann, W. G., Renold, A. E., and Rouiller, C., 1968, Structural evidence for glucagon producing cells in the intestinal mucosa of the rat, *Diabetologia* **4**:56.

Orci, L., Stauffacher, W., Renold, A. E., and Rouiller, C., 1970, The ultrastructural aspect of A-cells of non-ketotic and ketotic diabetic animals: Indications for stimulation and inhibition of glucagon production, *Acta. Isotopica* **10**:171.

Orci, L., Unger, R. H., and Renold, A. E., 1973, Structural coupling between pancreatic islet cell, *Experientia* **29**:1015.

Orci, L., Baetens, D., Dubois, M. P., and Rufener, C., 1975a, Evidence for the D-cell of the pancreas secreting somatostatin, *Horm. Metab. Res.* **7**:400.

Orci, L., Malaisse-Lagae, F., Amherdt, M., Ravazzola, M., Weisswange, A., Dobbs, R., Perrelet, A., and Unger, R., 1975b, Cell contacts in human islets of Langerhans, *J. Clin. Endocrinol. Metab.* **41**:841.

Orci, L., Malaisse-Lagae, F., Ravazzola, M., Rouiller, D., Renold, A. E., Perrelet, A., and Unger, R., 1975c, A morphological basis for intercellular communication between A- and B-cells in the endocrine pancreas, *J. Clin. Invest.* **56**:1066.

Orci, L., Baetens, D., Rufener, C., Amherdt, M., Ravazzola, M., Studer, P., Malaisse-Lagae, F., and Unger, R. H., 1976, Hypertrophy and hyperplasia of somatostatin-containing D-cells in diabetes, *Proc. Nat. Acad. Sci. U.S.A.* **73**:1338.

Orton, C. I., Segal, A. W., Bloom, S. R., and Clark, J., 1975, Hypersecretion of glucagon and gastrin in severely burnt patients, *Br. Med. J.* **2:**170.

Palmer, J. P., Bensen, J., Werner, P., and Ensinck, J. W., 1976, Glucagon secretion in a totally pancreatectomized patient, *Clin. Res.* **24:**119A.

Park, C. R., and Exton, J. H., 1972, Glucagon and the metabolism of glucose, *in: Glucagon: Molecular Physiology, Clinical and Therapeutic Implications* (P. J. Lefebvre and R. H. Unger, eds.), pp. 77–108, Pergamon Press, Oxford.

Parrilla, R., Jimenez, I., and Ayuso-Parrilla, M. S., 1975, Glucagon and insulin control in gluconeogenesis in the perfused isolated rat liver. Effects on cellular metabolite distribution, *Eur. J. Biochem.* **56:**375.

Pelletier, G., Leclerc, R., Arimura, A., and Schally, A. V., 1975, Immunohistochemical localization of somatostatin in the rat pancreas, *J. Histochem. Cytochem.* **23:**699.

Polak, J. M., Bloom, S., Coulling, I., and Pearse, A. G. E., 1971, Immunofluorescent localization of enteroglucagon cells in the gastrointestinal tract of the dog, *Gut* **12:**311.

Pollock, H. G., and Kimmel, J. R., 1975, Chicken glucagon: Isolation and amino acid sequence studies, *J. Biol. Chem.* **250:**9377.

Rabinovitch, A., and Dupré, J., 1974, Effects of gastric inhibitory polypeptide present in impure pancreozymin–cholecystokinin on plasma insulin and glucagon in the rat, *Endocrinology* **94:**1139.

Raskin, P., and Unger, R. H., 1976a, Effects of exogenous glucagon in insulin-treated diabetics, *Diabetes* (abstract) **25**(Suppl.):341.

Raskin, P., and Unger, R. H., 1976b, Effect of insulin and somatostatin on A-cell dysfunction in human diabetes, *Clin. Res.* (abstract), **24:**486A.

Raskin, P., Fujita, Y., and Unger, R. H., 1975, Effect of insulin–glucose infusions on plasma glucagon levels in fasting diabetics and nondiabetics, *J. Clin. Invest.* **56:**1132.

Rigopoulou, D., Valverde, I., Marco, J., Faloona, G., and Unger, R. H., 1970, Large glucagon immunoreactivity in extracts of pancreas, *J. Biol. Chem.* **245:**496.

Rocha, D. M., Faloona, G. R., and Unger, R. H., 1972, Glucagon stimulating activity of twenty amino acids in dogs, *J. Clin. Invest.* **51:**2346.

Rocha, D. M., Santeusanio, F., Faloona, G. R., and Unger, R. H., 1973, Abnormal pancreatic alpha cell function in bacterial infections, *N. Engl. J. Med.* **288:**700.

Rodbell, M., Krans, H. M., Pohl, S. L., and Birnbaumer, L., 1971, The glucagon-sensitive adenyl cyclase system in plasma membranes of rat liver. III. Binding of glucagon: Method of assay and specificity, *J. Biol. Chem.* **246:**1861.

Rodbell, M., Lin, M. C., and Salomon, Y., 1974, Evidence for interdependent action of glucagon and nucleotides on the hepatic adenylate cyclase system, *J. Biol. Chem.* **249:**59.

Rodbell, M., Lin, M. C., Salomon, Y., Londos, C., Harwood, J. P., Martin, B. L., Rendell, M., and Berman, M., 1975, Role of adenine and guanine nucleotides in the activity and response of adenylate cyclase systems to hormones: Evidence of multisite transition states, *in: Advances in Cyclic Nucleotide Research* (G. I. Drumond, P. Greengard, and G. A. Robison, eds.), pp. 3–30, Raven Press, New York.

Rosselin, G., Jarrousse, C., Rancon, R., and Portha, P., 1973, L'AMP cyclique médiateur de la sécrétion du glucagon due aux acides aminés, *C.R. Acad. Sci. Paris* **276**:1017.

Russell, R. C. G., Walker, C. J., and Bloom, S. R., 1975, Hyperglucagonemia in the surgical patient, *Br. Med. J.* **1**:10.

Sakurai, H., Dobbs, R., and Unger, R. H., 1974, Somatostatin-induced changes in insulin and glucagon secretion in normal and diabetic dogs, *J. Clin. Invest.* **54**:1395.

Sakurai, H., Dobbs, R. E., and Unger, R. H., 1975, The role of glucagon in the pathogenesis of the endogenous hyperglycemia of diabetes mellitus, *Metabolism* **24**:1287.

Salomon, Y., Lin, M. C., London, C., Rendell, M., and Rodbell, M., 1975, The hepatic adenylate cyclase system. I. Evidence for transition states and structural requirements for guanine nucleotide activation, *J. Biol. Chem.* **250**:4239.

Sasagawa, T., Kobayashi, S., and Fujita, T., 1973, Electron microscopy of human GEP endocrine cells, *in: Gastro-Entero-Pancreatic Endocrine System* (T. Fujita, ed.), p. 31, Igaku Shoin, Tokyo.

Sasaki, K., Dockerill, S., Adamiak, D. A., Tickle, I. J., and Blundell, T., 1975a, X-ray analysis of glucagon and its relationship to receptor binding, *Nature* **257**:751.

Sasaki, H., Rubalcava, B., Baetens, D., Blazquez, E., Srikant, C. B., Orci, L., and Unger, R. H., 1975b, Identification of glucagon in the gastrointestinal tract, *J. Clin. Invest.* **56**:135.

Schade, D. S., and Eaton, R. P., 1975a, Modulation of fatty acid metabolism by glucagon in man. I. Effects in normal subjects, *Diabetes* **24**:502.

Schade, D. S., and Eaton, R. P., 1975b, Modulation of fatty acid metabolism by glucagon in man. II. Effects in insulin-deficient diabetics, *Diabetes* **24**:510.

Sherwin, R. S., Hendler, R. G., and Felig, P., 1975, Effect of ketone infusions on amino acid and nitrogen metabolism in man, *J. Clin. Invest.* **55**:1382.

Sherwin, R. S., Fisher, M., Hendler, R., and Felig, P., 1976, Hyperglucagonemia and blood glucose regulation in normal, obese, and diabetic subjects, *N. Engl. J. Med.* **294**:455.

Srikant, C. B., McCorkle, K., and Dobbs, R. E., 1976, A biologically active "macro-'glucagon' (IRG)" in glucagon-secreting tissues of the dog, *Diabetes* (abstract) **25**:(Suppl.):325.

Staehelin, L. A., 1974, Structure and function of intercellular junctions, *Int. Rev. Cytol.* **39**:191.

Starzl, T. E., Porter, K. A., Kashiwagi, N., and Putnam, C. W., 1975, Portal hepatotrophic factors, diabetes mellitus, and acute liver atrophy, hypertrophy, and regeneration, *Surg. Gynecol. Obstet.* **141**:843.

Sundby, F., and Markussen, J., 1971, Isolation, crystallization, and amino acid composition of rat glucagon, *Horm. Metab. Res.* **3**:184.

Sundby, F., and Markussen, J., 1972, Rabbit glucagon: Isolation, crystallization, and amino acid composition, *Horm. Metab. Res.* **4**:56.

Sundby, F., Frandsen, E. K., Thomsen, J., Kristiansen, K., and Brundfeldt, K., 1972, Crystallization and amino acid sequence of duck glucagon, *FEBS Lett.* **26**:289.

Sutherland, E. W., and DeDuve, C., 1948, Origin and distribution of the hyperglycemic–glycogenolytic factor of the pancreas, *J. Biol. Chem.* **175**:663.

Tager, H. S., and Steiner, D. F., 1973, Isolation of a glucagon-containing peptide: Primary structure of a possible fragment of proglucagon, *Proc. Nat. Acad. Sci. U.S.A.* **70:**2321.

Thomsen, J., Kristiansen, K., Brunfeldt, K., and Sundby, F., 1972, The amino acid sequence of human glucagon, *FEBS Lett.* **21:**315.

Toyota, T., Sato, S., Kudo, M., Abe, K., and Goto, Y., 1975, Secretory regulation of endocrine pancreas: Cyclic AMP and glucagon secretion, *J. Clin. Endocrinol. Metab.* **41:**81.

Trakatellis, A. C., Tada, K., Yamaji, K., and Gardiki-Kouidou, P., 1975, Isolation and partial characterization of anglerfish proglucagon, *Biochemistry* **14**(8):1508.

Unger, R. H., 1971, Glucagon and the insulin: glucagon ratio in diabetes and other catabolic illnesses, *Diabetes* **20:**834.

Unger, R. H., 1976, Diabetes and the alpha cell (Banting Memorial Lecture), *Diabetes* **25:**136.

Unger, R. H., and Eisentraut, A. M., 1969, Entero-insular axis, *Arc. Intern. Med.* **123:**261.

Unger, R. H., and Orci, L., 1975, The essential role of glucagon in the pathogenesis of diabetes mellitus, *Lancet* **1:**14.

Unger, R. H., Ketterer, H., Dupré, J., and Eisentraut, A. M., 1967, The effects of secretin, pancreozymin, and gastrin on insulin and glucagon secretion in anesthetized dogs, *J. Clin. Invest.* **46:**630.

Unger, R. H., Ohneda, A., Aguilar-Parada, E., and Eisentraut, A. M., 1969, The role of aminogenic glucagon secretion in blood glucose homeostasis, *J. Clin. Invest.* **48:**810.

Unger, R. H., Aguilar-Parada, E., Müller, W. A., and Eisentraut, A. M., 1970, Studies of pancreatic alpha cell function in normal and diabetic subjects, *J. Clin. Invest.* **49:**837.

Unger, R. H., Madison, L. L., and Müller, W. A., 1972, Abnormal alpha cell function in diabetics: Response to insulin, *Diabetes* **21:**301.

Valverde, I., Villanueva, M. L., Lozano, I., and Marco, J., 1974, Presence of glucagon immunoreactivity in the globulin fraction of human plasma ("Big Plasma Glucagon"), *J. Clin. Endocrinol. Metab.* **39:**1090.

Valverde, I., Dobbs, R., and Unger, R. H., 1975, Heterogeneity of plasma glucagon immunoreactivity in normal, depancreatized, and alloxan diabetic dogs, *Metabolism* **24:**1021.

Valverde, I., Lemon, H. M., Kessinger, A., and Unger, R. H., 1976, Distribution of plasma glucagon immunoreactivity in a patient with a suspected glucagonoma, *J. Clin. Endocrinol. Metab.* **42:**804.

Vranic, M., Pek, S., and Kawamori, R., 1974, Increased "glucagon immunoreactivity" (IRG) in plasma of totally depancreatized dogs, *Diabetes* **23:**905.

Weir, G. C., Turner, R. C., Martin, D. B., 1973, Glucagon radioimmunoassay using antiserum 30K: Interference by plasma, *Horm. Metab. Res.* **5:**241.

Weir, G. C., Knowlton, S. D., and Martin, D. B., 1975, Nucleotide and nucleoside stimulation of glucagon secretion, *Endocrinology* **97:**932.

Willerson, J. T., Hutcheson, D. R., Leshin, S. J., Faloona, G. R., and Unger, R. H., 1974, Serum glucagon and insulin levels and their relationship to blood glucose values in patients with acute myocardial infarction and acute coronary insufficiency, *Am. J. Med.* **57:**747.

Wilmore, D. W., Lindsey, C. A., Faloona, G. R., Moylan, J. A., Pruitt, B. A., Unger, R. H., 1974, Hyperglucagonemia after burns, *Lancet* **1:**73.

Wise, J. K., Hendler, R., and Felig, P., 1973, Influence of glucocorticoids on glucagon secretion and plasma amino acid concentrations in man, *J. Clin. Invest.* **52:**2774.

Wollheim, C. B., Blondel, B., Rabinovitch, A., and Renold, A. E., 1973, Insulin and glucagon release in pancreatic monolayer cultures: Effects of cyclic nucleotides, *in: Eighth Congress of the International Diabetes Federation, Brussels,* p. 48, International Congress Series No. 280, Excerpta Medica, Abstracts.

Yoshinaga, T., Okuno, G., Shinji, Y., Tsujii, T., and Nishikawa, M., 1966, Pancreatic A-cell tumor associated with severe diabetes mellitus, *Diabetes* **15:**709.

Recent Developments in Body Fuel Metabolism

Philip Felig

4.1. Introduction

The major energy-yielding fuels ingested in the diet and found as normal body constituents are carbohydrate, fat, and protein. This review will focus on some recent advances in the disposal, production, and interconversion of these substrates. Emphasis will be placed on normal physiology, inasmuch as various disease states (e.g., diabetes, obesity, amino acid disorders) are covered in detail elsewhere in this volume. In addition, the fuel response to such conditions as starvation and exercise will also be reviewed.

4.2. Glucose Metabolism

4.2.1. Glucose Disposal

The disposal of an oral glucose load, as reflected by the blood glucose response on an oral glucose tolerance test, depends on insulin-mediated

PHILIP FELIG • Department of Internal Medicine; Section of Endocrinology, Yale University School of Medicine, New Haven, Connecticut 06510.

cellular uptake and metabolism of glucose. The precise tissue site of this uptake of glucose has, however, not been readily apparent. Although it is known that liver, muscle, and adipose cells are all insulin-responsive tissues, the quantitative distribution of glucose uptake between hepatic and nonhepatic tissues has only recently been delineated. Felig *et al.* (1975) addressed this question by examining splanchnic glucose exchange in normal subjects before and after ingestion of an oral glucose load. Since glucose absorption occurs by the portal route, the delivery of ingested glucose to peripheral tissues depends on its escape from the splanchnic bed. Over the 3-hr period following ingestion of 100 g glucose, a total of 40 g glucose was observed to enter the systemic circulation from the splanchnic bed. Of even greater interest was the observation that total splanchnic glucose delivery during this period exceeded the basal rate by only 15 g. It is well established that the basal rate of peripheral glucose utilization primarily represents uptake by non-insulin-dependent tissues, such as the brain and the blood cellular elements. Thus, the total amount of glucose made available for disposal as increased (above-basal) glucose utilization by peripheral, insulin-dependent tissues such as fat and muscle accounts for only 15% of the oral glucose load. From these data on splanchnic glucose balance, the changes in arterial glucose level, and the known basal rate of glucose uptake by non-insulin-dependent tissues, an estimate of the overall tissue disposal of an oral glucose load may be made. As shown in Table I, peripheral (extrahepatic) tissues can account for only 15% of the disposal of an oral glucose load via insulin-dependent pathways. Less that 5% of the glucose load remains in the tissue space. The remaining portion of the glucose ingested thus represents utilization along hepatic pathways. About 25% is used to meet the non-insulin-dependent glucose requirements of brain and blood cellular elements, thereby sparing liver glycogen. The remainder of the glucose load, approximately 55%, represents net hepatic glucose uptake for glycogen synthesis, triglyceride formation, and, to a much smaller extent, glycolysis.

In addition to providing evidence of net hepatic retention of glucose, these findings underscore the importance of hepatic glucose exchange in determining the height and shape of the oral glucose tolerance test. Thus, the peak rise in arterial blood glucose is proportional to the extent of splanchnic glucose escape. Furthermore, the early decline in blood glucose and the secondary elevation often observed at 2–3 hr after glucose ingestion coincide with an initial fall and delayed, secondary rise in splanchnic glucose delivery. The primacy of the liver as the site of glucose disposal can also account for the "flat glucose tolerance curve," as a normal variant. Previous studies have shown that in as many as 30% of healthy persons with no evidence of a malabsorption syndrome, the blood glucose response to oral glucose may at no time exceed 100 mg/100 ml. In such persons, the insulin increment is neither excessive nor diminished.

Table I. Sites of Disposal of a 100-g Oral Glucose Load in Normal Man[a]

Site	Disposal (%)
Unmetabolized	<5%
Glucose remaining in glucose space of body fluids	
Insulin-dependent peripheral Uptake	15%
Increased (above-basal) uptake by fat and muscle tissue	
Hepatic glycogen-sparing	25%
Peripheral delivery of ingested glucose to noninsulin-dependent tissues (e.g., brain), thereby sparing liver glycogen	
Hepatic glucose retention	55%
Glycogen synthesis	
Triglyceride formation	
Glycolysis	

[a]Based on the data of Felig *et al.* (1975).

The lack of a greater rise in blood glucose can be explained on the basis of a greater retention of the glucose load within the liver, rather than as an indication of malabsorption or hyperinsulinemia. Interestingly, Felig *et al.* (1975) noted that in some normal individuals, the increase in peripheral glucose delivery amounted to less than 5 g in 3 hr.

Concerning the mechanism responsible for the retention of the oral glucose load within the splanchnic bed, that glucose is absorbed by the portal circulation necessitates exposure of the absorbed glucose to the liver prior to systemic delivery. Of additional, and perhaps greater, importance are the higher concentrations of insulin in portal as compared to peripheral blood (Blackard and Nelson, 1970). Furthermore, transplantation of pancreatic islet cells to the peritoneum or thigh muscles of diabetic rats reduces hyperglycemia, but fails to restore blood glucose levels to normal (Ballinger and Lacy, 1972), while interportal transplantation of pancreatic islets results in complete amelioration of the diabetic syndrome (Kemp *et al.*, 1973; Amamoo *et al.*, 1974). These observations emphasizing the role of hepatic as compared to peripheral disposal of ingested glucose provide a possible rationale for the importance of normalizing portal–peripheral insulin gradients in attempting to ameliorate clinical diabetes by means of either islet cell transplantation or mechanical glucose-sensing, insulin-delivering devices.

It is of interest that the direct observations on splanchnic glucose balances after a glucose meal agree with indirect estimates of hepatic vs. peripheral glucose disposal. In studies comparing oral and intravenous glucose tolerance curves in rats (Scow and Cornfield, 1954) as well as in man (Perley and Kipnis, 1967), it has been estimated that no more than 30–40% of the orally ingested glucose enters the peripheral circulation. In addition, observations on uptake of glucose by peripheral forearm tissues also demonstrate that considerably less than half the glucose load is made available for extrahepatic disposal (Jackson et al., 1973). Thus, the evidence from measurements of splanchnic and peripheral glucose exchange, as well as indirect comparisons of oral and intravenous glucose tolerance curves, point to the liver as the major site of glucose disposal. Moreover, studies on the sensitivity of hepatic glucoregulatory mechanisms to small changes in insulin and alterations in hepatic glucose metabolism in states of insulin deficiency (diabetes) or insulin resistance (obesity) further underscore the role of the liver in glucose homeostasis (Felig and Wahren, 1975a).

4.2.2. Insulin–Glucagon Interaction in Glucose Disposal

In recent years, attention has been focused on the possibility that the metabolism of glucose does not depend solely on the insulin concentration, but depends on the relative concentrations of insulin and glucagon (Unger, 1971). This conclusion was derived in part from the demonstration that following a glucose meal, not only does the insulin level increase, but also the circulating glucagon concentration is reduced (Müller et al., 1970). In addition, in vitro studies have suggested the importance of insulin:glucagon ratios in regulating carbohydrate metabolism (Parilla et al., 1974). Inasmuch as glucagon is believed to be devoid of effects on glucose translocation in muscle or fat tissue, the demonstration that the liver is the major site of glucose disposal provides indirect evidence for bihormonal modulation of this phenomenon. The hypothesis that the insulin:glucagon ratio, rather than absolute alterations in insulin, and that suppression of glucagon secretion by glucose are essential elements for the normal metabolism of this substrate was tested in studies involving infusion of physiological doses of glucagon (Sherwin et al., 1976b). In their investigation, these workers examined the effects of a 6-hr infusion of glucagon at a dose of 3 ng/kg per min on the blood glucose response to ingestion of 100 g glucose by normal, healthy subjects. The glucagon infusion resulted in a plasma glucagon increment of approximately 300 pg/ml, which corresponds to the elevations observed in physiological circumstances such as protein ingestion (Unger, 1971), starvation (Unger, 1971), or prolonged exercise (Ahlborg et al., 1974), as well as to the hyperglucagonemia observed in such disease states as diabetic ketoacidosis (Müller et al., 1973), uremia (Sherwin et al., 1976a), and cirrhosis (Sherwin et al., 1974). Despite the sustained hyperglucagonemia, the blood glucose response to an oral glucose load administered after 3 hr of the glucagon infusion was no different from that observed in a saline control study (Fig. 1). Maintenance of normal glucose tolerance did not depend on compensatory hyperinsulinemia, inasmuch as the insulin levels were also precisely the same during the glucagon and the control infusion. These findings thus indicate that failure of suppression of glucagon secretion by glucose does not bring about a diabetic glucose tolerance curve. Furthermore, elevation of glucagon cannot of itself bring about a deterioration in glucose tolerance. These observations thus provide strong evidence that the key factor determining normal glucose disposal is not the insulin:glucagon ratio or the simultaneous suppression of glucagon, but is dependent on the increment in insulin secretion. Supporting the key role of insulin in the maintenance of normal glucose homeostasis was the further observation that in chemical diabetics and insulin-treated juvenile diabetics, sustained hyperglucagonemia could not of itself bring about worsening of diabetic control (Sherwin *et al.*, 1976b). Glucagon was capable of causing deterioration in glucose tolerance only in circumstances of acute insulin deficiency. Thus, it would appear that insulin secretion is the main factor determining normal glucose disposal, while insulin lack is the primary factor responsible for the diabetic state. The role of glucagon appears to be one of stimulating glucose production in the fasting state and in response to protein ingestion (Wahren *et al.*, 1976), and in accentuating the diabetic defect in circumstances of absolute insulin deficiency. However, final assessment of the relative importance of insulin and glucagon in diabetes must await further studies.

The relative importance of glucagon as compared to insulin in glucose disposal is also apparent from observations on the glucoregulatory response to small increments (10–15 mg/100 ml) in blood glucose (Felig and Wahren, 1975a). When blood glucose levels are raised by 10–15 mg/100 ml (by slow infusion of glucose: 2 mg/kg per min), glucose homeostasis is maintained by virtue of a 85% inhibition in hepatic glucose output (Felig and Wahren, 1971a). These changes in hepatic glucose balance are engendered by a 60–100% increment in insulin levels, but occur in the absence of measurable changes in plasma glucagon concentration (Felig *et al.*, 1974b; Felig and Wahren, 1975a). Thus, disposal of small glucose loads is not dependent on an inhibition in glucagon secretion, but appears to be entirely regulated by an increase in insulin secretion.

4.3. Protein and Amino Acid Metabolism

In recent years, a number of studies have clarified the pattern of interorgan amino acid exchange as it exists in the postabsorptive and prolonged fasting condition (Felig, 1975). As shown in Fig. 2, alanine and

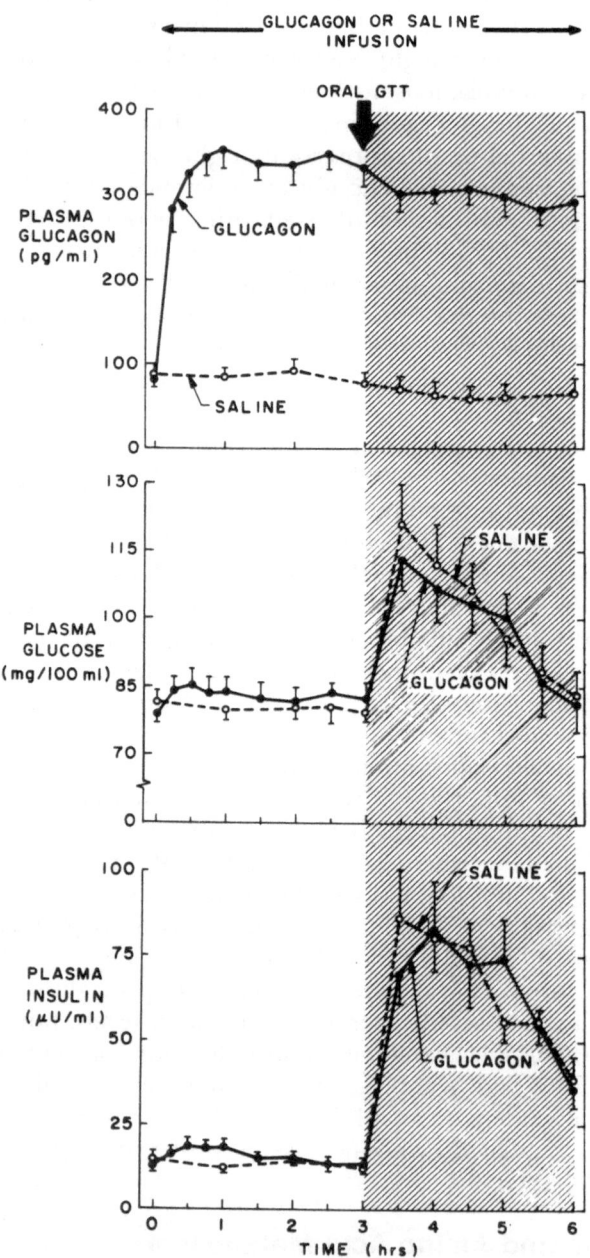

Fig. 1. Failure of sustained hyperglucagonemia to alter glucose tolerance in normal subjects. (Reproduced from Sherwin *et al.*, 1976b, with permission.)

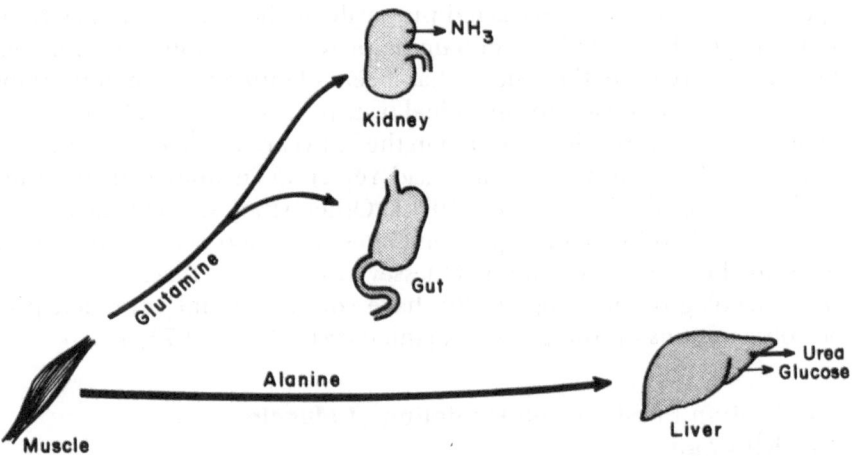

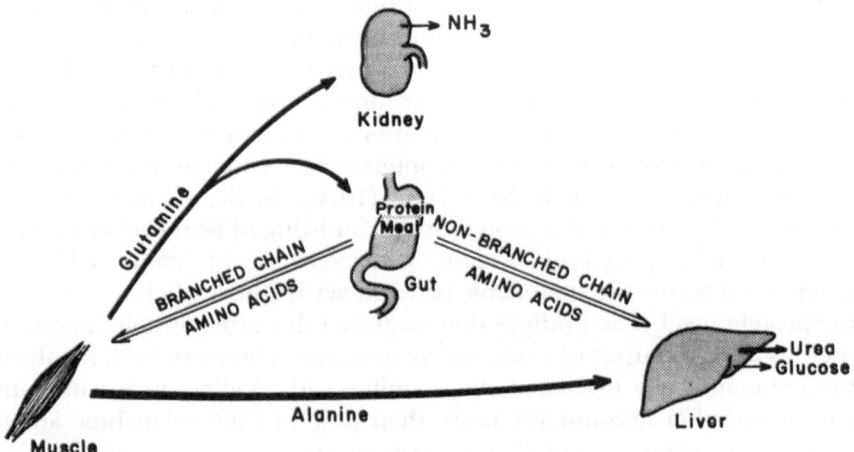

Fig. 2. Interorgan amino acid exchange in the fasted (postabsorptive) and the protein-fed state. Alanine and glutamine are continuously released during both fasting and feeding. Nitrogen repletion in muscle occurs via selective splanchnic escape and muscle uptake of branched-chain amino acids after protein feeding. The remainder of the amino acids are largely retained in the splanchnic bed.

glutamine have been identified as the quantitatively most important amino acids released by muscle tissue. In the case of alanine, the site of uptake of this amino acid is primarily the liver. Besides that released from muscle, additional alanine is made available to the kidney and gut. With respect to glutamine, it is extracted primarily by the kidney and gastrointestinal tissues. In the kidney, glutamine provides substrate for ammonia synthesis, whereas in the gut, it has been identified as an important energy-yielding substrate for intestinal transport processes (Windmueller and Spaeth, 1974). Studies reported in the last year have been undertaken to examine the pattern of amino acid repletion in muscle tissue after protein feeding (Wahren *et al.*, 1976). Other studies, focusing on the mechanism whereby alanine predominates in amino acid output from muscle in the fasting condition (Odessey *et al.*, 1974; Blackshear *et al.*, 1975; Palaiologos and Felig, 1976), have confirmed and extended previous observations on the glucose–alanine cycle (Felig, 1973, 1975).

4.3.1. Protein Feeding and Repletion of Muscle Nitrogen

It has been recognized that following the ingestion of a mixed protein meal, there are marked variations in the increments of individual amino acids observed in peripheral blood (Frame, 1958). The largest elevations, amounting to 2-fold increments or more, are observed for the branched-chain amino acids (valine, leucine, and isoleucine), which remain elevated for as long as 8 hr. In contrast, other amino acids such as alanine show little change in plasma concentration after protein feeding. Most recently, the effects of protein ingestion on interorgan exchange of amino acids have been examined by Wahren *et al.* (1976). In these studies, normal healthy subjects ingested a protein meal consisting of lean beef consumed in a dose of 3 g/kg body weight. Net exchange of amino acids was determined across the splanchnic bed and across the leg before and after the protein meal. The findings demonstrated that after protein ingestion, there is a large output of amino acids from the splanchnic bed, involving predominantly the branched-chain amino acids. Valine, isoleucine, and leucine together account for more than 60% of total splanchnic amino acid output, even though they contribute only 20% of the total amino acids in the protein meal. Simultaneously with the output of amino acids from the splanchnic bed, leg exchange of most amino acids reverted from a net output in the basal state to a net uptake after protein feeding. As in the case of splanchnic exchange, the uptake of amino acids across the leg was most marked for the branched-chain amino acids. The latter accounted for more than half the total peripheral amino acid uptake in the first hour, and for 90–100% at 2–3 hr. Most interestingly, alanine and glutamine were observed to be continuously released by the leg tissues after the protein meal. In addition, there was continuous net extraction of these amino acids by the splanchnic bed, confirming the direct observation of ongoing release of alanine and glutamine from an extrahepatic (muscle) site.

These findings thus indicate a special role for the branched-chain amino acids in body nitrogen metabolism after protein feeding (see Fig. 2). The primacy of these amino acids in protein-stimulated amino acid output from the splanchnic bed suggests a unique tendency for these amino acids to escape hepatic uptake or metabolism or both after intestinal absorption. These observations are in keeping with the relative unimportance of the liver in branched-chain amino acid metabolism (Miller, 1962). In contrast, the relatively minor increments in arterial concentration and splanchnic escape of other amino acids suggest a major role for the liver in the uptake and utilization of most amino acids ingested in a protein meal. Complementing the pattern of splanchnic amino acid output, the branched-chain amino acids are responsible for most of the amino acid uptake by muscle tissue after a protein meal. Underscoring this finding is the observation that alanine and glutamine are continuously released from the leg and transported to the splanchnic bed in the protein-fed as well as in the fasted state. Thus, the branched-chain amino acids are the major source for repletion of muscle nitrogen after protein intake. Furthermore, since the branched-chain amino acids comprise only 20% of the amino acid residues in muscle proteins (Kominz *et al.*, 1954; Odessey *et al.*, 1974), it is likely that these amino acids are not solely utilized for protein synthesis, but are largely catabolized within muscle, thereby providing an *in situ* source of energy for muscle. These relationships in interorgan amino acid exchange and the key role of the branched-chain amino acids in the protein-fed state are shown in Fig. 2. A nitrogen "shuttle" is suggested, whereby branched-chain amino acids provide for nitrogen repletion in muscle tissue in the fed state, and in which, in the fed as well as the fasted state, alanine and glutamine are continuously released from muscle.

These observations on protein feeding and amino acid metabolism in normal subjects have been extended by observations in the diabetic state (Wahren *et al.*, 1976). In insulin-dependent diabetics, the elevation in branched-chain amino acids in arterial concentration after protein feeding is exaggerated. In addition, their uptake by muscle tissue is reduced, particularly 2–3 hr after protein feeding. Furthermore, an exaggerated peripheral output of alanine is seen in the diabetics. Thus, the findings suggest that nitrogen repletion in muscle tissue is insulin-dependent, and is diminished in the diabetic state, thus providing evidence that diabetes is a disorder of protein tolerance as well as glucose tolerance.

4.3.2. Amino Acid Output from Muscle in the Fasting State

A major question regarding muscle amino acid metabolism concerns the predominance of alanine in the output of amino acids from muscle tissue in fasted subjects. Studies obtained over the last several years have shown a close relationship between alanine and pyruvate availability and output from muscle tissue, suggesting that pyruvate provides the carbon skeleton for alanine synthesis (Felig *et al.,* 1970; Felig and Wahren, 1971b; Felig, 1973). On the basis of these findings in intact man, it has been suggested that glucose-derived pyruvate provides 60–70% of the carbon skeletons for alanine production (Felig, 1973). More recent *in vitro* studies with isolated diaphragm employing isotopically labeled glucose have in fact demonstrated that 60–70% of the carbon skeletons in alanine released from rat diaphragm are derived from glucose (Odessey *et al.,* 1974). Similar conclusions have been reached from observations in hepatectomized rats (Blackshear *et al.,* 1975). With respect to the nitrogen source for alanine synthesis, a special role for the branched-chain amino acids was demonstrated with the observation that physiological increments of valine, leucine, and isoleucine have a specific effect (not shared by other amino acids) in stimulating alanine output from diaphragm muscle (Odessey *et al.,* 1974; Palaiologos and Felig, 1976). While other investigators have suggested that a variety of amino acids can stimulate alanine output from isolated muscle (Garber *et al.,* 1976), such studies have been criticized on the basis of the unphysiologically high concentrations of amino acids used (Odessey *et al.,* 1974). On the other hand, the recent demonstration that inhibition of decarboxylation can interfere with valine- and isoleucine-stimulated output of alanine does raise the possibility that these amino acids contribute carbon skeletons as well as nitrogen to alanine synthesis (Snell, 1976; Garber *et al.,* 1976). Regardless of the source of the carbon skeletons for alanine, the data derived from *in vitro* observations with the isolated muscle, as well as those involving protein feeding in intact man (Wahren *et al.,* 1976), support a special role for the branched-chain amino acids in alanine formation, in the repletion of nitrogen in muscle tissue, and as energy-yielding fuel for muscle during prolonged exercise (see Section 4.5).

The regulation of amino acid metabolism in the fasting state has also been extended with recent observations on the effect of ketones on alanine output from muscle (Sherwin *et al.,* 1975). Hyperketonemia induced by infusion of ketone bodies has been demonstrated to have a specific effect in lowering blood alanine levels and in decreasing nitrogen catabolism in muscle tissue (Sherwin *et al.,* 1975). This interplay between ketones and amino acids may constitute an important mechanism for protein conservation in prolonged fasting. It is discussed in greater detail in Section 4.4.4.

4.4. Fatty Acid and Ketone Metabolism

Adipose tissue and its constituent triglycerides represent the most important storage form of body fuel, accounting for 85% of the stored calories in the body cell mass. Utilization of stored fat initially requires mobilization of free fatty acids (FFA), which can subsequently undergo terminal oxidation in a variety of tissues (skeletal muscle, heart, liver), reconversion to triglyceride (in liver or adipose tissue), or partial oxidation (in the liver) to the ketone acids, β-hydroxybutyrate, and acetoacetate. Inasmuch as adipose tissue physiology and lipoprotein metabolism are covered elsewhere (see Chapters 5 and 6), this discussion will focus primarily on ketone metabolism.

4.4.1. Substrate and Enzymatic Factors in Ketogenesis

For many years, it was believed that the prime factor regulating accelerated ketogenesis in starvation and diabetes was the circulating level of free fatty acids. The exquisite sensitivity of adipose tissue to the antilipolytic actions of insulin provided an explanation for the importance of substrate in determining ketogenic rates (Cahill et al., 1966). In the last five years, a variety of in vivo and in vitro studies have indicated that alterations in hepatic metabolism independent of fatty acid mobilization are equally important in the regulation of ketogenesis (Foster, 1967; McGarry et al., 1973). These observations implicating the metabolic set of liver as a prime control point in ketogenesis have received added impetus from recent studies in intact man as well as further in vitro observations on the biochemical mechanism and hormonal factors influencing ketone formation.

Studying normal healthy subjects, Grey et al. (1974) demonstrated that elevations in FFA induced in fed subjects by a fat meal–heparin regimen so as to achieve concentrations comparable to those observed after a 7-day fast (1500 μEq/liter) resulted in minimal elevations in ketone acids (10% of starvation levels). When fed and fasted subjects were compared at any given level of FFA, ketone acid concentrations were up to 10-fold greater in the fasted subjects. Furthermore, the fall in ketone levels accompanying a reduction in plasma FFA levels (induced by the antilipolytic agent pyrazole) was greater in subjects made hyperinsuli-nemic with dexamethasone than in control subjects. These findings thus provide evidence in intact man that in addition to influencing FFA availability, insulin-mediated alterations in the metabolic set of the liver are equally important in determining the rate of ketogenesis.

The metabolic site within the liver that is responsible for this activa-tion of ketogenesis has been suggested to reside at the carnitine acyltrans-ferase reaction (McGarry et al., 1973; McGarry and Foster, 1974). This enzyme catalyzes the transfer of long-chain fatty acids across the mito-chondrial membrane. Since β-oxidation of fatty acids occurs solely within the mitochondria, accelerated transfer of FFA across the membrane results in augmented fatty acid oxidation and acetyl CoA production. The marked increase in acetyl CoA availability exceeds the capacity for its oxidation to CO_2 via the Krebs cycle, resulting in condensation of acetyl CoA molecules to form ketone acids (Fig. 3). Interestingly, direct assays of carnitine acyltransferase activity fail to reveal significant increments in enzyme activity in liver mitochondria prepared from ketotic rats (McGarry and Foster, 1974; DiMarco and Hoppel, 1975). On the other hand, studies with (−)-octanoylcarnitine (a medium-chain fatty acid esteri-fied to carnitine) in the perfused liver have provided evidence of increased activity of the carnitine acyltransferase reaction in ketotic livers (McGarry and Foster, 1974). The failure to observe this phenomenon in isolated mitochondria has been attributed to changes incident to disrup-tion of cellular integrity in the isolation process (McGarry and Foster, 1974).

4.4.2. Hormonal Regulation of Ketogenesis

The nature of the signal to the liver that alters the acyltransferase reaction has been examined by McGarry et al. (1975b) in studies involving the use of antiinsulin serum and glucagon. These authors demonstrated that within 1 hr of in vivo administration of either antiinsulin serum or glucagon, livers from fed rats rapidly increased their rates of ketogenesis and their ability to oxidize long-chain fatty acids and (−)-octanoylcarni-tine. These findings thus suggest hormonal activation of the carnitine acyltransferase system. Interestingly, while antiinsulin serum induced a marked rise in circulating FFA and ketones, this effect was not observed in the glucagon-treated animals. While the authors attribute this lack of an in vivo ketonemic effect to endogenous insulin secretion induced by large amounts of glucagon, administration of smaller amounts of glucagon that fail to raise insulin levels also failed to induce a ketonemic state. The authors nevertheless do provide evidence that activation of hepatic keto-

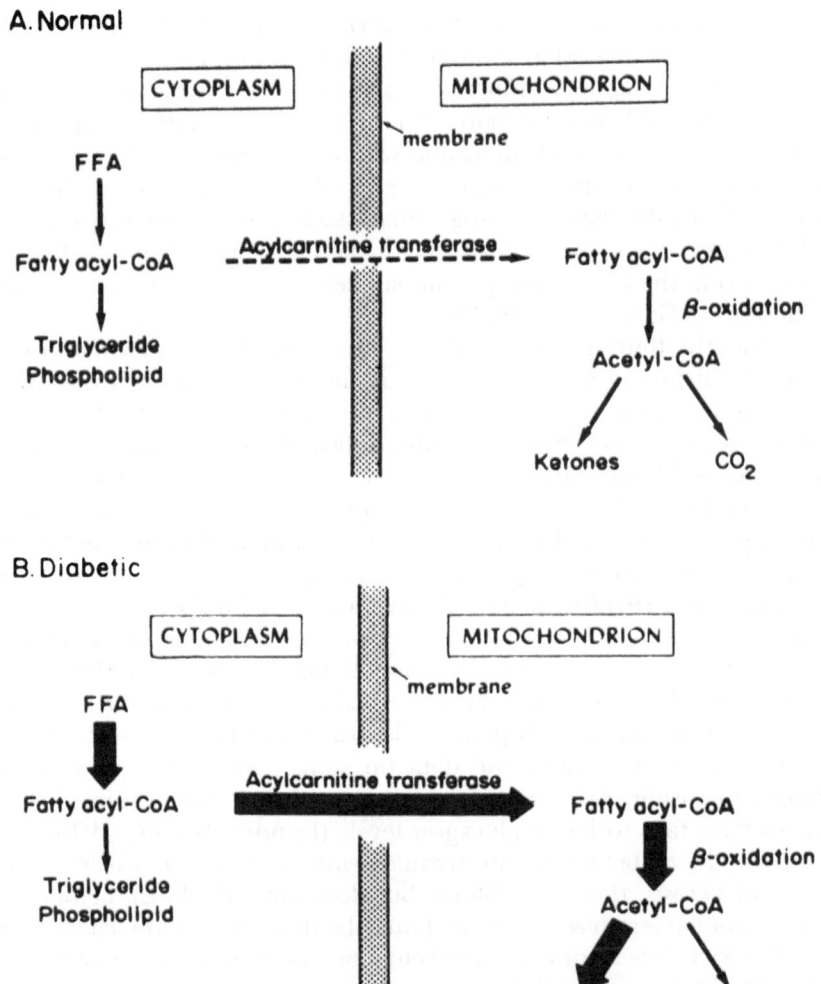

Fig. 3. Regulatory sites of ketogenesis in diabetes. In the diabetic, delivery of FFA is increased and oxidation is accelerated through activation of the carnitine acyltransferase step. (Reproduced from McGarry and Foster, 1973, with permission.)

genesis in the isolated liver is a bihormonally mediated process dependent on changes in glucagon as well as insulin (McGarry *et al.*, 1975b).

Evidence supporting a role for glucagon in the regulation of ketogenesis also derives from studies with somatostatin (Gerich *et al.*, 1975). This tetradecapeptide, isolated from the hypothalamus as the growth hormone release–inhibiting factor, also inhibits the secretion of glucagon and insulin. In insulin-withdrawn diabetics, Gerich *et al.* (1975) reported that treatment with somatostatin markedly inhibited the rate of ketone acid elevation. This inhibitory influence of somatostatin was not dependent on alterations in FFA mobilization. Schade and Eaton (1975) reported a greater rise in ketone acids in insulin-withdrawn diabetics when glucagon was administered in the face of elevated FFA levels than when saline was infused. Thus, the data involving somatostatin or glucagon infusion suggest that the glucagon-sensitive step in ketogenesis in human diabetics resides within the liver, findings compatible with the data in experimental animals of McGarry *et al.* (1975b).

While the findings discussed above have implicated glucagon excess as well as insulin deficiency as essential in the pathogenesis of ketosis, other studies point to insulin lack as the primary hormonal factor in ketogenesis, much the same as insulin deficiency is the primary factor in the glucose intolerance in diabetes (Sherwin *et al.*, 1976b). As noted above, *in vivo* administration of glucagon (in pharmacological or physiological doses) fails to raise blood ketone levels in experimental animals, whereas a prompt rise in ketones follows the administration of antiinsulin serum (McGarry *et al.*, 1976b). Similarly, in insulin-treated diabetics, a 3-fold rise in glucagon levels induced by infusion of this hormone cannot of itself raise blood ketone levels (Sherwin *et al.*, 1976b). Furthermore, 10–30-fold elevations in plasma glucagon are observed in patients with the glucagon-oma syndrome; yet, in such patients, ketosis is conspicuous by its absence (Mallinson, 1974). Finally, the data on somatostatin also point to the primacy of insulin deficiency. In patients with already manifest ketosis, somatostatin fails to lower glucagon levels (Lundbaek *et al.*, 1976). Furthermore, in diabetic patients treated with somatostatin earlier in the course of ketosis, this agent blunts but does not fully block ketone acid accumulation (Gerich *et al.*, 1975). Thus, the data suggest, on balance, that the primary factor responsible for ketogenesis is insulin lack, which acts to augment lipolysis as well as to accelerate intrahepatic ketogenesis. In circumstances of insulin lack (but not in the absence of insulin lack), glucagon accelerates further the intrahepatic formation of ketone acids.

With respect to the mechanism whereby either or both insulin and glucagon alter ketogenesis, it is noteworthy that neither antiinsulin serum nor glucagon can stimulate hepatic gluconeogenesis when added directly to the perfused liver (McGarry *et al.*, 1975b). The requirement for *in vivo* administration of these agents thus raised the possibility that their action is mediated via extrahepatic production of a factor that stimulates the carnitine acyltransferase reaction in the liver. Reasoning on theoretical grounds that the concentration of carnitine within the liver could influence the flux of fatty acids across the mitochondrial membrane, McGarry *et al.* (1975a) examined carnitine levels in livers from animals rendered ketogenic by antiinsulin serum, glucagon, alloxan, and starvation. In all circumstances, increased ketogenesis was accompanied by a proportional rise in tissue carnitine levels. Furthermore, when added to the perfusion medium, carnitine directly stimulated hepatic ketogenesis. These observations suggest that the augmentation in ketogenesis associated with hypoinsulinemia is mediated via augmented hepatic accumulation of carnitine (McGarry *et al.*, 1975a). It remains to be established whether either or both insulin and glucagon influence muscle release of carnitine, hepatic extraction of carnitine, or both processes.

4.4.3. Ketone Accumulation in Starvation

During starvation, ketone bodies progressively accumulate, reaching levels after 3 weeks of starvation of 8–10 mM (Owen *et al.*, 1969). This increase in ketone bodies represents an imbalance in ketone production and utilization rates, rather than an ongoing increase in ketone production. The rate of ketogenesis during starvation increases rapidly, reaching values of 115 g/day within 72 hr (Garber *et al.*, 1974). Despite a further increase in blood ketone acid levels from 2.5 mM to 8–10 mM over the ensuing 3–6 weeks of starvation, hepatic ketone production shows no further increase from the 3-day-fasted rates (Garber *et al.*, 1974; Owen *et al.*, 1969). Thus, a fall in the rate of ketone-body removal by peripheral tissues is a key factor in the development of the hyperketonemia of prolonged starvation. Although utilization of ketones by brain increases in starvation (Owen *et al.*, 1967), uptake by muscle tissue (Owen and Reichard, 1971; Hagenfeldt and Wahren, 1971) and total body turnover of ketone bodies decline as starvation continues for prolonged periods (Owen *et al.*, 1973; Reichard *et al.*, 1974). In addition to the saturation of ketone utilization processes in muscle, prolonged starvation is characterized by increased renal tubular reabsorption of acetoacetate and β-hydroxybutyrate (Sapir and Owen, 1975). After a prolonged fast, these tubular reabsorptive processes account for the conservation of approximately 500 mmole of ketone acids per day. Thus, both decreased muscle utilization and augmented renal tubular reabsorption of ketone acids contribute to the progressive rise and maintenance of hyperketonemia in starvation. Inasmuch as uptake of ketone acids by tissues other than muscle, notably brain, is directly proportional to arterial concentration, the processes contributing to hyperketonemia may be viewed as mechanisms designed to augment cerebral ketone utilization, thereby lessening the requirements for gluconeogenesis during starvation.

SUBJECT V.Z.

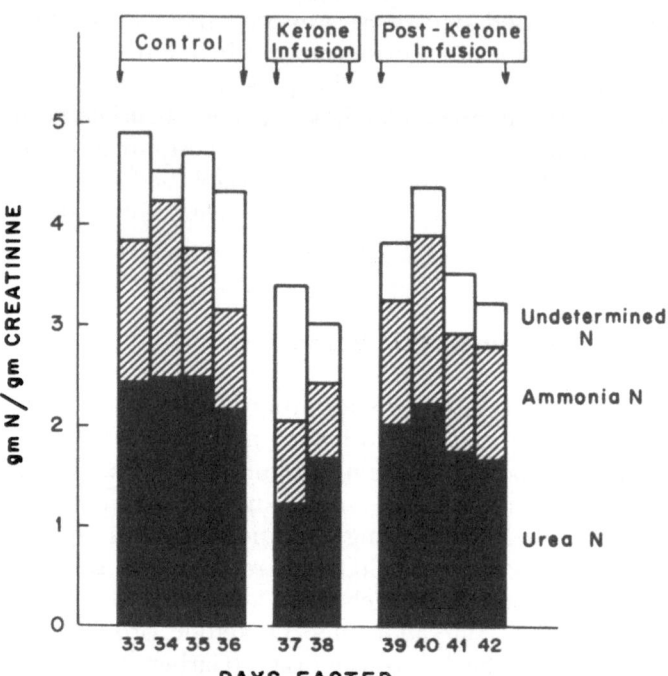

Fig. 4. Influence of ketone infusion on nitrogen balance during starvation. Administration of ketones resulted in a decrease in nitrogen wasting, which reverted to preinfusion control levels after cessation of the infusion. (Based on the data of Sherwin *et al.*, 1975.)

4.4.4. Ketone–Alanine Interactions

In addition to the role of ketones in starvation as a substrate for the brain, recent studies indicate that they have an important influence on protein breakdown and precursor availability for gluconeogenesis (Sherwin *et al.*, 1975). During prolonged fasting, hepatic gluconeogenesis, and concomitantly the rate of protein breakdown, decline progressively (Owen *et al.*, 1969). The diminution in hepatic gluconeogenesis is mediated by a reduction in circulating glucogenic amino acids, particularly alanine, and a decrease in the outflow of these amino acids from muscle (Felig *et al.*, 1969, 1970). With respect to the mechanism of these changes, neither the fall in insulin nor the transient increase in glucagon or growth hormone provides an explanation of the hypoalaninemia and reduction in protein catabolism. Sherwin *et al.* (1975), employing infusions of β-hydroxybutyrate, have provided evidence that ketones may be the mediator of this response to starvation.

In postabsorptive subjects infused with ketones, a specific decline in plasma alanine that simulated the hypoalaninemia of starvation was achieved. When ketones were infused to prolonged fasted subjects whose plasma alanine levels had already fallen by 40% below prefast levels, the increment induced in blood ketone acids was accompanied by an additional 30% reduction in plasma alanine. Furthermore, during prolonged infusions of ketones in subjects fasted 5–10 weeks, urinary nitrogen excretion fell by 30%, returning to baseline after cessation of the infusions (Fig. 4). That this effect of ketones is mediated via an action on muscle tissue is suggested by *in vitro* observations. In the isolated diaphragm, addition of ketones results in decreased protein and amino acid catabolism, and a specific reduction in net outflow of alanine (Palaiologos and Felig, 1976).

These findings indicate that increased ketone acid levels are of central importance in the hypoalaninemia and nitrogen conservation of starvation. Ketones are thus postulated to have a dual role in the metabolic adaptation to starvation (Fig. 5). Ketones substitute for glucose as substrate for the brain, thereby reducing total glucose utilization. Simultaneously, they inhibit protein catabolism and alanine outflow from muscle, thereby limiting precursor availability for hepatic gluconeogenesis. In this manner, the twin goals of glucose homeostasis and protein conservation are achieved in prolonged fasting (Fig. 5) (Felig and Saudek, 1976).

These observations on ketone–alanine interactions may also provide an explanation for the beneficial effects on nitrogen balance reported with amino acid infusions in the absence of glucose. Blackburn *et al.* (1973) and Hoover *et al.* (1975) have noted that peripherally infused mixtures of amino acids provide more positive nitrogen balance in postoperative patients than is observed when 5% dextrose is infused with the amino

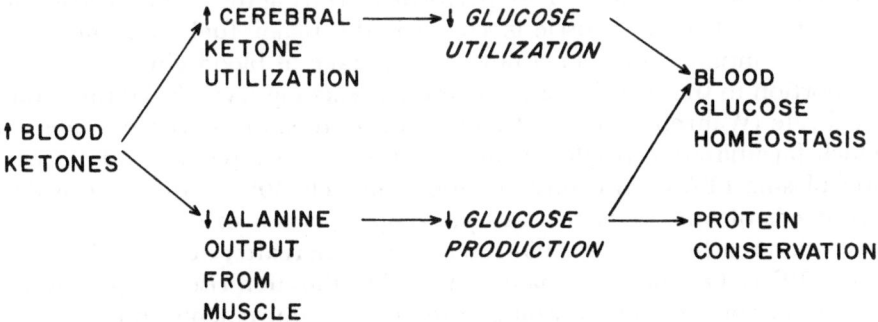

Fig. 5. Postulated mechanism by which glucose homeostasis and protein conservation are achieved in prolonged fasting. Ketones play a central role, as substrate for the brain and as a signal to muscle by which alanine output and protein catabolism are reduced. (From Felig and Saudek, 1976.)

acids. The greater effectiveness of the pure amino acid mixture may reflect the action of endogenous hyperketonemia in sparing body protein stores in the face of exogenous amino acids. On the other hand, it should be emphasized that in the absence of exogenous amino acids, infusion of glucose will result in less nitrogen wasting than is observed in the totally fasted patient (O'Connell *et al.*, 1974; Aoki *et al.*, 1975). Thus, while ketonemia may provide a protein-sparing mechanism in prolonged fasting and in association with amino acid administration, it should not be considered a desirable goal in the patient on short-term treatment with parenteral, electrolyte-containing fluids. Such patients should receive glucose (100–200 g/day) in the infusate.

4.5. Fuel Metabolism in Exercise

In the resting state, uptake of glucose by muscle accounts for less than 10% of the total oxygen consumption by muscle, and for less than 10% of the total body turnover of glucose. The major fuels consumed by resting muscle are FFA, while the major site of glucose consumption in the resting state is brain. During exercise, the increased consumption of oxygen necessitates marked changes in the magnitude and pattern of fuel utilization. The latter is in turn influenced by the hormonal milieu, as is evident from studies in normal as well as diabetic subjects (Felig and Wahren, 1975b).

4.5.1. Brief and Prolonged Exercise in Normal Subjects

The pattern of fuel utilization in normal man depends on the duration and severity of the exercise performed. During the earliest phases of exercise (5–10 min), muscle glycogen is the major fuel consumed. As exercise continues and blood flow rises, uptake of blood glucose rises in proportion to the severity of the exercise, reaching levels 7–20 times the basal rate (Wahren *et al.*, 1971). Thus, in contrast to the resting state, in which fat utilization predominates, by 40 min of exercise, blood glucose and plasma FFA each contribute approximately 40% of the total oxidative needs of muscle. With more prolonged periods of exercise, glucose utilization reaches a peak at 90–180 min, and thereafter declines (Ahlborg *et al.*, 1974). On the other hand, fatty acid utilization rises progressively, accounting by 4 hr for over 60% of total fuel requirements and for twice the contribution provided from glucose. The primary factor regulating fatty acid uptake is the rate of its delivery. In addition to fatty acid utilization, bloodborne amino acids, particularly the branched-chain amino acids, emerge as energy-yielding fuels for muscle in prolonged exercise. Thus, after 4 hr of exercise, a net flow of valine, leucine, and isoleucine from liver to the exercising leg is observed (Ahlborg et al., 1974). This situation contrasts markedly with the resting state, in which there is a net output of amino acids from muscle, and with short-term exercise, in which there is no significant uptake or output of branched-chain amino acids from liver or muscle (Felig and Wahren, 1971b).

The overall pattern of fuel utilization in muscle during exercise may thus be characterized as triphasic. Initially, muscle glycogen predominates, thereafter bloodborne glucose and FFA contribute equally, while in prolonged exercise, FFA increase in quantitative importance, and endogenous branched-chain amino acids serve as an auxiliary fuel.

Inasmuch as exercise is associated with augmented glucose utilization, maintenance of glucose homeostasis in exercise necessitates an increase in glucose production. As in the case of glucose uptake by muscle, glucose output from the liver rises in direct proportion to the intensity of the exercise performed (Wahren et al., 1971). The total glucose released during short-term (10–40-min) heavy exercise amounts to 18–20 g, and represents primarily (85–90%) glycogenolysis; uptake of gluconeogenic precursors is unchanged from the resting state (Wahren et al., 1971). In contrast, during more prolonged exercise (4 hr) and in association with depletion of liver glycogen stores, uptake of gluconeogenic precursors rises 3-fold above basal levels, accounting for 40–50% of total hepatic glucose production (Ahlborg et al., 1974). This increment in gluconeogenesis is primarily a result of augmented hepatic fractional extraction of glucose precursors.

With respect to the mechanism of these changes in glycogenolysis and gluconeogenesis, hypoinsulinemia, hyperglucagonemia (in prolonged or severe exercise), and increased circulating levels of epinephrine and norepinephrine have been observed (Felig and Wahren, 1975b). None of these factors, however, may be essential for exercise-induced stimulation of glucose output. For example, prevention of the fall in insulin by infusion of glucose fails to abolish the rise in hepatic glucose output (Felig et al., 1974a). During mild, prolonged exercise, augmented glucose production occurs in advance of changes in plasma glucagon (Ahlborg et al., 1974), and in the absence of demonstrable increments in plasma catecholamines (Galbo et al., 1975). The rise in glucose output during exercise, as with other glucopenic states, may thus be primarily mediated via intrahepatic neurogenic influences (Brodows et al., 1975).

4.5.2. Exercise in Diabetes Mellitus

A salutary effect of exercise on diabetes has generally been recognized by clinicians as manifested by a diminution in insulin requirements and improved glucose tolerance. This interaction between diabetes and

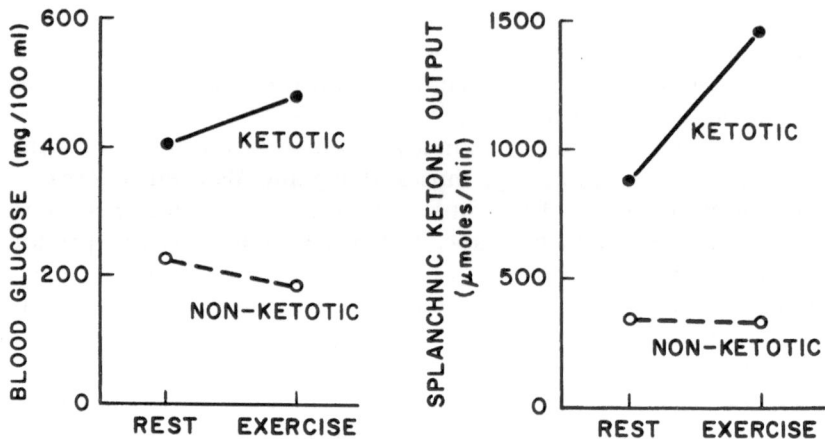

Fig. 6. Influence of the status of diabetic "control" on the metabolic response to starvation. In patients with glucose levels of 250 mg/100 ml or less, exercise results in a fall in blood glucose and unchanged ketone production rates. In contrast, in more severely hyperglycemic patients, blood glucose levels rise and ketogenesis increases during exercise. (Based on the data of Wahren *et al.*, 1975.)

exercise is better understood, however, in the context of overall fuel utilization and production (Felig and Wahren, 1975b).

In the diabetic, glucose uptake by the exercising leg is comparable to that in controls, indicating that augmented glucose utilization in exercise is not dependent on increased availability of insulin (Wahren *et al.*, 1975; Sanders *et al.*, 1964). On the other hand, the contribution of FFA is 50% greater than in normals, reflecting the higher circulating levels of FFA and the depletion of muscle glycogen stores in the diabetics. In addition, in the diabetic group, hepatic uptake of gluconeogenic precursors rises 2–3-fold during short-term exercise, in contrast to the unchanged rates of precursor uptake in short-term exercise in normal controls. Furthermore, in the diabetics, a substantial muscle uptake of branched-chain amino acids is observed within the first 40 min (Wahren *et al.*, 1975). Thus, the overall effect of diabetes is to accelerate the metabolic response to exercise. The greater dependence on fatty acids, the absolute rise in hepatic gluconeogenesis, and the consumption by muscle of branched-chain amino acids, none of which is observed until 4 hr in normal subjects (Ahlborg *et al.*, 1974), are demonstrable within 40 min in diabetics (Wahren *et al.*, 1975).

Concerning the effect of exercise on "diabetic control," the response is largely determined by the extent of insulin deficiency, as manifested by hyperglycemia and hyperketonemia at the time exercise is initiated (Wahren *et al.*, 1975). In diabetic patients with blood glucose levels of 200–300 mg/100 ml or less, moderate exercise performed 24 hr after the last insulin dose results in a 30–50 mg/100 ml decline in blood glucose (Fig. 6).

In such patients, ketone production by the liver is not stimulated. In contrast, in patients with more severe hyperglycemia (blood glucose >350 mg/100 ml) and mild to moderate ketonemia (blood ketones 2–3 mM), exercise results in a 50–100 mg/100 ml rise in blood glucose. In addition, ketone production increases 2–3-fold above basal, resting levels (Fig. 6). Thus, in such poorly controlled patients, exercise may intensify rather than ameliorate the hyperglycemic, gluconeogenic, and ketogenic effects of diabetes (Wahren *et al.*, 1975).

References

Ahlborg, G., Felig, P., Hagenfeldt, L., Hendler, R., and Wahren, J., 1974, Substrate turnover during prolonged exercise in man: Splanchnic and leg metabolism of glucose, free fatty acids, and amino acids, *J. Clin. Invest.* **53:**1080.

Amamoo, D. G., Woods, J. E., and Donovan, J. L., 1974, Preliminary experience with pancreatic islet-cell implantation, *Mayo Clin. Proc.* **49:**289.

Aoki, T. T., Müller, W. A., Brennan, M. F., and Cahill, G. F., Jr., 1975, Metabolic effects of glucose in brief and prolonged fasted man, *Amer. J. Clin. Nutr.* **28:**507.

Ballinger, W. F., and Lacy, P. E., 1972, Transplantation of intact pancreatic islets in rats, *Surgery* **72:**175.

Blackard, W. G., and Nelson, N. C., 1970, Portal and peripheral vein immunoreactive insulin concentrations before and after glucose infusion, *Diabetes* **19:**302.

Blackburn, G. L., Flatt, J. P., Clowes, G. H. A., and O'Donnell, T. E., 1973, Peripheral intravenous feeding with isotonic amino acid solutions, *Amer. J. Surg.* **125:**447.

Blackshear, P. J., Holloway, P. A. H., and Alberti, K. G. M. M., 1975, Factors regulating amino acid release from extrasplanchnic tissues in the rat. Interactions of alanine and glutamine, *Biochem. J.* **150:**379.

Brodows, R. G., Pi-Sunyer, F. X., and Campbell, R. G., 1975, Sympathetic control of hepatic glycogenolysis during glucopenia in man, *Metabolism* **24:**617.

Cahill, G. F., Jr., Herrera, M. G., Morgan, A. P., Soeldner, J. S., Steinke, J., Levy, P. L., Reichard, G. A., and Kipnis, D. M., 1966, Hormone–fuel interrelationships during fasting, *J. Clin. Invest.* **45:**1751.

DiMarco, J. P., and Hoppel, C., 1975, Hepatic mitochondrial function in ketogenic states: diabetes, starvation, and after growth hormone administration, *J. Clin. Invest.* **55:**1237.

Felig, P., 1973, The glucose–alanine cycle, *Metab. Clin. Exp.* **22:**179.

Felig, P., 1975, Amino acid metabolism in man, *Annu. Rev. Biochem.* **44:**933.

Felig, P., and Saudek, C. D., 1976, The metabolic events of starvation, *Amer. J. Med.* **60:**117.

Felig, P., and Wahren, J., 1971a, Influence of endogenous insulin secretion on splanchnic glucose and amino acid metabolism, *J. Clin. Invest.* **50:**1702.

Felig, P., and Wahren, J., 1971b, Amino acid metabolism in exercising man, *J. Clin. Invest.* **50:**2703.

Felig, P., and Wahren, J., 1975a, Symposium I: hormone fuel interactions in normal and diabetic man. The liver as site of insulin and glucagon action in normal, diabetic and obese humans, *Isr. J. Med. Sci.* **11**:528.

Felig, P., and Wahren, J., 1975b, Fuel homeostasis in exercise, *N. Engl. J. Med.* **293**:1078.

Felig, P., Owen, O. E., Wahren, J., and Cahill, G. F., Jr., 1969, Amino acid metabolism during prolonged starvation, *J. Clin. Invest.* **48**:584.

Felig, P., Pozefsky, T., Marliss, E., and Cahill, G. F., Jr., 1970, Alanine: Key role in gluconeogenesis, *Science* **167**:1003.

Felig, P., Wahren, J., and Hendler, R., 1974a, Sensitivity of hepatic glucoregulatory mechanisms in exercising man, presented at the 56th Annual Meeting of the Endocrine Society, Atlanta, Georgia, June 12–14, 1974.

Felig, P., Wahren, J., Hendler, R., and Brundin, T., 1974b, Splanchnic glucose and amino acid metabolism in obesity, *J. Clin. Invest.* **53**:582.

Felig, P., Wahren, J., and Hendler, R., 1975, Influence of oral glucose ingestion on splanchnic glucose and gluconeogenic substrate metabolism in man, *Diabetes* **24**:468.

Foster, D. W., 1967, Studies in the ketosis of fasting, *J. Clin. Invest.* **46**:1283.

Frame, E. G., 1958, The levels of individual free amino acids in the plasma of normal man at various intervals after a high-protein meal, *J. Clin. Invest.* **37**:1710.

Galbo, H., Holst, J. J., and Christensen, N. J., 1975, Glucagon and plasma catecholamine responses to graded and prolonged exercise in man, *J. Appl. Physiol.* **38**:70.

Garber, A. J., Menzel, P. H., Boden, G., and Owen, O. E., 1974, Hepatic ketogenesis and gluconeogenesis in humans, *J. Clin. Invest.* **54**:981.

Garber, A. J., Karl, I. E., and Kipnis, D. M., 1976, Alanine and glutamine synthesis and release from skeletal muscle. II. The precursor role of amino acids in alanine and glutamine synthesis, *J. Biol. Chem.* **251**:836.

Gerich, J. E., Lorenzi, M., Bier, D. M., Schneider, V., Tsalikian, E., Karam, J. H., and Forsham, P. H., 1975, Prevention of human diabetic ketoacidosis by somatostatin: Evidence for an essential role of glucagon, *N. Engl. J. Med.* **292**:985.

Grey, N. J., Karl, I., and Kipnis, D. M., 1975, Physiologic mechanisms in the development of starvation ketosis in man, *Diabetes* **24**:10.

Hagenfeldt, L., and Wahren, J., 1971, Human forearm muscle metabolism during exercise. VI. Substrate utilization in prolonged fasting, *Scand. J. Clin. Lab. Invest.* **27**:299.

Hoover, H. C., Jr., Grant, J. P., Gorschboth, M. S., and Ketcham, A. S., 1975, Nitrogen-sparing intravenous fluids in postoperative patients, *N. Engl. J. Med.* **293**:172.

Jackson, R. A., Peters, N., Advani, U., Perry, G., Rogers, J., Brough, W. H., and Pilkington, T. R. E., 1973, Forearm glucose uptake during the oral glucose tolerance test in normal subjects, *Diabetes* **22**:442.

Kemp, C. B., Knight, M. J., Scharp, D. W., Lacy, P. E., and Ballinger, W. F., 1973, Transplantation of isolated pancreatic islets into the portal vein of diabetic rats, *Nature* **244**:447.

Kominz, D. R., Hough, A., Symonds, P., and Laki, K., 1954, The amino acid composition of actin, myosin, tropomyosin and the meromyosins, *Arch. Biochem. Biophys.* **50**:148.

Lundbaek, K., Christensen, S. F., Hansen, A. P., Iversen, J., Orskov, H., Seyer-Hansen, K., Alberti, K. G. M. M., and Whitefoot, R., 1976, Failure of somatostatin to correct manifest diabetic ketoacidosis, *Lancet* **1**:215.

Mallinson, C. N., Bloom, S. R., Warin, A. P., Salmon, P. R., and Cox, B., 1974, A glucagonoma syndrome, *Lancet* **2**:1.

McGarry, J. D., and Foster, D. W., 1973, Acute reversal of experimental diabetic ketoacidosis in the rat with (+)-decanoylcarnitine, *J. Clin. Invest.* **52**:877.

McGarry, J. D., and Foster, D. W., 1974, The metabolism of (−)-octanoylcarnitine in perfused livers from fed and fasted rats. Evidence for a possible regulatory role of carnitine acyltransferase in the control of ketogenesis, *J. Biol. Chem.* **249**:7984.

McGarry, J. D., Meier, J. M., and Foster, D. W., 1973, The effects of starvation and refeeding on carbohydrate and lipid metabolism *in vivo* and in the perfused rat liver, *J. Biol. Chem.* **248**:270.

McGarry, J. D., Robles-Valdes, C., and Foster, D. W., 1975a, Role of carnitine in hepatic ketogenesis, *Proc. Nat. Acad. Sci. U.S.A.* **72**:4385.

McGarry, J. D., Wright, P. H., and Foster, D. W., 1975b, Hormonal control of ketogenesis. Rapid activation of hepatic ketogenic capacity in fed rats by anti-insulin serum and glucagon, *J. Clin. Invest.* **55**:1202

Miller, L. L., 1962, The role of the liver and nonhepatic tissues in the regulation of free amino acid levels in the blood, *in: Amino Acid Pools, Distribution, Formation and Function of Free Amino Acids* (J. T. Holden, ed.), pp. 708–728, Elsevier, Amsterdam.

Müller, W. A.. Faloona, G. R., Aguilar-Parada, E., and Unger, R. H., 1970, Abnormal alpha-cell function in diabetes: response to carbohydrate and protein ingestion, *N. Engl. J. Med.* **283**:109.

Müller, W. A., Faloona, G. R., and Unger, R. H., 1973, Hyperglucagonemia in diabetic ketoacidosis: Its prevalence and significance, *Amer. J. Med.* **54**:52.

O'Connell, R. C., Morgan, A. P., Aoki, T. T., Ball, M. R., and Moore, F. D., 1974, Nitrogen conservation in starvation: Graded responses to intravenous glucose, *J. Clin. Endocrinol. Metab.* **39**:555.

Odessey, R., Khairallah, E. A., and Goldberg, A. L., 1974, Origin and possible significance of alanine production by skeletal muscle, *J. Biol. Chem.* **249**:7623.

Owen, O. E., and Reichard, G. A., Jr., 1971, Human forearm metabolism during progressive starvation, *J. Clin. Invest.* **50**:1536.

Owen, O. E., Morgan, A. P., Kemp, H. G., Sullivan, J. M., Herrera, M. G., and Cahill, G. F., Jr., 1967, Brain metabolism during fasting, *J. Clin. Invest.* **46**:1589.

Owen, O. E., Felig, P., Morgan, A. P., Wahren, J., and Cahill, G. F., Jr., 1969, Liver and kidney metabolism during prolonged starvation, *J. Clin. Invest.* **48**:574.

Owen, O. E., Reichard, G. A., Jr., Markus, H., Boden, G., Mozzoli, M. A., and Shuman, C. R., 1973, Rapid intravenous sodium acetoacetate infusion in man: metabolic and kinetic responses, *J. Clin. Invest.* **52**:2606.

Palaiologos, G., and Felig, P., 1976, Effects of ketone bodies on amino acid metabolism in isolated rat diaphragm, *Biochem. J.* **154**:709.

Parrilla, R., Goodman, M. N., and Toews, C. J., 1974, Effect of glucagon:insulin ratios on hepatic metabolism, *Diabetes* **23**.725.

Perley, M. J., and Kipnis, D. M., 1967, Plasma insulin responses to oral and intravenous glucose: Studies in normal and diabetic subjects, *J. Clin. Invest.* **46**:1954.

Reichard, G. A., Jr., Owen, O. E., Haff, A. C., Paul, P., and Bortz, W. M., 1974, Ketone-body production and oxidation in fasting obese humans, *J. Clin. Invest.* **53**:508.

Sanders, C. A., Levinson, G. E., Abelmann, W. H., and Freinkel, N., 1964, Effect of exercise on the peripheral utilization of glucose in man, *N. Engl. J. Med.* **271**:220.

Sapir, D. G., and Owen, O. E., 1975, Renal conservation of ketone bodies during starvation, *Metabolism* **24**:23.

Schade, D. S., and Eaton, R. P., 1975, Glucagon regulation of plasma ketone body concentration in human diabetes, *J. Clin. Invest.* **56**:1340.

Scow, R. L., and Cornfield, J., 1954, Quantitative relations between oral and intravenous glucose tolerance curves, *Amer. J. Physiol.* **179**:435.

Sherwin, R., Joshi, P., Hendler, R., Felig, P., and Conn, H. O., 1974, Hyperglucagonemia in Laennec's cirrhosis: The role of portal–systemic shunting, *N. Engl. J. Med.* **290**:239.

Sherwin, R. S., Hendler, R. G., and Felig, P., 1975, Effect of ketone infusions on amino acid and nitrogen metabolism in man, *J. Clin. Invest.* **55**:1382.

Sherwin, R. S., Bastl, C., Finkelstein, F. O., Fisher, M., Black, H., Hendler, R., and Felig, P., 1976a, Influence of uremia and hemodialysis on the turnover and metabolic effects of glucagon, *J. Clin. Invest.* **57**:722.

Sherwin, R. S., Fisher, M., Hendler, R., and Felig, P., 1976b, Hyperglucagonemia and blood glucose regulation in normal, obese and diabetic subjects, *N. Engl. J. Med.* **294**:455.

Snell, K., 1976, Alanine release by rat hemidiaphragm muscle *in vitro, Biochem. Soc. Trans.* **4**:287.

Unger, R. H., 1971, Glucagon physiology and pathophysiology, *N. Engl. J. Med.* **285**:443.

Wahren, J., Felig, P., Ahlborg, G., and Jorfeldt, L., 1971, Glucose metabolism during leg exercise in man, *J. Clin. Invest.* **50**:2715.

Wahren, J., Hagenfeldt, L., and Felig, P., 1975, Splanchnic and leg exchange of glucose, amino acids, and free fatty acids during exercise in diabetes mellitus, *J. Clin. Invest.* **55**:1303.

Wahren, J., Felig, P., and Hagenfeldt, L., 1976, Effect of protein ingestion on splanchnic and leg metabolism in normal man and patients with diabetes mellitus, *J. Clin. Invest.* **57**:987.

Windmueller, H. G., and Spaeth, A. E., 1974, Uptake and metabolism of plasma glutamine by the small intestine, *J. Biol. Chem.* **249**:5070.

5

Recent Endocrine and Metabolic Investigations Relevant to Obesity

Jules Hirsch and Bruce S. Schneider

5.1. Introduction

It will not be the objective of this report to provide a comprehensive review of current research on obesity. Such reviews have appeared periodically, a recent excellent example being the published report of a conference held under the auspices of the Fogarty International Health Center (Bray, 1973). The purpose of this review is to describe several recent developments in obesity research, which have excited the interest of those involved in the study of human obesity and which have particular relevance to diabetes and metabolism.

At present, there is a consensus that the etiology of all obesity is most likely not to be found in any single enzymatic or metabolic defect, nor is it the result of any single psychogenic factor. Obesity in man appears to be

JULES HIRSCH and BRUCE S. SCHNEIDER • Rockefeller University, New York, New York 10021.

of multifactorial origin, and is perhaps best viewed as one or more of a series of possible defects in a complex regulatory system that governs the normal sequestration of calories as a reserve in adipose tissues. It has been helpful to consider this regulated system of fat storage as an interaction between the level of stored calories and some "set point" for normal or optimal caloric storage. The final pathway or locus of the "set point" control is presumed to be in the CNS. Various mathematical and computer-based models of food intake and fat-storage regulation have been based on such theoretical considerations (Hirsch, 1972), and the "active" compartments in such models are almost always the CNS, adipose tissue, and the gastrointestinal tract. It is assumed that a variety of neural and humoral mechanisms operate to link these systems in a coordinated manner. Needless to say, the potential hormonal links for these various compartments have been under careful scrutiny, and perhaps no hormone has been so much implicated in obesity and the control of food intake as has insulin.

5.2. Insulin

It is undoubtedly true that insulin plays a central role in caloric storage. The ingestion of any type of foodstuff will trigger insulin release, since not only glucose, but also amino acids and fatty acids, can lead to prompt pancreatic release of insulin. Furthermore, starvation is characteristically accompanied by exceedingly low levels of serum insulin in both man and animals. Thus, the special role of insulin as a potential controller of food intake and in the production of obesity has been of particular interest in recent years, and such work is described in several categories below.

5.2.1. Carbohydrate Resistance in Obesity

Although obese subjects without a family history of diabetes or stigmata of diabetes usually have normal or near-normal carbohydrate tolerance, it has been recognized for many years that insulin levels following a glycemic stimulus are exceedingly high in obese subjects (Karam *et al.*, 1963). This hyperinsulinemia is not the only manifestation of peripheral resistance to carbohydrate metabolism. It has been shown (Olefsky *et al.*, 1974) that under conditions in which endogenous insulin release is pharmacologically suppressed, there is an "impedance" to glucose metabolism in peripheral tissues that is ameliorated by weight reduction. In fact, it is reasonable to assume that carbohydrate tolerance is kept within normal or near-normal bounds in the nondiabetic obese only at the expense of pancreatic hyperfunction and high insulin levels. The hyper-insulinemia of obesity has been thought to be a frequent cause of hyper-triglyceridemia, perhaps the result of hepatic overproduction of triglycer-ide under excess insulin stimulation (Reaven *et al.*, 1967).

Although the pathogenesis of the hyperinsulinemia of obesity remains unclear, several studies in recent years have been helpful in evaluating this endocrinologic disturbance. To begin with, it can be shown that with weight reduction, hyperinsulinemia abates. Furthermore, Sims *et al.* (1973) have demonstrated that the production of obesity by experimental means evokes hyperinsulinemia. When normal, nondiabetic and nonobese young males were force-fed, slow weight gain occurred over time, and moderate obesity was produced. In this circumstance, both impaired glucose utilization and hyperinsulinemia occur as obesity develops. It seems unlikely, therefore, that hyperinsulinemia is ordinarily antecedent to obesity.

It has been proposed that the mechanism for hyperinsulinemia and tissue resistance to carbohydrate may be as follows:

excess   → pancreatic   → chronic insulin   → insulin
carbohydrate   hyperfunction   excess in   resistance
intake (a   peripheral
concomitant of   tissues
hyperphagia in
obese subjects)

If this were the explanation, then one might expect that the greater the degree of obesity in any series of subjects, the higher would be the insulin levels. Yet, better correlations of serum insulin levels in obesity have been found, not with total mass of stored fat, but rather with adipocyte size (Stern *et al.*, 1972), indicating the possibility of some special role of adipocyte size in either insulin resistance or pancreatic hyperfunction.

A more direct test of the pathogenetic sequence above has been made using an experimental model of obesity in the rat. The Zucker obese rat or "fatty" possesses genetically determined obesity, the result of an autosomal, recessive mutation. Obese animals are hyperinsulinemic, show carbohydrate resistance, and also are hypertriglyceridemic; nonobese littermates show none of these abnormalities. It has been shown that when these animals become obese on either high-carbohydrate or high-fat intake, all develop hyperinsulinemia. In fact, when obese animals were permitted ad-lib feeding of fat, but were carefully pair-fed the same amount of carbohydrate as was taken by nonobese, nonhyperinsulinemic controls, hyperinsulinemia still developed in the obese, and *in vitro* measures of insulin release from pancreatic islets remained abnormally high

(Stern *et al.*, 1975). Clearly, obesity provoked hyperinsulinemia by some mechanism other than high-carbohydrate intake.

These findings lead one to speculate on the possibility that some aspect of the overfed or overfilled adipose depot can provoke pancreatic hyperfunction without assuming the necessity for high-carbohydrate intake. The aforementioned correlation of adipocyte size with serum insulin level is tantalizing, as is the well-documented finding that enlarged human or rat adipocytes are less responsive to insulin action than smaller adipocytes. Since overfeeding can produce many changes other than adipocyte enlargement, e.g., alterations in muscle and liver metabolism, and since adipose tissue metabolizes only a small fraction of ingested glucose, it is hard to be certain of any unique role of adipose tissue in producing hyperinsulinemia. This could only occur via some as yet unspecified mechanism. Recently, the study of insulin receptors in adipocytes, as well as in cells other than adipocytes, has provided new data on the disturbance of insulin metabolism in obesity.

5.2.2. Studies on Insulin Receptors

In the recent past, a novel approach to the study of insulin metabolism has been widely applied. The theoretical basis of this approach is that insulin, like other polypeptide hormones, exerts its action by binding to specific receptors located on the surface of target cells. The hormone need not enter the cells, but can produce its intracellular effects via secondary messengers that are activated (or perhaps inhibited) when the hormone is bound to its receptor. Since the binding of a polypeptide hormone to a tissue receptor represents the first step in hormone action, and since this binding is a necessary (but not sufficient) condition for hormone action, then a quantitative analysis of tissue receptors might provide some insight into normal and abnormal endocrine physiology.

With the use of ^{125}I-labeled insulin as a tracer for *in vitro* studies, the kinetics of insulin binding to suspensions of adipocytes and other intact cells and membrane preparations have been studied. By determining the total insulin bound and the ratio of bound to free insulin, it has been possible to estimate both the apparent affinity constants of the insulin receptors and the number of receptors per cell. A variety of underlying assumptions, such as the binding of only one molecule of insulin per receptor site, are necessary for these analyses, yet interesting comparisons of similar cell preparations from patients or animals in different pathological states have been made, and these data are less dependent on specific assumptions. The laboratories of Cuatrecasas, Katzen, and Roth have pioneered in these studies, and to date, some intriguing findings that are highly relevant to both obesity research and our general understanding of the mode of action of peptide hormones have been made.

The kinetics of receptor affinity for insulin have been studied not only in adipocytes, but also in liver cell membranes and monocytes. Originally, it was felt that adipocytes, both large and small, have a fixed number of receptors (Amatruda *et al.*, 1975). The insulin insensitivity of the large adipocyte was due, it was reasoned, to the possible separation of a fixed number of receptor sites over a wider surface. In other investigations, it was found that adipocytes as well as hepatocytes of genetically obese mice had fewer than the normal complement of insulin receptors. Both genetically obese mice and mice made obese by treatment with gold thioglucose were shown to have fewer receptors located on the hepatocyte membranes, and with food-intake restriction, the number of receptors increased (Soll *et al.*, 1975). The finding that cells other than adipocytes share in the receptor deficiency of obesity had also prompted a study of insulin binding to circulating monocytes in obese humans. It was found (Archer *et al.*, 1975) that a decrease in the concentration of monocyte receptors with a possible decrease in receptor affinity is characteristic of obese man. But with weight reduction and a decline in hyperinsulinemia, the receptor number and insulin affinity became more normal. The suggestion has been made that the waxing and waning of receptor number as insulin increases or decreases is a secondary manifestation of the exposure of the receptor cell to high or low hormone levels (Roth *et al.*, 1975). To date, a number of laboratories have been able to relate the number of receptors per cell to the level of insulin in plasma. It remains to be shown, however, which event is primary and which is secondary in the pathogenesis of the tissue resistance of obesity. In addition, the relationship between *in vitro* binding phenomena and subsequent metabolic events remains to be established. Work now in progress in several laboratories suggests that there may be a reduction in insulin binding in circumstances in which glucose metabolism is actually increasing.

That receptor studies may reveal other previously unsuspected abnormalities in hormone action that have direct application to understanding human disease is shown in a recent publication from the Roth laboratory. Human subjects with acanthosis nigricans and hyperinsulinemia (Kahn *et al.*, 1976) have been separated into those with diminished receptor affinity, perhaps on genetic grounds, from a group of patients who have circulating substances that diminish peptide-binding by competing with insulin for receptor-binding. Such receptor "antibodies" may be a significant element in insulin resistance in states other than acanthosis nigricans. Thus, discriminating tools are now available for a careful investigation of the insulin insensitivity of obesity. It will be of extreme importance to know to what degree abnormalities of receptor-binding are ever antecedent to hyperinsulinemia and, in general, the degree to which receptor changes can primarily affect insulin levels. It appears unlikely that these detailed receptor studies will show that receptor-binding is only a simple function of the insulin level. The studies with acanthosis nigricans surely suggest that this matter is more complex, and may well yield clinically useful data.

5.2.3. Insulin as a Controller of Appetite and Hunger

A regulated system of fat storage would operate most elegantly and simply if there were a single sensor of the level of fat storage. The sensor should ideally relay information to feeding centers in the CNS and maintain control over fat storage by regulating food intake. Woods and Porte (1976) have suggested that insulin may be the sought-for substance that accomplishes just these physiological functions. There are reasons for and against this possibility:

1. Insulin can provoke obesity in experimental animals. When protomine zinc insulin is administered chronically to animals, considerable hyperphagia and obesity will occur (MacKay *et al.*, 1940). One might reason that insulin is thereby established as a prime candidate for the "hunger hormone." If, on the other hand, insulin levels were a measure of the degree of fat storage, one might suppose that a sudden increase in insulin levels would give false information as to the level of fat storage; i.e., high insulin is an index of fat storage, and exogenously administered insulin would give the erroneous information that fat stores are excessive, and the insulin would thereby act to suppress further food intake. A more likely sequence of events would be that insulin acts to stimulate food intake only indirectly. By creating hypoglycemia and inaugurating a train of other metabolic events similar to starvation, such as gastric hypermotility, the animal is "misled" into overeating.

In the obese state in both man and experimental animals, there is no evidence that insulin operates to create hunger. Indeed, hyperinsulinemia is so invariably geared to peripheral tissue resistance to insulin action that hypoglycemia and its attendant effects are not seen in the hyperinsulinemic obese. For this reason, insulin-lowering agents such as biguanides do not help the moderately obese diabetic to reduce any more than do sulfonylurea compounds, which enhance insulin levels. Thus, the excess insulin of the obese may not be as effective in promoting appetite and hunger as equivalent amounts of exogenously administered insulin.

2. Rats made obese by ventromedial hypothalamic lesions develop hyperinsulinemia (Hales and Kennedy, 1964). The highest levels of insulin occur as obesity becomes massive, so the insulin elevations might be though to be secondary to the obesity. However, it has been shown that animals develop hyperinsulinemia within a brief time following hypothalamic lesioning and before overeating is allowed to occur (Frohman *et al.*, 1969). Thus, there is a centrally induced effect on insulin levels in lesioned

animals. Whether insulin resistance and glucose intolerance develop at the same time is not clear, although hypoglycemia has not been described in such experimental animals. One could argue, as above, that only high and effective insulin concentrations, such as to produce hypoglycemia, could promote hyperphagia.

3. Animals made diabetic by alloxan are resistant to hypothalamic injury by gold-thioglucose (Debons *et al.*, 1968). Gold-thioglucose administration is a form of chemical hypothalamic lesioning, which is believed to operate by localizing neurocytotoxic gold in hypothalamic glucoreceptors. The loss of affinity for glucose by these receptors in the diabetic animal, and the restoration of the lesioning capability of gold-thioglucose when insulin is given (Debons *et al.*, 1969), suggest that insulin is needed to promote glucose transport into those vital hypothalamic areas that control satiety and food intake. These are complex experimental observations, yet they lend support to the idea that insulin is actively involved in CNS metabolism, particularly in those portions of the hypothalamus that are of importance in the control of food intake.

4. What speaks strongly against a special role for insulin in sensing fat storage and promoting human obesity is the sequence of events following weight reduction in obese patients. With resumption of normal weight, insulin level and carbohydrate metabolism achieve normal levels, yet it is in just this circumstance that the formerly obese manifest their greatest degrees of hyperphagia. It is not unusual for the reduced obese to fall victim to massive hyperphagia at levels of 6000–8000 kcal/day and there is thereby rapid restoration of the lost triglyceride in adipocytes. Indeed, it is just this phenomenon that makes the treatment of massive obesity by starvation or prolonged hospitalization on low-calorie diets so rarely successful in the long run. Something other than measurable plasma levels of insulin must be the initiator of this type of hyperphagia. Perhaps spinal fluid levels of insulin, as hypothesized by Woods and Porte (1976), may be a more important measure of the fed or starved. Unfortunately, measures of spinal fluid insulin in obese, formerly obese, or even normal subjects have not yet been reported in any systematic studies.

5.3. Thermogenesis and Thyroid Function

Two standard and widely accepted dicta concerning the cause and proper treatment of obesity are: (1) Calories are not utilized in a superefficient manner by the obese, nor do any nonobese, except during the most dire disorders, uncouple oxidative phosphorylation so as to waste calories as heat. Thus, "calories are calories," and the anecdotes of the neighbor or relative who consumes huge amounts of food and yet remains thin are simply inaccurate observations. (2) Thyroid function is normal in the vast majority of obese patients. Unfortunately, patients sometimes receive thyroid medication for obesity, but it is a rare occurrence when documented hypothyroidism that requires treatment and obesity coexist.

Probably these dicta are still correct, but some current findings suggest that a reassessment of the situation is in order. It may well be that differences in thermogenesis or in subtleties of thyroid function vary from one person to another, and although these may be small variations in energy metabolism, if they are persistently active for years, they could explain some fraction of the unwanted stored calories of the obese.

Sims (1976) has recently extended his observations on the experimental production of obesity in man to include studies in which young males are placed on hypercaloric feedings rich in carbohydrate. Supplements of carbohydrate of roughly 2000 kcal/day were added to basal caloric needs. These subjects gained less weight than those placed on feedings equivalent in caloric excess, but with less carbohydrate and more fat. Most interestingly, one group of subjects force-fed high-carbohydrate meals in this manner showed greater increases in body temperature, both following feeding and during overnight measures of temperature, than did subjects fed the same number of calories, but with less carbohydrate. Although the observed increases in thermogenesis were small, and could account for only a fraction of the lost calories that failed to be accumulated as excess fat storage, these findings echo the *luxuskonsumption* referred to by clinicians of past generations.

More than 50 years ago, it was suggested that body weight and body fat storage resist the day-to-day variations of caloric intake in such a way that over a broad range, excess calories can be disposed of as heat (*luxuskonsumption*), and deficient caloric intake can be resisted by greater efficiency of caloric utilization (Neumann, 1902). This reviewer hastens to add that in his experience, he has never found massively obese individuals who are not also massive caloric consumers; on diets of 2000 or even 2500 kcal/day, all lose weight. Nevertheless, the finding that there are definite variations in the mode of caloric utilization in different nonobese individuals suggests that small differences integrated over time may be a factor in the assumption of obesity.

Perhaps even more at variance with current teaching has been the finding that nutritional influences can lead to subtle modifications in thyroid function, again reminiscent of *luxuskonsumption*. T_4 is peripherally altered to T_3 and 3,3',5'-triiodothyronine, or reverse T_3. Reverse T_3 is less calorigenic than T_3, and so the ratio of these two hormones could, to some small degree, affect the metabolic consequences and heat production of equal amounts of T_4 released by the thyroid. Fortunately, T_3 and reverse T_3 can be measured by specific radioimmunoassays.

The subjects of Sims who were fattened on high-carbohydrate diets and developed less fatness than was anticipated showed small but definite changes in the direction that might be surmised: T_3 rose from 137 ± 4 to 169 ± 9 ng/100 ml, and the less calorigenic, reverse T_3 declined from 33 ± 4 to 21 ± 4 ng/100 ml. Opposite effects have been reported in undernourished individuals. Adults suffering from protein-caloric malnutrition in Calcutta, India, had high reverse T_3 and low T_3 levels (Chopra *et al.*, 1975), a situation favoring caloric conservation, or at least less calorigenicity of the products of T_4 metabolism. These abnormalities disappeared when adequate calories were consumed.

It is too early to know what these findings mean in relationship to spontaneous human obesity. Yet, for the first time, there appears to be a glimmer of experimental evidence favoring the folk wisdom that individuals vary in their propensities to "put on fat," even with the same caloric intake, and also that calories from different foodstuffs may not be precisely equivalent. Clearly, none of these findings can be taken to mean that thyroid hormones, T_3 or T_4, should be given to any obese subjects unless there is clear evidence for hypothyroidism on the basis of standard clinical laboratory tests and clinical evaluation.

5.4. The Gastrointestinal Tract

It has been useful to consider food intake behavior in two categories: (1) appetitive behavior, or the factors that lead to the onset of a meal; and (2) satiety behavior, or the factors that terminate a meal. It is not at all clear which aspect of behavior is faulty in obese man. There is much evidence incriminating satiety, but a good case can also be made for errors in appetite or hunger. In some experimentally obese rodents, such as hypothalamically lesioned animals in the dynamic or markedly hyperphagic phase, one regularly observes both larger and more frequent meals (Becker and Kissileff, 1974). But in some types of obesity, satiety and appetitive aspects of behavior may vary in other directions; thus, animals receiving insulin will eat smaller meals, but at more frequent intervals (Panksepp, 1973).

Gastric distention is surely one mechanism by which satiety can be provoked, but it is not possible to explain human food-intake behavior exclusively on the basis of variable distensibility of the gastrointestinal tract or any similar mechanical factor such as gastrointestinal length. Recently, two new developments have entered this area of consideration: (1) the increasing use of jejunoileal shunting for the treatment of obesity, and (2) the demonstration that a gut hormone, cholecystokinin, may have important effects on satiety, at least in rats and monkeys.

5.4.1. Jejunoileal Shunts

For roughly two decades, the production of jejunoileal shunts has been advocated for the treatment of massive obesity. Undoubtedly, several thousand obese patients have received shunts in this country. There is a consensus that this is not a procedure without hazard, and thus should be reserved for those with so-called "morbid" obesity, in whom the obesity is demonstrably life-threatening in a proximate sense, e.g., the presence of hypercapnia and hypoxia, and also in whom repeated efforts at more conservative management have proven unsuccessful.

Shunting carries with it a high morbidity for immediate postoperative problems of wound injection and dehiscence. With the passage of time, oxalate stones, hepatic dysfunction, arthropathy, and electrolyte imbalances can constitute severe threats to life, which may require reestablishment of normal intestinal contiguity. Often, the surgical repair of a shunt is done at a time when complications are menacing; hence, the surgical mortality and morbidity following repair can be exceedingly high. There is evidence that the incidence of some complications may be lessened by careful attention to nutritional details following surgery. For example, oxalate stone formation could be lessened by following a diet low in oxalate (Earnest et al., 1974), and the hepatic disorder may be ameliorated by assuring that the patient continuously adheres to a diet adequate in proteins. This latter recommendation may require special supplementation with protein hydrolysates or synthetic amino acid mixtures (Ames et al., 1976).

One of the most fascinating observations on these patients, an observation particularly germane to this review, is that most patients usually experience a relative degree of anorexia following shunting. The hyperphagia that was present before surgery seems to subside thereafter. A new caloric equilibrium is established in which patients can consume a 2000–2500 kcal diet of foods that do not provoke steatorrhea or other gastrointestinal discomfort without experiencing the food drives so typically found after weight reduction. At this level of food intake, body fat stores come into an equilibrium such that the patient remains moderately obese, usually at a body weight of 150–200 pounds (Salmon, 1971).

This relative anorexia after shunting may be in part the result of "learning" just how much food can be consumed with discomfort. In some instances, progressive deterioration of hepatic function might produce anorexia. Fortunately, such degrees of hepatic dysfunction are not typical. Thus, observation of these patients brings up the question whether a more specific and perhaps physiologically based alteration in appetite or perhaps satiety has been induced by the surgery. This is of particular interest, since it has been shown recently that at least one gut hormone does have definite effects on prompt satiety.

5.4.2. Cholecystokinin and Satiety

In a series of elegant and carefully controlled experiments, Smith, Gibbs, and their colleagues have demonstrated a clear connection between gut hormones and prompt satiety (Gibbs *et al.*, 1973). Rats with gastric fistulas so arranged that ingested food was promptly ejected via the fistula would, under appropriate experimental conditions, continue to eat huge amounts of food as though no satiety signal were perceived. When the food was placed in the duodenum, there was prompt cessation of further food intake. These investigators showed that intraduodenal installation of food was not perceived by the rat as an aversive stimulus (Liebling *et al.*, 1975). In searching for the explanation for these findings, they showed that cholecystokinin, a peptide of intestinal origin, was a potent inhibitor of food intake when administered to the gastrostomized rat parenterally. Interestingly, a synthetic octapeptide identical in composition to a fragment of the 33-amino-acid cholecystokinin gave the same results when administered in equivalent quantities. Furthermore, gastrin, which shares a portion of this potent octapeptide sequence, had an effect, albeit a weaker one, in inhibiting feeding in the gastrostomized animal (Smith *et al.*, 1974). Secretin and glucagon were found to have no such effects. Very recently, it has been shown that a partially purified preparation of cholecystokinin given intravenously to monkeys inhibited the intake of a meal of solid food presented to the animals following an overnight fast (Gibbs *et al.*, 1976). The purified octapeptide also had this effect when given in equivalent amounts, as did the intragastric administration of l-phenylalanine, a releaser of endogenous cholecystokinin. The d-form, which is known to be a much weaker releaser of the hormone, had no such effects.

It is, of course, tempting to believe that the metabolism of gut hormone is so altered in jejunoileal shunting that the satiety mechanism is enhanced, perhaps due to rapid gastrointestinal transit of food and thus the rapid presentation of food to a jejunal surface, which hypertrophies markedly following surgery. Bray *et al.* (1976) have recently shown that the output of gastrin after a standard meal rose after surgery from 5.3 to 6.8 ng-min/ml. This rise, of course, could be due to a primary excess of gastrin production, or to less inhibition from inhibiting peptides produced in the upper small intestine. Unfortunately, radioimmunoassays of cholecystokinin have not been simple to devise. For this reason, there have as yet been no measurements of this intestinal peptide before and after surgery. This is a high priority of investigation, and it is to be hoped that adequate assays will be forthcoming shortly.

5.5. Appetite and Substrate Utilization

It is clear from many different types of investigations that the ultimate fuel for oxidation by muscle and other organs is different from the mix of fat and carbohydrate in the diet. Thus, studies of FFA metabolism (Frederickson and Gordon, 1958) clearly indicate that a large fraction of ingested carbohydrate is first transformed to free or unesterified fatty acids prior to oxidation. In the obese state, there is a distinct enhancement of FFA flux, and a large proportion of ingested carbohydrate is transformed to fatty acids (Nestel and Whyte, 1968). Whether this enhanced fatty acid formation is a reflection of the resistance to carbohydrate metabolism already discussed, or whether the increased FFA production provokes the phenomenon of carbohydrate intolerance, similar to that found on a low-carbohydrate intake, remains unclear.

Since both glucose and FFA have been implicated as possible signals for hunger and appetite, the availability and utilization of these substrates is of considerable potential importance in understanding the hyperphagia of obesity. Two recent lines of investigation have provided somewhat discordant yet interesting probes into these possibilities.

5.5.1. Protein-Sparing and Ketogenic Diets

Blackburn and Flatt (1973) and Genuth *et al.* (1974) have used similar diets for rapid weight reduction in obese subjects. The Genuth diet is 45 g casein calcium and 30 g glucose. The Blackburn and Flatt diet is similarly low in calories, with abundant protein as lean beef, but severely restricted in carbohydrate and calories. The relatively high-protein intakes, compared to carbohydrate and fat, are used to provide some hedge against the loss of nitrogen and lean body mass that accompanies such semistarvation. The low carbohydrate is presumed to be of value for maintaining low insulin levels and a high rate of production of ketone bodies. The ketosis is in itself somewhat protein-sparing, and the low insulin levels assure that there will be no antilipolytic effects of insulin inhibiting free fatty acid liberation from adipose tissue and ketone formation in the liver (Flatt and Blackburn, 1974). The low insulin level, it has been noted, may also prevent the appetite or hunger that might be produced by higher insulin levels, as discussed above.

Whatever biochemical rationale there may be for such diets, the clinical observations of these groups are such as to suggest that these diets may have advantages for weight reduction when compared with the ordinary 900–1200-kcal diet with a more typical mix of foodstuffs. Implicit is the claim that adherence to these diets is better than with more usual diets, and thus there may be some aspect of ketosis or protein-sparing that is also appetite-sparing. There are as yet no conclusive data to permit a final judgment on this matter. A very different type of alteration in substrate availability has recently been found to provoke anorexia in rats, as is described in the following section.

5.5.2. Inhibition of Fatty Acid Synthesis

Sullivan *et al.* (1974) have observed that hydroxycitrate given orally to rats will inhibit food intake. Hydroxycitrate is a competitive inhibitor of the enzyme ATP citrate lyase, which provides acetyl CoA for lipogenesis. The substrate for this enzyme is citrate, which is produced in the mitochondrion and passed into the cytoplasm. Studies have shown that hydroxycitrate markedly reduces lipogenesis, and also has very marked effects on food intake. It has been difficult to show that the effects of hydroxycitrate on appetite are not some nonspecific drug toxicity. Ordinary citrate in equivalent amounts has no effect on appetite in the rat, and Sullivan and Triscari (1976) have argued cogently for the absence of such nonspecific appetite-suppressant effects of hydroxycitrate.

Interestingly, one of the biochemical effects of hydroxycitrate is an increase in hepatic glycogen synthesis. To some degree, this effect can be viewed as a result of directing calories away from lipogenesis and into carbohydrate synthesis. This situation is not exactly the reciprocal of ketosis, but it is certainly a totally different metabolic situation from the unbridled lipolysis and low hepatic glycogen synthesis found in ketosis. Yet both states have been suggested to be anorexigenic. In the case of the hydroxycitrate effect, recent work of Russek (1963) may be useful in attempting to find some theoretical basis for the anorexia. Russek has theorized that glucose concentration in liver cells may stimulate hepatic glucoreceptors, which can modulate hunger. Russek's ideas stem from studies in which he has shown that intraportal administration of glucose to a fasting animal has anorexic effects not shared by intraportal injection of saline or intrajugular injections of glucose. Novin *et al.* (1974) have also shown greater effects of glucose on appetite when given intraportally than in controlled injections in other sites. A variety of other studies that lend credence to the concept that hepatic glucoreceptors may have a role in hunger have recently been reviewed by Russek (1976). Although many of these studies are yet to be confirmed, it is clear that an examination of metabolic substrates and their effects on liver and other organs may yet provide some clues as to the interactions of peripheral metabolism and centrally mediated appetitive and satiety behavior.

References

Amatruda, J. M., Livingston, J. N., and Lockwood, D. H., 1975, Insulin receptor: Role in the resistance of human obesity to insulin, *Science* **188:**264.

Ames, F. C., Copeland, E. M., Leeb, D. C., Moore, D. L., and Dudrick, S. J., 1976, Liver dysfunction following small-bowel bypass for obesity—Nonoperative treatment of fatty metamorphosis with parenteral hyperalimentation, *J. Amer. Med. Assoc.* **235:**1249.

Archer, J. A., Gorden, P., and Roth, J., 1975, Defect in insulin binding to receptors in obese man—Amelioration with calorie restriction, *J. Clin. Invest.* **55:**166.

Becker, E. E., and Kissileff, H. R., 1974, Inhibitory controls of feeding by the ventromedial hypothalamus, *Amer. J. Physiol.* **226:**383.

Blackburn, G. L., and Flatt, J. P., 1973, Preservation of lean body mass during acute weight reduction, *Fed. Proc. Fed. Amer. Soc. Exp. Biol.* **32:**916.

Bray, G. A., 1973, *Obesity in Perspective* (G. A. Bray, ed.), DHEW Publication No. (NIH) 75-708, Fogarty International Center Series on Preventive Medicine, Vol 2, Part 2, U.S. Government Printing Office, Washington, D.C.

Bray, G. A., Barry, R. E., and Benfield, J. R., 1976, Intestinal bypass surgery for obesity: Risks and mechanisms, *Clin. Res.* **24:**484A.

Chopra, I. J., Chopra, U., Smith, S. R., Reza, M., and Solomon, D. H., 1975, Reciprocal changes in serum concentrations of 3,3′,5′-triiodothyronine (reverse T_3) and 3,3′,5-triiodothyronine (T_3) in systemic illnesses, *J. Clin. Endocrinol. Metab.* **41:**1043.

Debons, A. F., Krimsky, I., Likuski, H. J., From, A., and Cloutier, R. J., 1968, Gold thioglucose damage to the satiety center: Inhibition in diabetes, *Amer. J. Physiol.* **214:**652.

Debons, A. F., Krimsky, I., From, A., and Cloutier, R. J., 1969, Rapid effects of insulin on the hypothalamic satiety center, *Amer. J. Physiol.* **217:**1114.

Earnest, D. L., Johnson, G., Williams, H. E., and Admirand, W. H., 1974, Hyperoxaluria in patients with ileal resection: An abnormality in dietary oxalate absorption, *Gastroenterology* **66:**1114.

Flatt, J. P., and Blackburn, G. L., 1974, The metabolic fuel regulatory system: Implications for protein-sparing therapies during caloric deprivation and disease, *Amer. J. Clin. Nutr.* **27:**175.

Frederickson, D. S., and Gordon, R. S., Jr. 1958, Transport of fatty acids, *Physiol. Rev.* **38:**585.

Frohman, L. A., Bernardis, L. L., Schnatz, J. D., and Burek, L., 1969, Plasma insulin and triglyceride levels after hypothalamic lesions in weanling rats, *Amer. J. Physiol.* **216:**1496.

Genuth, S. M., Castro, J. H., and Vertes, V., 1974, Weight reduction in obesity by outpatient semistarvation, *J. Amer. Med. Assoc.* **230**:987.

Gibbs, J., Young, R. C., and Smith, G. P., 1973, Cholecystokinin elicits satiety in rats with open gastric fistulas, *Nature* **245**:323.

Gibbs, J., Falasco, J. D., and McHugh, P. R., 1976, Cholecystokinin—Decreased food intake in rhesus monkeys, *Amer. J. Physiol.* **230**:15.

Hales, C. N., and Kennedy, G. C., 1964, Plasma glucose, non-esterified fatty acid and insulin concentrations in hypothalamic–hyperphagic rats, *Biochem. J.* **90**:620.

Hirsch, J., 1972, Discussion, *in: Advances in Psychosomatic Medicine*, Vol. 7 (F. Reichsman, ed.), pp. 229–242, Karger, Basel.

Kahn, C. R., Flier, J. S., Bar, R. S., Archer, J. A., Gorden, P., Martin, M. M., and Roth, J., 1976, The syndromes of insulin resistance and acanthosis nigricans—Insulin-receptor disorders in man, *N. Engl. J. Med.* **294**:739.

Karam, J. H., Grodsky, G. M., and Forsham, P. H., 1963, Excessive insulin response to glucose in obese subjects as measured by immunochemical assay, *Diabetes* **12**:197.

Liebling, D. S, Eisner, J. D., Gibbs, J., and Smith, G. P., 1975, Intestinal satiety in rats, *J. Comp. Physiol. Psychol.* **89**:955.

Mackay, E. M., Callaway, J. W., and Barnes, R. H., 1940, Hyperalimentation in normal animals produced by protamine insulin, *J. Nutr.* **20**:59.

Nestel, P. J., and Whyte, H. M., 1968, Plasma free fatty acid and triglyceride turnover in obesity, *Metabolism* **17**:1122.

Neumann, R. O., 1902, Experimentelle Beiträge zur Lehre von dem täglichen Nahrungsbedarf des Menschen unter besonderer Berücksichtigung der Notwendigen Eiweifsmenge, *Arch. Hyg.* **45**:1.

Novin, D., Sanderson, J. D., and Vanderweele, D. A., 1974, The effect of isotonic glucose on eating as a function of feeding condition and infusion site, *Physiol. Behav.* **13**:3.

Olefsky, J., Reaven, G. M., and Farquhar, J. W., 1974, Effects of weight reduction on obesity. Studies of lipid and carbohydrate metabolism in normal and hyperlipoproteinemic subjects, *J. Clin. Invest.* **53**:64.

Panksepp, J., 1973, Reanalysis of feeding patterns in the rat, *J. Comp. Physiol. Psychol.* **82**:78.

Reaven, G. M., Lerner, R. L., Stern, M. P., and Farquhar, J. W., 1967, Role of insulin in endogenous hypertriglyceridemia, *J. Clin. Invest.* **46**:1756.

Roth, J., Kahn, C. R., Lesniak, M. A., Gorden, P., De Meyts, P., Megyesi, K., Neville, D. M., Jr., Gavin, J. R., Soll, A. H., III, Freychet, P., Goldfine, I. D., Bar, R. S., and Archer, J. A., 1975, Receptors for insulin, NSILA-S, and growth hormone: Applications to disease states in man, *Recent Prog. Horm. Res.* **31**:95.

Russek, M., 1963, Participation of hepatic glucoreceptors in the control of intake of food, *Nature* **197**:79.

Russek, M., 1976, A conceptual equation of intake control, *in: Hunger: Basic Mechanisms and Clinical Implications* (D. Novin, W. Wyrwicka, and G. A. Bray, eds.), pp. 327–347, Raven Press, New York.

Salmon, P. A., 1971, The results of small intestine bypass operations for the treatment of obesity, *Surg. Gynecol. Obstet.* **132:**965.

Sims, E. A. H., 1976, Experimental obesity, dietary-induced thermogenesis, and their clinical implications, *in: Clinics in Endocrinology and Metabolism* (M. J. Albrink, ed.), W. B. Saunders Co. Ltd., London (in press).

Sims, E. A. H., Danforth, E., Jr., Horton, E. S., Bray, G. A., Glennon, J. A., and Salans, L. B., 1973, Endocrine and metabolic effects of experimental obesity in man, *Recent Prog. Horm. Res.* **29:**457.

Smith, G. P., Gibbs, J., and Young, R. C., 1974, Cholecystokinin and intestinal satiety in the rat, *Fed. Proc. Fed. Amer. Soc. Exp. Biol.* **33:**1146.

Soll, A. H., Kahn, C. R., Neville, D. M., Jr., and Roth, J., 1975, Insulin receptor deficiency in genetic and acquired obesity, *J. Clin. Invest.* **56:**769.

Stern, J. S., Hollander, N., Batchelor, B. R., Cohn, C. K., and Hirsch, J., 1972, Adipose-cell size and immunoreactive insulin levels in obese and normal-weight adults, *Lancet* **2:**948.

Stern, J. S., Johnson, P. R., Batchelor, B. R., Zucker, L. M., and Hirsch, J., 1975, Pancreatic insulin release and peripheral tissue resistance in Zucker obese rats fed high- and low-carbohydrate diets, *Amer. J. Physiol.* **228:**543.

Sullivan, A. C., Triscari, J., Hamilton, J. G., and Miller, O. N., 1974, Effect of (−)-hydroxycitrate upon the accumulation of lipid in the rat: II. Appetite, *Lipids* **9:**129.

Sullivan, A. C., and Triscari, J., 1976, Possible interrelationship between metabolite flux and appetite, *in: Hunger: Basic Mechanisms and Clinical Implications* (D. Novin, W. Wyrwicka, and G. A. Bray, eds.), pp. 115–125, Raven Press, New York.

Woods, S. C., and Porte, D., Jr., 1976, Insulin and the set-point regulation of body weight, *in: Hunger: Basic Mechanisms and Clinical Implications* (D. Novin, W. Wyrwicka, and G. A. Bray, eds.), pp. 273–280, Raven Press, New York.

6

Disorders of Lipid and Lipoprotein Metabolism

DeWitt S. Goodman

6.1. Introduction

It is the aim of this chapter to review the major advances that occurred during 1975 with regard to our knowledge about the metabolism of the major plasma lipids and lipoproteins, and about clinical abnormalities in lipid transport, with particular emphasis on the hyperlipidemias. In addition, some recent major developments that occurred before 1975 will be reviewed briefly in order to provide important background information. The well-established association between the presence of hyperlipidemia and an increased risk of the development of coronary heart disease (Kannel *et al.*, 1961, 1971; Carlson and Böttiger, 1972) has served to stimulate both biochemists and clinicians to focus considerable research efforts on this area.

DEWITT S. GOODMAN • Department of Medicine, College of Physicians and Surgeons of Columbia University, New York, New York 10032.

A detailed review of the world epidemiology of coronary heart disease was recently presented by Keys (1975).

6.2. Lipoprotein Structure and Metabolism

6.2.1. Introduction

Lipids are not soluble in water, and they circulate in plasma in association with certain specific proteins in the form of plasma lipoproteins. Four classes of specific lipoproteins circulate in plasma; their characteristics are summarized in Table I. Two of these classes, chylomicrons and VLDL, are composed predominantly of triglyceride and represent, respectively, the transport form of exogenous (dietary) and endogenous triglyceride. Chylomicrons are normally not present in postabsorptive plasma after an overnight fast. The LDL (or (β-lipoprotein) contains cholesterol as its major component, and normally represents the circulating form of most of the plasma cholesterol.

The chemistry and metabolism of the lipoproteins have been the subjects of intensive research activity in many laboratories during the past few years, and a great deal of information is being developed about these macromolecules. It has been shown that the protein portions of the VLDL and HDL are heterogeneously comprised of a number of small- to medium-sized polypeptide moieties (called *apolipoproteins*), and that the four classes of lipoproteins share several apolipoprotein components in common. Two excellent reviews on the structure, function, and metabolism of the human plasma lipoproteins appeared in 1975 (Morrisett *et al.*, 1975; Eisenberg and Levy, 1975).

6.2.2. Very-Low-Density Lipoproteins

The VLDL are produced mainly by the liver, and represent the vehicle for transport of triglyceride fatty acid (as endogenous triglyceride) from the liver to tissue sites, particularly to adipose tissue for storage. VLDL are also produced by the intestine. VLDL triglyceride is largely removed from the blood by a lipolytic process, probably involving lipoprotein lipase. VLDL are heterogeneous with regard to size (about 30–80 nm in diameter), density (0.95–1.006 g/ml), and flotation rate (see Table I). VLDL protein is comprised of several different apolipoproteins, including apoB (the protein moiety of LDL), three small (mol. w. approximately 6000–10,000) apoproteins designated apoC-I, apoC-II, and apoC-III, and an arginine-rich apoprotein also called the "high arg" protein. The apoproteins apoC-I, apoC-II, and apoC-III have also been referred to in

Table I. The Plasma Lipoproteins[a]

	Chylomicrons	VLDL[b]	LDL[b]	HDL[b]
Density	<1.006	<1.006	1.019–1.063	1.063–1.21
Electrophoretic mobility	(origin)	pre-β	β	α_1
Size (diam., nm)	75–300	30–80	20	7–10
Gofmann terminology	$S_f > 400$	S_f 20–400	S_f 0–20	(HDL)
Composition (%)[c]:				
Protein	2	10	25	50
TG	88	60	10	5
Cholesterol	5	12	50	20
PL	5	18	15	25
Major apoproteins	(uncertain)	B; C-I, C-II, C-III; "High Arg"	B	A-I, A-II

[a]Modified from Levy *et al.* (1974).
[b]VLDL: very-low-density lipoproteins; LDL: low-density lipoproteins; HDL: high-density lipoproteins.
[c]The percentage compositions are approximations.

the literature in terms of their carboxy-terminal residues, as apoLP-Ser, apoLP-Glu, and apoLP-Ala, respectively. Information is rapidly growing about the chemical structures and the physiological or structural roles of the individual apolipoproteins. Thus, for example, apoC-II is a potent activator of lipoprotein lipase.

The complete amino acid sequence of apoC-I, consisting of a single polypeptide chain of 57 residues, has been reported recently (Jackson *et al.*, 1974; Shulman *et al.*, 1975). The primary structure of apoC-III, consisting of 79 residues, has also been reported (Brewer *et al.*, 1974). The amino acid sequence of apoC-II has not yet been reported.

The total chemical synthesis of apoC-I was reported in abstract form late in 1975 (Sigler et al., 1975). Both the synthetic polypeptide and the native apoC-I were found to activate the enzyme lecithin–cholesterol acyltransferase (LCAT).

Methods for the quantitation of the major apoproteins of human VLDL have been developed by Kane et al. (1975). The mean content of apolipoprotein B in 43 samples from normolipidemic subjects was $36.9 \pm 1.2\%$ ($\pm$S.E.M.) of the total protein. Three subspecies of apoC-III together comprised a mean of 63% of the remaining apoproteins, with the mean ratios of apoC-I to apoC-II to apoC-III (sum of three subspecies) to the arginine-rich peptide being 1:2:12:4. The distribution of the apoproteins was found to be a function of particle diameter when VLDL were fractionated according to size. Thus, in fractions below 70–80 nm diameter, apoB comprised an increasing percentage of the total protein with decreasing particle diameter. Among the other apoproteins, the percentage of the arginine-rich and apoC-I peptides increased, and that of apoC-II declined, progressively with decreasing particle size.

6.2.3. Low-Density Lipoproteins

Most of the plasma cholesterol normally circulates as part of LDL. Because of the relatively small size of LDL, plasma containing even greatly increased levels of LDL appears clear. In contrast, plasma containing elevated concentrations of VLDL appears uniformly cloudy or turbid, particularly after overnight storage in the refrigerator. Plasma containing chylomicrons appears turbid when drawn; after overnight storage, the chylomicrons float to the top of the tube, where they appear as a "cream-like" chylo layer.

Recent studies have demonstrated that LDL originates mainly as part of the structure of the VLDL, and is largely formed as the product of VLDL metabolism (rather than being independently produced by the liver) (Eisenberg et al., 1973; Sigurdsson et al., 1975). In order to quantitate the interrelationship between apolipoprotein B in VLDL and in LDL, Sigurdsson et al. (1975) simultaneously measured the turnover and synthetic rates of radioiodinated apoB in VLDL and LDL in both normo- and hyperlipidemic subjects. The results were consistent with the view that most, if not all, of VLDL apoB is converted into LDL apoB, and that most, if not all, of LDL apoB is derived from VLDL apoB in normotriglyceridemic subjects. The site(s) of LDL catabolism is not clearly known, although many peripheral cell types have been shown capable of such catabolism (as discussed in Section 6.4).

6.2.4. High-Density Lipoproteins

The HDL are composed of approximately half protein and half lipid. HDL are independently produced and secreted by the liver. HDL serve as the major substrate for the plasma LCAT reaction, which is responsible for the formation and turnover of plasma cholesteryl esters (Glomset and Norum, 1973). The protein moiety of HDL is made up mainly of two apolipoproteins called apoA-I and apoA-II. ApoA-I, the major protein constituent of HDL, is a single polypeptide chain of 245 amino acids, the sequence of which was reported in 1975 (Baker et al., 1975). The amino acid sequence of ApoA-II, which consists of a dimer of two identical polypeptides of 77 amino acids each, was reported in 1972 (Lux et al., 1972). HDL also contains small amounts of the C apoproteins, and can serve as an important reservoir of these via either or both exchange and transfer between VLDL and HDL.

6.3. Hyperlipidemias—Definition and Classification

6.3.1. "Normal" Levels of Plasma Lipids

Normal levels of plasma lipids cannot be defined precisely, since coronary risk rises continuously with cholesterol levels over a wide concentration range. In addition, it is necessary to interpret a given serum lipid level in terms of age, since the serum concentrations of cholesterol and triglyceride increase as a population becomes older. The mean ($\pm$S.D.) concentrations of cholesterol in a study in Seattle (Goldstein *et al.*, 1973a) were found to rise from 192 ± 33 mg/dl in men aged 20–29 to a level of 239 ± 42 in men in their fifties, and to decline thereafter. The decline in cholesterol concentrations in the older age groups may reflect the higher death rate and earlier death of younger persons with high cholesterol concentrations.

One approach to the problem of determining which values should be considered abnormal has been to determine the serum cholesterol and triglyceride concentrations that separate the upper 5% of the population from the lower 95% (the 95th percentile values). Values above the 95th percentile (for a given age and sex) are considered as clearly elevated, and hence are defined as hyperlipidemic.

6.3.2. Classification by Lipid Elevation

Patients with hyperlipidemia can be classified as having hypercholesterolemia, hypertriglyceridemia, or mixed hyperlipidemia (hypercholesterolemia and -triglyceridemia) by measurement of total serum cholesterol and triglyceride levels. This classification is sufficient for the clinical management of most patients. If hypertriglyceridemia is present, the presence or absence of chylomicrons can be determined by observation of the serum after storage overnight in the refrigerator (see Section 6.2.3).

6.3.3. Classification by Type of Hyperlipoproteinemia

Since an elevated lipid level means that there is an elevated level of one or more lipoproteins, hyperlipidemia can be translated into hyperlipoproteinemia by classifying patients according to which lipoprotein is elevated. The distribution of lipoproteins seen after serum is subjected to electrophoresis on paper or agarose gel was the basis of a system of classification for hyperlipidemia proposed by Fredrickson *et al.* (1967). This typing system, as adopted by the World Health Organization (Beaumont *et al.*, 1970), divided serum lipid disorders (elevations) into 6 types (designated I, IIa, IIb, III, IV, and V), depending on which lipoproteins were elevated. The hyperlipoproteinemias commonly observed are: type IIa (hyperbetalipoproteinemia, and hence hypercholesterolemia); type IIb (hyperbetalipoproteinemia plus hyperprebetalipoproteinemia, and hence hypercholesterolemia plus -triglyceridemia); and type IV (hyperprebetalipoproteinemia, and hence endogenous hypertriglyceridemia). Although the typing on the basis of lipoprotein electrophoresis does give a phenotypic description of the lipoprotein pattern at the time of sampling, recent family and genetic studies (Hazzard *et al.*, 1973; Goldstein *et al.*, 1973b; Rose *et al.*, 1973; Nikkilä and Aro, 1973) suggest that lipoprotein phenotyping may have limited, if any, usefulness in the clinical management of patients with hyperlipidemia (Fredrickson, 1975; Havel, 1975). In most patients, the lipoprotein phenotype can be accurately assessed by determination of the fasting serum cholesterol and triglyceride levels, together with observation of the serum after overnight storage.

6.3.4. Genetic Classification

Fasting total serum cholesterol and triglyceride concentrations alone have proved useful in genetic studies. The frequency of hyperlipidemia in 500 survivors of acute myocardial infarction and in relatives of hyperlipidemic survivors was determined in a large study in Seattle (Goldstein *et al.*, 1973a,b). Hyperlipidemia was arbitrarily defined as values of either or both cholesterol and triglyceride exceeding the 95th percentile for the control group (spouse controls of infarct survivors). Hyperlipidemia was found in 31% of the infarct survivors. Family studies showed that the majority of the hyperlipidemic survivors appeared to have genetic abnormalities, and, in fact, 54% were classified as having one of three conditions consistent with a monogenic pattern of inheritance. The most common genetic abnormality (30% of families of hyperlipidemic survivors) was "familial combined hyperlipidemia," in which family members had elevated serum levels of either cholesterol or triglyceride or both. Familial hypertriglyceridemia was found in 14% of the hyperlipidemic survivors, and familial hypercholesterolemia in 10%. In this project, lipoprotein phenotypes were compared with the genetic analysis [based on serum lipid levels in relatives (Hazzard *et al.*, 1973)]. On an individual basis, no lipoprotein pattern (among the types studied, which were IIa, IIb, IV, and V) proved to be specific for any particular genetic lipid disorder. Furthermore, no genetic disorder was specified by any one of the lipoprotein patterns. Hence, the lipoprotein patterns presumably do not provide a classification according to specific pathogenetic defects.

The practical conclusion from these studies is that in order to diagnose genetic disease it is necessary—since we lack specific genetic markers for the several conditions—to measure cholesterol and triglyceride concentrations on the first degree relatives of an individual with hyperlipidemia. This offers families the benefit of having younger members with hyperlipidemia identified before they have symptomatic ischemic heart disease. Diagnosing genetic hyperlipidemia may also have prognostic value. In familial hypercholesterolemia, Slack (1969) calculated the chance of a first attack of ischemic heart disease in males was 5.4% by the age of 30, 51% by age 50, and 85% by age 60. For women, the risks were lower, at 0, 12%, and 57%, respectively. Stone et al. (1974) showed a similar cumulative probability of ischemic heart disease of 16% in males with familial hypercholesterolemia at age 40 years with a rise to 52% by age 60. As in Slack's study, the risk was lower in females with the risk from the disorder lagging 20 years behind the risk in males. Familial hyperlipidemic individuals, then, merit maximum intervention therapy. It has been estimated that of the order of 1 in 150 individuals in the general population may be a carrier of a gene predisposing to one of the three major familial lipid disorders.

6.4. Familial Hypercholesterolemia

6.4.1. Introduction

Familial hypercholesterolemia (FH) is well established to be a single-gene mutation, transmitted as an autosomal dominant trait in humans. The prevalence of the disorder is approximately 1 in 500 persons in the general American population. Affected heterozygotes show a 2- to 3-fold elevation in the plasma cholesterol level from early childhood, and a high frequency of tendinous xanthomas and premature coronary heart disease as adults. In the rare subjects who are homozygous for the FH gene, the clinical syndrome is much more severe. These subjects demonstrate 4- to 6-fold elevations in LDL, with total plasma cholesterol values often exceeding 800 mg/dl, together with the early appearance of xanthomas and of atherosclerotic vascular disease, with death from myocardial infarction often occurring in the second or third decade of life.

Major developments occurred during 1975 dealing with the pathogenesis, the diagnosis and classification, and the treatment of patients with FH.

6.4.2. Pathogenesis

Insight into the pathogenetic defect in FH has been obtained from studies with skin fibroblasts in culture *in vitro*. The results of studies reported before 1975 have been effectively summarized by Goldstein, Brown, and their colleagues (Goldstein and Brown, 1975; Brown *et al.*,

1975a). These studies demonstrated that normal human fibroblasts possess receptors on their cell surfaces that bind LDL with high affinity and specificity. Binding of LDL to these receptors was found to lead to at least two major metabolic consequences: (1) cholesterol synthesis by the cell was suppressed by suppression of the activity of the key regulatory enzyme 3-hydroxy-3-methylglutaryl coenzyme A reductase (HMG CoA reductase); and (2) the bound LDL was degraded by proteolysis.

When fibroblasts from patients homozygous for FH were studied, major differences from normal were seen. The fibroblasts from the FH homozygotes showed a nearly complete inability to bind LDL over a wide concentration range. As a result, these cells did not suppress HMG CoA reductase activity in the presence of LDL, and hence synthesized cholesterol at a much higher rate than did normal cells in the presence of LDL. In addition, the cells of FH homozygotes showed a severe deficiency in their ability to degrade LDL. It was postulated that the primary genetic defect in FH resides in a gene the product of which is necessary for the production of a high-affinity cell-surface receptor for LDL.

Consistent with genetic considerations, fibroblasts from FH heterozygotes contained approximately half the normal number of LDL receptors. This shortage resulted in a situation in which a normal degree of suppression of HMG CoA reductase activity and a normal rate of LDL degradation could be attained only in the presence of a 2-3-fold elevation in extracellular LDL levels.

When cholesterol was added directly (in a small volume of ethanol) to the culture medium of either normal cells or homozygote FH cells, similar suppression of HMG CoA reductase activity was observed in both kinds of cells. Thus, the LDL receptor could be bypassed by direct addition of the sterol, and the effects of this addition were manifested in the FH cells, which lack the LDL receptor. Of 47 steroid compounds tested by direct addition for their ability to suppress HMG CoA reductase activity in cultured human fibroblasts, 11 were more potent than cholesterol (Brown and Goldstein, 1974). All these compounds had similar effects on fibroblasts from a homozygote with FH. 7-Ketocholesterol, which was 100 times more potent than cholesterol on a weight basis, suppressed HMG CoA reductase activity in normal cells by more than 90% in 2 hr. In fact, when normal cells were cultured in the presence of 7-ketocholesterol but in the absence of lipoproteins, the suppression of endogenous cholesterol synthesis by 7-ketocholesterol resulted in a marked inhibition of cell growth. This inhibition of cell growth was prevented by the presence in the culture medium of either cholesterol or mevalonate. Thus, cholesterol is absolutely required for the survival and multiplication of human cells.

Further studies of the role of the LDL receptor in the normal metabolism of human fibroblasts demonstrated that binding of LDL to its receptor leads to the transfer of LDL cholesterol into the cell (receptor-mediated uptake) (Brown *et al.*, 1975b). This transfer in turn leads to several related enzymatic events, including: (1) suppression of HMG CoA reductase activity; (2) LDL catabolism; and (3) stimulation of intracellular cholesterol esterification. All these events were virtually absent in fibroblasts from patients with the homozygous form of FH. It was concluded that LDL–receptor interactions constitute an important biochemical mechanism for the regulation of the cholesterol content of normal human fibroblasts.

Studies of the details of this mechanism indicated that the cellular uptake of cholesterol from LDL appears to involve the internalization of receptor-bound LDL by endocytosis, followed by fusion of the endocytotic vesicles with lysosomes. The essential role of the lysosome in mediating the subsequent events was shown by an elegant series of studies by Goldstein, Brown, and their colleagues (Goldstein *et al.*, 1975a,c). Within the lysosome, the protein component of the LDL is rapidly degraded by proteases, and the cholesteryl ester component of the LDL is hydrolyzed by a lysosomal acid lipase. The resulting unesterified cholesterol is transferred to the cellular compartment, where it suppresses HMG CoA reductase and activates an acyl-CoA:cholesterol acyltransferase (thus activating its own esterification).

In addition, very recent studies have demonstrated that the LDL receptor itself is under feedback regulation, so that its activity (and hence the amount of cholesterol that enters the cell) is inversely proportional to the cellular content of cholesterol (Brown and Goldstein, 1975). Thus, cultured fibroblasts can obtain cholesterol by increasing the number of receptors, and, conversely, they protect themselves against an overaccumulation of the sterol by suppressing the synthesis of LDL receptors. This appears to be an important part of the balance of regulatory processes by which normal fibroblasts maintain a fairly constant intracellular concentration of cholesterol.

Studies have also been made of the rate of sterol synthesis, from radioactive acetate and mevalonate, of human leukocytes isolated from fresh defibrinated blood from normal subjects and from patients with the heterozygous form of FH (Fogelman *et al.*, 1975). When leukocytes are incubated in a medium containing lipid-free serum, synthesis of sterols from acetate, but not from mevalonate, is much enhanced. It was shown that this increased synthesis resulted from increased levels of HMG CoA reductase activity in the cells. A comparison was made of the activation of sterol synthesis from acetate in leukocytes from normals and from heterozygote FH patients. The FH leukocytes responded to incubation in lipid-free sera with a significantly higher activation (correlated with a higher induction of HMG CoA reductase) than did normal leukocytes. Moreover, the leukocytes from a FH heterozygote were found to release into a lipid-free incubation medium more endogenously synthesized sterol than the cells of a normal person. It was pointed out that leukocytes, as well as cultured fibroblasts, are useful and readily accessible human cells for exploring the normal and abnormal control of sterol biosynthesis in man.

Measurements of the turnover *in vivo* of the apoprotein of LDL in patients with homozygous FH were carried out (Simons *et al.*, 1975; Bilheimer *et al.*, 1975). A decreased fractional rate of catabolism and an increased (as compared to normal) absolute rate of synthesis of the apoprotein of LDL were found in the homozygous FH patients. In the 4 FH patients studied by Simons *et al.* (1975), autologous LDL and LDL from a normal subject were found to be metabolized at the same fractional and absolute rates. In addition, in the circulation of a normal subject, LDL from a normal subject and that from a patient with FH were metabolized at the same rates.

6.4.3. Diagnosis and Classification

The diagnosis of FH can be made in the research laboratory by carrying out studies with skin fibroblasts in culture derived from the patient under evaluation. As described above, fibroblasts from patients heterozygous (or homozygous) for FH differ from normal fibroblasts by showing less suppression of HMG CoA reductase activity and less stimulation of cholesterol esterification on addition of LDL to lipoprotein-deficient culture medium. Using this approach, the simplest method appears to be the study of the rate of incorporation of ^{14}C-labeled oleate into cholesteryl esters under standardized conditions. It has also been proposed that the rate of incorporation of radioactive acetate into digitonin-precipitable sterols might be useful as an assay for the diagnosis of FH (Khachadurian *et al.*, 1975).

Evidence has been obtained for the existence of genetic heterogeneity within the FH syndrome. Goldstein et al. (1975b) reported that within the group of patients classified clinically as homozygous FH, there exist at least two biochemically distinct subgroups. One group, called *receptor-negative FH*, comprises patients whose fibroblasts fail to show specific LDL binding at any concentration of LDL, and thus manifest virtually complete absence of the biochemical functions mediated by the LDL receptor. These mutant cells appear to lack functional LDL receptors. The cells of the other group of FH homozygotes, called *receptor-defective FH*, possess a low, but detectable, level of LDL receptor function. At high levels of LDL, this class of mutant cells, unlike the receptor-negative cells, is capable of esterifying cholesterol and suppressing HMG CoA reductase activity. For fibroblasts from 3 patients who possess the receptor-defective mutation, it was calculated that their degree of function could be achieved if they possessed only about 10% of the normal binding of LDL.

Evidence for biochemical heterogeneity that could be correlated with clinical heterogeneity in patients with homozygous FH was presented by Breslow *et al.* (1975). As pointed out by these workers, some patients with homozygous FH are completely resistant to conventional forms of therapy such as diet and lipid-lowering drugs, whereas other patients derive considerable lowering of plasma cholesterol from such therapy. Studies were carried out with fibroblasts from 2 patients with homozygous FH unresponsive to therapy (plasma cholesterol levels in the range 700–900 mg/dl) and with fibroblasts from 4 patients who responded to diet plus drug therapy. The average plasma cholesterol level in the latter group of patients was 701 mg/dl before treatment and 318 mg/dl after vigorous therapy. In fibroblasts from the therapy-responsive patients, LDL suppressed HMG CoA reductase activity to $41\pm12\%$ of control (without LDL), whereas fibroblast enzyme activity from the 2 therapy-unresponsive patients was not suppressed. LDL binding to fibroblasts from both groups was defective as compared to normal controls, but fibroblasts from therapy-responsive patients did show a low level of specific binding of LDL, significantly greater than that seen with therapy-unresponsive fibroblasts. It was suggested that the biochemical differences may help explain the variable response to therapy seen in patients with homozygous FH. As discussed, the genetic possibilities for FH include either one gene locus with at least three alleles (normal, moderately deficient, severely deficient or defective) or two gene loci, each with two or more alleles, at least one of which controls LDL binding to the cell.

6.4.4. Portacaval Shunt Surgery and Homozygous Familial Hypercholesterolemia

In 1973, Starzl *et al.* (1973) reported that they had performed an end-to-side portacaval shunt in a 12-year-old girl with homozygous FH that had been refractory to medical treatment, and that this procedure had resulted in a marked and persistent decrease in plasma cholesterol levels, resolution of xanthomata, and apparent improvement in coronary blood flow. Although this patient died suddenly 1½ years after shunt surgery (Starzl *et al.*, 1974), the sustained lowering of plasma cholesterol level achieved by the surgical procedure has aroused a great deal of interest among clinicians and investigators interested in the problem of FH. Information about 6 other patients with homozygous FH subjected to portacaval shunt surgery has recently been reported (Stein *et al.*, 1975; Krogh and Wickens, 1974; Bilheimer *et al.*, 1975). In 5 of the patients, sustained reductions in plasma total and LDL cholesterol levels were observed; most of the patients also demonstrated clinical improvement with regard to signs and symptoms related to FH. One patient, a 6-year-old girl, was metabolically studied in detail before and after shunt surgery (Bilheimer *et al.*, 1975). Before surgery, this patient showed elevated rates of production of both cholesterol and LDL, together with a reduced fractional catabolic rate of LDL. Five months after shunt surgery, the rate of LDL synthesis had declined by 48%, and this decline caused a 39% drop in the plasma LDL cholesterol level, despite a 17% reduction in the fractional catabolic rate of LDL. The rate of total body synthesis of cholesterol fell by 62%, as compared with the preoperative value.

The mechanism whereby portacaval shunt surgery leads to the observed changes in homozygous FH patients remains to be defined. Since this procedure is not without risks, it should be viewed with caution before being recommended for any given patient. It has, furthermore, been recommended that FH patients who are to undergo this procedure be studied intensively before and after surgery (Ahrens, 1974; Mitchell and Levy, 1974). The National Heart and Lung Institute has offered to act as an initial focus or registry for information exchange on current or planned shunt procedures for this condition (Mitchell and Levy, 1974).

6.4.5. Other Therapy

The use of plasma exchange in the management of homozygous FH was reported by Thompson et al. (1975). Two young women with homozygous FH and coronary and aortic atheroma were treated by repeated plasma exchange using a continuous-flow blood-cell separator for 4 and 8 months. A pronounced reduction in plasma cholesterol and LDL concentrations was achieved by exchanging each patient's plasma with cholesterol-free plasma protein fraction at 3-weekly intervals on an outpatient basis. By prelabeling the patients' cholesterol with carbon-14 and comparing the specific activity of the cholesterol in adipose tissue with that in plasma, evidence was obtained of an influx of tissue cholesterol into plasma after each exchange. There were no side effects, and both patients lost their angina. It was suggested that plasma exchange may offer a new and practical approach to the long-term management of this lethal disorder, and may also provide information about the possible reversibility of human atheroma.

For more short-term management, intravenous hyperalimentation has been found to significantly lower plasma cholesterol and LDL levels in patients with homozygous FH (Stein et al., 1975; Torsvik et al., 1975). The mechanism of this effect is unknown.

6.5. Type III Hyperlipoproteinemia

Type III hyperlipoproteinemia was first identified by Fredrickson et al. (1967) by the application of lipoprotein electrophoresis to the study of the familial hyperlipoproteinemias. In this disease, which is also referred to as *broad-beta disease, floating-beta disease,* and *dysbetalipoproteinemia,* there is a change in the composition of the abnormal lipoprotein ("floating-beta VLDL") the concentration of which is increased. Many patients with this type III disorder show palmar xanthomas along with tuberous or tendon xanthomas elsewhere. Patients with type III hyperlipoproteinemia have been of special interest because of a high incidence of premature vascular disease, and because of rapid response of their hyperlipidemia to diet and clofibrate.

Fredrickson *et al.* (1975) recently compared two methods of defining type III hyperlipoproteinemia, namely, the presence of "floating beta" lipoproteins compared to an estimate of the relative content of cholesterol and triglyceride in lipoproteins of density less than 1.006 (VLDL). They concluded that the ratio of VLDL cholesterol to plasma triglyceride concentration was a more satisfactory way of diagnosing type III hyperlipoproteinemia. In a large group of subjects with primary hyperlipidemia and their relatives, the ratio gave a large symmetrical peak between 0.1 and 0.25. It was felt that ratios above 0.30 signify type III hyperlipoproteinemia, and that the diagnosis should be suspected if the ratio is between 0.25 and 0.30. Evidence for the usefulness of this lipid ratio in the diagnosis of the type III disorder was also provided by Mishkel *et al.* (1975).

The clinical and biochemical features of type III hyperlipoproteinemia in 49 patients from 23 to 70 years of age were described (Morganroth *et al.,* 1975). An increase in VLDL of abnormal chemical composition was the basis for diagnosis. The untreated patients all had hypercholesterolemia and hypertriglyceridemia and, on the average, decreased concentrations of both LDL and HDL; 74% had xanthomas, and classic "xanthoma striata palmaris" was found in more than half; 37% had ischemic heart disease, detected earlier in men than in women; and 27% had peripheral vascular disease (compared to 4% of subjects with type II hyperlipoproteinemia). Of 35 subjects, 25 achieved normal lipid levels with dietary therapy alone. Analysis of 29 kindreds showed hyperlipidemia in half of adult blood relatives; half of these had type III, the remainder usually a simple endogenous hypertriglyceridemia (type IV). Only 2 of 55 children less than 20 years of age were affected, both with type IV. It was pointed out that the inheritance of the type III disorder is not clear, but it was felt that most patients with type III probably represent a disorder due to the presence of a single mutant autosomal allele with incomplete and variable expression or "penetrance," regulated in part by age-related factors.

A study of the occurrence of type III in a single, large kindred of 108 members spanning 4 generations has also provided evidence for an autosomal dominant mode of inheritance (Hazzard *et al.,* 1975). At least 1 member of the first generation pair was normal, at least 5 of their 9 children had type III patterns, and at least 2 of these (whose spouses were normal) transmitted this pattern to their offspring. It was suggested that in this kindred, the common occurrence of hypertriglyceridemia (in a type IV pattern) might represent either a variable phenotypic expression of the gene for broad-beta disease or the coexistence of a second, independent genetic lipid disorder.

Evidence has been presented that the unusual floating-beta VLDL that is found in type III hyperlipoproteinemia represents the abnormal accumulation of normal intermediates in the metabolism of triglyceride-rich lipoproteins (chylomicrons and VLDL). Studies were carried out by Hazzard and Bierman (1975b) in which VLDL from subjects with endogenous hypertriglyceridemia (type IV pattern) or broad-beta disease (type III) were analyzed under varying dietary and pharmacological conditions following starch block electrophoresis. In other studies, the effects of exogenous and endogenous triglyceride on the levels, composition, and distribution of chylomicrons and VLDL in endogenous hypertriglyceridemia and broad-beta disease were compared (Hazzard and Bierman, 1975a). The results observed were consistent with the hypothesis that the slower (beta) migrating, triglyceride-poor VLDL found in the type III patients are normal intermediate (or remnant) forms in a continuous catabolic process. The concentration of these remnants is dwarfed by that of the faster, triglyceride-rich species of VLDL in subjects with endogenous hypertriglyceridemia. In subjects with the type III disorder, however, the "remnants" accumulate (as the beta-VLDL characteristic of this disorder), most likely as a result of a relative blockade in their further catabolism. Evidence that the floating-beta VLDL that is found in postabsorptive patients with type III hyperlipoproteinemia represents an "intermediate" lipoprotein that accumulates because of an impaired catabolism of VLDL to LDL has also been reported by Patsch et al. (1975). The nature and anatomical locus of the defect in the catabolic processing of chylomicron and VLDL remnants in type III patients remain to be defined.

6.6. Familial Lecithin: Cholesterol Acyltransferase Deficiency

Since 1967, 7 patients from 3 different Scandinavian families have been described with a syndrome characterized by diffuse corneal opacities, normochromic anemia, and proteinuria with late renal insufficiency (Glomset and Norum, 1973). The anemia was found to have a hemolytic component associated with approximately 2-fold increases in erythrocyte unesterified cholesterol and lecithin, and with the presence of lipid vacuoles in the cells of the bone marrow and spleen. Proteinuria has been associated with intra- and extracellular lipid in the glomeruli.

The enzyme LCAT could not be detected in the plasma of these patients, and all the patients had abnormal plasma lipids and lipoproteins. Thus, the lipoproteins all contained very low proportions of cholesteryl ester and high proportions of unesterified cholesterol and lecithin. In these patients, the VLDL have beta mobility on electrophoresis, and often contain high concentrations of very large particles. The LDL include abnormally large particles, rich in unesterified cholesterol and lecithin, intermediate-sized particles similar to those found in obstructive jaundice (the so-called lipoprotein-X), and normal-sized particles that contain about 10 times the normal amount of triglyceride. The HDL include abnormally large and small particles of unusual electrophoretic mobility and appearance on electron microscopy. These and other abnormalities presumably depend on the LCAT deficiency, although the pathogenetic mechanisms remain to be fully defined. It has been felt that although familial LCAT deficiency is a rare condition, studies of the patients with this disorder can provide considerable valuable information about the normal metabolic role of the LCAT reaction in man.

Glomset, Norum, and their colleagues recently reported studies aimed at exploring the origin of the abnormal lipoproteins, their metabolic interrelationships, and the changes induced in them by the LCAT reaction. *In vivo* studies were performed to explore the possibility that some of the lipoproteins in the patients' plasma are related to chylomicrons (Glomset *et al.*, 1975). Four patients with familial LCAT deficiency were given successive diets that differed in triglyceride, carbohydrate, or cholesterol content, and after each dietary period, the lipoproteins were analyzed by a variety of methods. The results suggested that the concentrations of the large VLDL and LDL, the intermediate-sized LDL, and the small HDL are related to the absorption and subsequent transport of dietary fatty acids. Since these lipoproteins are rich in unesterified cholesterol and lecithin, two polar lipids that form a large part of the surfaces of chylomicrons, it was suggested that components of chylomicron surfaces may accumulate in the patients' plasma following enzymic removal of chylomicron triglyceride and contribute to several of the abnormal lipoproteins.

The effects of incubating the patients' plasma lipoproteins with partially purified LCAT *in vitro* were studied (Norum *et al.*, 1975). They observed a variety of changes that showed that the LCAT reaction can alter the apolipoprotein content and physical properties as well as the lipid content of the patients' lipoproteins.

Studies on the genetics of LCAT deficiency were reported recently (Teisberg *et al.*, 1975). The genetic basis of the disorder seems to be the presence of a LCAT deficiency gene in double dose. This gene was felt to probably be the result of a single mutational event. Gene linkage studies revealed nonrandom assortment between LCAT deficiency and serum haptoglobin (H_p) types. Association was found between the LCAT deficiency gene and the $H_p{}^{1S}$ gene. It was proposed that the LCAT gene is situated close to the α-haptoglobin locus on chromosome number 16.

6.7. Chronic Renal Failure and Hyperlipidemia

It has been known for several years that hypertriglyceridemia is common in patients with nonnephrotic uremia (Bagdade *et al.*, 1968). The development of hypertriglyceridemia was recently studied in 38 patients who were at different deteriorative stages of chronic renal insufficiency (McCosh *et al.*, 1975), as measured by corrected creatinine clearance. Patients in the mild stages of chronic renal insufficiency showed no change in plasma triglyceride levels, whereas in the moderate and severe stages, plasma triglycerides were significantly elevated. Patients undergoing chronic hemodialysis showed still higher levels of triglyceride (214 ± 36 mg/dl, mean $\pm$ S.E.M.). Even higher levels of triglyceride (276 ± 250 mg/dl, mean $\pm$ S.D.) were previously reported by Bagdade *et al.* (1968) in patients undergoing chronic hemodialysis. In both of these studies, reduced postheparin lipolytic activity was observed in the patients with renal insufficiency and hypertriglyceridemia, suggesting that impaired triglyceride removal from plasma may be the mechanism involved in the hyperlipidemia.

Patients on prolonged maintenance hemodialysis manifest accelerated atherosclerosis and premature atherosclerotic vascular disease. The survival experience of 39 patients receiving long-term regular hemodialysis in Seattle since 1960 was studied (Lindner *et al.*, 1974). The mean ($\pm$S.D.) age was 37 ± 9.5 years for the group at the start of dialysis. The mean duration of treatment was 6.5 years (range 1–13 years). Overall mortality was 56.4% at the end of the 13-year follow-up period, and 14 of 23 deaths could be attributed to atherosclerotic complications. Myocardial infarction was responsible for 8 deaths, stroke for 3, and refractory congestive heart failure for 3. The incidence of these complications in these patients was many times higher than for normal and hypertensive groups of comparable age, and was similar to rates found in patients with familial hypercholesterolemia. These findings indicate that accelerated atherosclerosis is a major risk to long-term survivors on maintenance hemodialysis.

Although a number of factors may play a role in causing the accelerated atherosclerosis seen in these patients, it is likely that hypertriglyceridemia is one of the important factors. Accordingly, interest has developed in exploring possible treatment approaches in order to reduce or eliminate hyperlipidemia in patients with chronic renal insufficiency. Drug treatment in such patients requires very close surveillance. Thus, it was recently reported that muscle weakness and tenderness, together with a rise in serum creatine kinase, were noted in 5 uremic patients treated with 1–2 g clofibrate/day because of hyperlipidemia (Pierides *et al.*, 1975). Drug toxicity was associated with excessively high levels of the unesterified acid form of clofibrate (the form normally found in the circulation) in serum. Since clofibrate is normally excreted from the body mainly as the glucuronide conjugate in the urine, it can be anticipated that patients with chronic renal failure might require relatively small doses of clofibrate in order to achieve lipid-lowering effects without drug toxicity.

Different results have been seen in different clinics with regard to the incidence of hyperlipidemia in renal failure patients after successful renal transplantation. Casaretto *et al.* (1974) reported a high incidence of hyperlipidemia in 41 renal transplant patients. In contrast, Beaumont *et al.* (1975) reported that most (78%) of 42 patients with a successful renal transplant had a normal serum lipid profile. The possible role of corticosteroid immunosuppressive therapy in affecting serum lipid levels in these patients was commented on in both reports. Further data are needed with regard to serum lipid levels and other metabolic and pharmacological parameters in renal transplant patients.

6.8. Diabetes Mellitus and Hyperlipidemia

Hyperlipidemia, particularly hypertriglyceridemia, commonly occurs in patients with inadequately treated diabetes mellitus when blood sugar levels are high and the disease is uncontrolled. In many instances, the hypertriglyceridemia appears to be a consequence of insulin deficiency, with associated reduced activity of lipoprotein lipase. With better blood glucose control, however, lower levels of plasma lipids are observed.

Kaufmann *et al.* (1975) measured plasma lipids, blood glucose, and urinary glucose excretion in 270 juvenile diabetic children on admission to and throughout periods of summer camping, during which the effects of a "usual" and a "modified" diabetic diet were assessed. The usual diabetic diet contained 700–1500 mg cholesterol/day, with a polyunsaturated:saturated (P:S) ratio of 0.1; the modified diet limited cholesterol to 300 mg/day, with a P:S ratio of 1.0. Both diets maintained calories with 40% as fat, 40% as carbohydrate, and 20% as protein. Analysis of fasting blood glucose, glucose excretion, and body weight indicated that the groups were comparable except for the diet used. Elevated mean levels of cholesterol and triglyceride were approximately equally distributed in diabetic children of both sexes on admission to camp, with 24% demonstrating hyperlipidemia. Thus, the plasma lipids in these juvenile diabetics were elevated when first observed. On admission, the frequency of observed lipoprotein phenotypes was: 11% type II, 10% type IV, and 3% type V. After following the usual diet, 21% were type II, 1% type IV, and none type V, with almost no reduction in the overall incidence of hyperlipoproteinemia, despite lower triglyceride and glucose levels. After the modified diet, however, the incidence of hyperlipoproteinemia was reduced to 5%, with 4% type II and 1% type IV. Thus, control of blood sugar levels along with a diabetic diet containing low cholesterol and higher polyunsaturated fat significantly reduced the incidence of hyperlipidemia, more effectively than control of blood sugar levels alone.

Evidence has been reported that diabetes mellitus and the genetic forms of hypertriglyceridemia appear to be inherited as separate disorders (Brunzell *et al.*, 1975). Among 91 patients whose diagnosis of a genetic type of hypertriglyceridemia was based on family studies, 27% had diabetes. To determine whether the familial forms of hypertriglyceridemia and genetic diabetes mellitus are inherited together or independently, the adult first-degree relatives of these patients were investigated for the presence of diabetes. The frequency of diabetes in first-degree relatives of the 25 diabetic patients with a familial form of hypertriglyceridemia was identical, whether such relatives were hyperlipidemic or not (13% vs. 14.7%). The frequency of diabetes in both the hyperlipidemic and the normolipidemic relatives of the 66 nondiabetic hypertriglyceridemic index cases also was not significantly different (6.2% vs. 4.0%). These results indicate that while diabetes is frequently associated with hypertriglyceridemia, genetic hypertriglyceridemia, *per se,* does not carry an increased risk of diabetes. Following treatment of diabetes, elevated triglyceride levels in index cases with both familial hypertriglyceridemia and untreated diabetes returned to lower, but still elevated, levels. Thus, the interaction of untreated diabetes and a familial form of hypertriglyceridemia determines the level of plasma triglyceride in a patient with both disorders.

6.9. Treatment of Hyperlipidemia

6.9.1. Diet

Treatment of hyperlipidemia is based on the assumption that lowering the coronary risk factor will result in a commensurate lowering of coronary risk itself. Definitive evidence that changing a coronary risk factor will reduce coronary risk is available only for the case of cigarette smoking. Thus, the Framingham study has shown that persons who stop smoking have a coronary risk close to that of persons who never smoked. For the factor of hyperlipidemia, however, such proof is not now available, although large-scale clinical trials aimed at trying to obtain such evidence are in progress.

Management of hyperlipidemia first involves the modification of the diet so as to lower the serum cholesterol level or the triglyceride level or both. It is known that the plasma cholesterol concentration is influenced by the amount of cholesterol in the diet, and also by the amounts of saturated and polyunsaturated fat in the diet. In one study, Mattson et al. (1972) fed increasing amounts of cholesterol to human volunteers, and found consistent dose-related increases in serum cholesterol levels. Moreover, Connor et al. (1964) have shown that the effect of dietary cholesterol is independent of that of dietary fat. Numerous studies have shown that polyunsaturated fat has a hypocholesterolemic effect, whereas saturated fats in the diet have an opposite effect.

On the basis of these and other observations, the American Heart Association has described and recommended therapy with a fat-controlled diet limited in cholesterol and saturated animal fat, with caloric intake appropriate for the patient to achieve and maintain an ideal body weight. Weight reduction is stressed in overweight patients, particularly in those with hypertriglyceridemia. Dietary cholesterol is limited to less than 300 mg/day, the fat content to 35% of total calories, and the saturated fat to less than 10% of calories. With such a diet, one can anticipate a 10–20% reduction in serum cholesterol concentration (Wilson et al., 1971; Lees and Wilson, 1971). Studies conducted with this diet have also demonstrated reductions in serum triglyceride concentration (Wilson et al., 1971; Hall et al., 1972), particularly in patients who are both hypertriglyceridemic and overweight. It was concluded (Hall et al., 1972) that "a low carbohydrate diet is seldom required to achieve significant lowering of serum triglyceride in middle-aged, obese, hypertriglyceridemic men, with or without hypercholesterolemia, provided that weight loss is accomplished and sustained and intake of saturated fat and cholesterol is low." The importance of weight reduction in hypertriglyceridemic men who are only very slightly overweight has recently been emphasized (Blacket et al., 1975). It was concluded that, ideally, no weight should be gained after reaching maturity.

Mattson et al. (1975) studied the effects of trans isomers of unsaturated fatty acids on the plasma lipid levels of men. The problem was addressed because partially hydrogenated vegetable oils sold in the United States have significant contents of such trans fatty acids. It was felt important to determine whether the isomeric structure of an unsaturated acid alters the effect of that acid on the blood lipid levels. A group of 33 men was fed for 21 days a formula diet that supplied 38% of their calories as fat. The fatty acid composition of the diet was 25% saturates, 16% polyunsaturates, and 58% monounsaturates. All the unsaturated acids were in the *cis* configuration. The subjects were then divided into two groups. One group of 17 men continued on the same diet. In the other group, 80% of the dietary fat was replaced with a hydrogenated fat in which 50–60% of the mono- and polyunsaturated fatty acids were in the *trans* configuration. Except for the presence or absence of *trans* acids, the fatty acid intakes of the two groups were the same. Over the 4-week period that the two diets were consumed, the group receiving the hydrogenated fat showed no change in plasma cholesterol or triglyceride levels, compared to the subjects consuming the unhydrogenated fat. Thus, the effect of a hydrogenated fat on blood lipid levels is determined by its fatty acid composition, and this effect is not altered by the isomeric form of the unsaturated acids.

6.9.2. The Coronary Drug Project

Many patients will remain hyperlipidemic despite dietary therapy, and in these patients, the question of the desirability of drug treatment to lower serum lipid levels must then be considered. It is often difficult to decide whether a given patient warrants treatment with lipid-lowering drugs. Many clinical investigators in this field currently believe that the benefit/risk ratio is high enough in the high-risk patients (lipid values above the 95th percentile) to warrant such treatment. This is particularly true for those patients who manifest other risk factors or who have a familial form of hyperlipidemia. Several multicenter primary prevention clinical trials, designed to evaluate the effectiveness of treatment in reducing coronary risk in patients without clinical heart disease, are currently in progress (see below).

A large, long-term secondary prevention clinical trial, the Coronary Drug Project, was completed recently (The Coronary Drug Project Research Group, 1975). The major objective of this trial was to test the efficacy and safety of several lipid-lowering drugs, compared to placebo, in the long-term therapy of coronary heart disease in men with proven previous myocardial infarction. The study population comprised men, originally 30–64 years of age, who had recovered from one or more verified episodes of myocardial infarction. From 1966 to 1969, the 53 clinical centers collaborating in this project recruited 8341 patients who were randomly assigned to 6 treatment groups. The 6 treatment regimens were: conjugated estrogens, 2.5 mg/day; conjugated estrogens, 5.0 mg/day; dextrothyroxine sodium, 6.0 mg/day; clofibrate 1.8 g/day; niacin, 3.0

g/day; and a lactose placebo, 3.8 g/day. The allocation schedule was designed to assure approximately 5 patients in the placebo group for every 2 patients in any of the other groups. Approximately 1100 men were allocated to each of the 5 active drug-treatment groups, and 2789 men to the placebo group. The study was double-blind in the sense that neither the patient nor the clinic staff was informed of the patient's drug allocation, except in the rare event of a medical emergency.

Three of the Coronary Drug Project treatment regimens were discontinued before the scheduled completion of the project. First, the 5.0-mg/day estrogen regimen was discontinued in 1970, chiefly because of an excess number of nonfatal cardiovascular events in this group when compared with placebo and lack of evidence of efficacy with respect to the primary endpoint, total mortality. Dextrothyroxine sodium was discontinued late in 1971, primarily because of an excess number of deaths in this treatment group compared with the placebo group, particularly among men with certain risk factors at entry. Finally, the 2.5-mg/day estrogen regimen was discontinued in 1973, chiefly due to a suggestion of both excess incidence of thromboembolism and excess mortality from cancer, along with a small excess in total mortality as compared with the placebo group.

The patients in the three groups that were continued to the scheduled completion of the project (clofibrate, niacin, and placebo) had their study medication terminated during June through August 1974. The mean length of time from randomization of these patients to cessation of drug treatment was 74 months. All the surviving patients were in the study for at least 54 months, and 96% for at least 5 years.

The primary endpoint established for determination of drug efficacy in the project was total mortality. Other major endpoints included cause-specific mortality, particularly coronary mortality and sudden death, and nonfatal cardiovasulcar events, such as recurrent myocardial infarction, acute coronary insufficiency, development of angina pectoris, congestive heart failure, stroke, pulmonary embolism, and arrhythmias.

With regard to clofibrate, no evidence was obtained for significant efficacy of clofibrate as concerns total mortality or cause-specific mortality. The 5-year total mortalities were 20.0% for clofibrate and 20.9% for placebo, a small difference that did not approach statistical significance. No subgroups of the study population were identified in which clofibrate showed clear benefit with regard to mortality. There were somewhat, but not statistically significant, lower rates in the clofibrate group with respect to coronary death and the combination of coronary death or definite, nonfatal myocardial infarction.

With regard to toxicity, there was a statistically significant excess incidence in the clofibrate group as compared to the placebo group of the following: thromboembolism (5-year rate of 5.2% vs. 3.2%); new angina pectoris (52.2% vs. 44.7% in 5 years); new intermittent claudication (21.0% vs. 16.9% in 5 years); and cardiac arrhythmias (5-year rates of 33.3% vs. 28.2%). There was also an excess incidence of the endpoint of any definite or suspected nonfatal cardiovascular event in the clofibrate as compared with the placebo group. In addition, there was a statistically highly significant increase in clinically apparent gallstones among patients taking clofibrate (3.0% vs. 1.3% in the placebo group in 5 years). An increased incidence of clinically apparent gallstones has also been observed in the W.H.O. Cooperative Trial of the primary prevention of ischemic heart disease using clofibrate that is being carried out in Europe (Cooper *et al.*, 1975). It was concluded that the Coronary Drug Project provides no evidence on which to recommend the use of clofibrate in the treatment of persons with coronary heart disease.

For the niacin treatment group, there was also no evidence of efficacy of drug treatment with regard to total mortality and cause-specific mortality. No subgroup of patients was identified in which niacin showed a definite beneficial effect with respect to 5-year mortality. The niacin group did experience a statistically significant lower incidence of definite, nonfatal myocardial infarction than the placebo group (5-year rates of 8.9% vs. 12.2%). On the other hand, the incidence of atrial fibrillation and of other cardiac arrhythmias was statistically significantly higher among men taking niacin than in the placebo group. Data from the study confirmed previously reported findings of increased incidence of dermatological and gastrointestinal problems and elevated levels of serum enzymes, serum uric acid, and glucose in men taking niacin. The long-term clinical significance, if any, of these chemical changes is unknown.

The results of the Coronary Drug Project indicate that treatment of myocardial infarction survivors with the drugs tested is in general not warranted. Unfortunately, the results of the project do not provide information relevant to the question of whether treatment of hyperlipidemic persons without clinical heart disease with these (or other) lipid-lowering drugs would be beneficial in preventing the development of coronary heart disease. The Coronary Drug Project conclusions are highly limited, because the project was not restricted to hyperlipidemic patients and because it can be expected that men with already far-advanced coronary atherosclerosis (previous myocardial infarction) would be the least amenable to preventive therapy. Thus, the primary prevention trials in hyperlipidemic men that are now in progress have been more appropriately designed to address the question of the clinical efficacy of preventive treatment with lipid-lowering drugs.

6.9.3. Primary Prevention of Ischemic Heart Disease

Information about the presence of asymptomatic coronary artery disease in apparently healthy subjects with various forms of hyperlipidemia was reported by Carlson *et al.* (1975). Evidence for such asymptomatic coronary artery disease was sought by recording ECGs before and during exercise stress testing in hyperlipidemic men. In order to obtain a suitable study population, serum cholesterol and triglyceride levels were measured in approximately 12,000 men attending a screening center. A group of 130 symptom-free men (ages 35–65) was selected from the top 2% with the highest lipid values. This group and 59 normolipidemic controls were subjected to exercise stress-testing. The frequency of so-called ischemic ECG changes (ST-segment depressions, Minnesota code 4.1–4.4) increased with age in both the controls and the hyperlipidemic group. Ischemic ECG changes were significantly more common in all types of hyperlipidemia (lipoprotein phenotypes IIa, IIb, III, and IV) than in the controls. The high frequency of the exercise ECG changes in symptom-free men with hyperlipidemia was felt to reinforce the argument for early treatment of hyperlipidemia to prevent ischemic heart disease.

The question of whether treatment of hyperlipidemia with lipid-lowering drugs can prevent the development of ischemic heart disease is being addressed by two major collaborative clinical trials that are now in progress. One of these, an ongoing study by Oliver and his colleagues being conducted in Edinburgh, Prague, and Budapest, is a primary prevention trial using clofibrate to lower hyperlipidemia in men of ages 30–59 at entry. The other is the Lipid Research Clinic's primary prevention trial of cholestyramine resin in type II hyperlipoproteinemic men being sponsored by the National Heart and Lung Institute. A related clinical trial is the Multiple Risk Factor Intervention Trial, which will assess the effectiveness of measures to reduce elevated serum cholesterol (by diet), high blood pressure (by diet and drugs), and cigarette smoking. It is hoped that these studies will, in time, provide definitive evidence that intervention programs directed at known coronary risk factors, and specifically at hyperlipidemia, can indeed reduce coronary risk.

References

Ahrens, E. H., Jr., 1974, Homozygous hypercholesteremia and the portacaval shunt: The need for a concerted attack by surgeons and clinical researchers, *Lancet* **2**:449–451.

Bagdade, J. D., Porte, D., Jr., and Bierman, E. L., 1968, Hypertriglyceridemia: A metabolic consequence of chronic renal failure, *N. Engl. J. Med.* **279**:181–185.

Baker, H. N., Gotto, A. M., Jr., and Jackson, R. L., 1975, The primary structure of human plasma high density apolipoprotein glutamine I (ApoA-I). II. The amino acid sequence and alignment of cyanogen bromide fragments IV, III, and I, *J. Biol. Chem.* **250**:2725–2738.

Beaumont, J. L., Carlson, L. A., Cooper, G. R., Fejfar, Z., Fredrickson, D. S., and Strasser, T., 1970, Classification of hyperlipidemias and hyperlipoproteine-mias, *Bull. W. H. O.* **43**:891–915.

Beaumont, J. E., Luke, R. G., Galla, J. H., Rees, E. D., and Siegel, R. R., 1975, Normal serum-lipids in renal-transplant patients, *Lancet* **1**:599–601.

Bilheimer, D. W., Goldstein, J. L., Grundy, S. M., and Brown, M. S., 1975, Reduction in cholesterol and low density lipoprotein synthesis after portaca-val shunt surgery in a patient with homozygous familial hypercholesterole-mia, *J. Clin. Invest.* **56**:1420–1430.

Blacket, R. B., Leelarthaepin, B., Woodhill, J. M., and Palmer, A. J., 1975, Type-IV hyperlipidemia and weight-gain after maturity, *Lancet* **2**:517–520.

Breslow, J. L., Spaulding, D. R., Lux, S. E., Levy, R. I., and Lees, R. S., 1975, Homozygous familial hypercholesterolemia: A possible biochemical explana-tion of clinical heterogeneity, *N. Engl. J. Med.* **293**:900–903.

Brewer, H. B., Jr., Shulman, R., Herbert, P., Ronan, R., and Wehrly, K., 1974, The complete amino acid sequence of alanine apolipoprotein (apoC-III), an apolipoprotein from human plasma very low density lipoproteins, *J. Biol. Chem.* **249**:4975–4984.

Brown, M. S., and Goldstein, J. L., 1974, Suppression of 3-hydroxy-3-methyl-glutaryl coenzyme A reductase activity and inhibition of growth of human fibroblasts by 7-ketocholesterol, *J. Biol. Chem.* **249**:7306–7314.

Brown, M. S., and Goldstein, J. L., 1975, Regulation of the activity of the low density lipoprotein receptor in human fibroblasts, *Cell* **6**:307–316.

Brown, M. S., Brannan, P. G., Bohmfalk, H. A., Brunschede, G. Y., Dana, S. E., Helgeson, J., and Goldstein, J. L., 1975a, Use of mutant fibroblasts in the analysis of the regulation of cholesterol metabolism in human cells, *J. Cell. Physiol.* **85**:425–436.

Brown, M. S., Faust, J. R., and Goldstein, J. L., 1975b, Role of the low density lipoprotein receptor in regulating the content of free and esterified choles-terol in human fibroblasts, *J. Clin. Invest.* **55**:783–793.

Brunzell, J. D., Hazzard, W. R., Motulsky, A. G., and Bierman, E. L., 1975, Evidence for diabetes mellitus and genetic forms of hypertriglyceridemia as independent entities, *Metabolism* **24**:1115.

Carlson, L. A., and Böttiger, L. E., 1972, Ischemic heart disease in relation to fasting values of plasma triglycerides and cholesterol, *Lancet* **1**:865–868.

Carlson, L. A., Ekelund, L. G., and Olsson, A. G., 1975, Frequency of ischemic exercise E.C.G. changes in symptom-free men with various forms of primary hyperlipemia, *Lancet* **2**:1–3.

Casaretto, A., Goldsmith, R., Marchioro, T. L., and Bagdade, J. D., 1974, Hyperli-pidemia after successful renal transplantation, *Lancet* **1**:481–484.

Connor, W. E., Stone, D. B., and Hodges, R. E., 1964, The interrelated effects of dietary cholesterol and fat upon human serum lipid levels, *J. Clin. Invest.* **43**:1691–1696.

Cooper, J., Geizerova, H., and Oliver, M. F., 1975, Clofibrate and gallstones, *Lancet* **1**:1083.

The Coronary Drug Project Research Group, 1975, Clofibrate and niacin in coronary heart disease, *J. Amer. Med. Assoc.* **231**:360–381.

Eisenberg, S., and Levy, R. I., 1975, Lipoprotein metabolism, *in: Advances in Lipid Research*, Vol. 13 (R. Paoletti and D. Kritchevsky, eds.), pp. 1–89, Academic Press, New York.

Eisenberg, S., Bilheimer, D. W., Levy, R. I., and Lindgren, F. T., 1973, On the metabolic conversion of human plasma very low density lipoprotein to low density lipoprotein, *Biochim. Biophys. Acta* **326**:361–377.

Fogelman, A. M., Edmond, J., Seager, J., and Popják, G., 1975, Abnormal induction of 3-hydroxy-3-methylglutaryl coenzyme A reductase in leukocytes from subjects with heterozygous familial hypercholesterolemia, *J. Biol. Chem.* **250**:2045–2055.

Fredrickson, D. S., 1975, Editorial: It's time to be practical, *Circulation* **51**:209–211.

Fredrickson, D. S., Levy, R. I., and Lees, R. S., 1967, Fat transport in lipoproteins—An integrated approach to mechanisms and disorders, *N. Engl. J. Med.* **276**:34.

Fredrickson, D. S., Morganroth, J., and Levy, R. I., 1975, Type III hyperlipoproteinemia: An analysis of two contemporary definitions, *Ann. Intern. Med.* **82**:150–157.

Glomset, J. A., and Norum, K. R., 1973, The metabolic role of lecithin:cholesterol acyltransferase: Perspectives from pathology, *Adv. Lipid Res.* **11**:1–65.

Glomset, J. A., Norum, K. R., Nichols, A. V., King, W. C., Mitchell, C. D., Applegate, K. R., Gong, E. L., and Gjone, E., 1975, Plasma lipoproteins in familial lecithin:cholesterol acyltransferase deficiency: Effects of dietary manipulation, *Scand J. Clin. Lab. Invest.* **35**(Suppl. 142):3–30.

Goldstein, J. L., and Brown, M. S., 1975, Hyperlipidemia in coronary heart disease: A biochemical genetic approach, *J. Lab. Clin. Med.* **85**:15–25.

Goldstein, J. L., Hazzard, W. R., Bierman, E. L., Schrott, H. G., and Motulsky, A. G., 1973a, Hyperlipidemia in coronary heart disease. I. Lipid levels in 500 survivors of myocardial infarction, *J. Clin. Invest.* **52**:1533–1543.

Goldstein, J. L., Schrott, H. G., Hazzard, W. R., Bierman, E. L., and Motulsky, A. G., 1973b, Hyperlipidemia in coronary heart disease. II. Genetic analysis of lipid levels in 176 families and delineation of a new inherited disorder, combined hyperlipidemia, *J. Clin. Invest.* **52**:1544–1568.

Goldstein, J. L., Brunschede, G. Y., and Brown, M. S., 1975a, Inhibition of the proteolytic degradation of low density lipoprotein in human fibroblasts by chloroquine, concanavalin A, and Triton WR 1339, *J. Biol. Chem.* **250**:7854–7862.

Goldstein, J. L., Dana, S. E., Brunschede, G. Y., and Brown, M. S., 1975b, Genetic heterogeneity in familial hypercholesterolemia: Evidence for two different mutations affecting functions of low-density lipoprotein receptor, *Proc. Nat. Acad. Sci. U.S.A.* **72**:1092–1096.

Goldstein, J. L., Dana, S. E., Faust, J. R., Beaudet, A. L., and Brown, M. S., 1975c, Role of lysosomal acid lipase in the metabolism of plasma low density lipoprotein: Observations in cultured fibroblasts from a patient with cholesteryl ester storage disease, *J. Biol. Chem.* **250:**8487–8495.

Hall, Y., Stamler, J., Cohen, D. B., Mojonnier, L., Epstein, M. B., Berkson, D. M., Whipple, I. T., and Catchings, S., 1972, Effectiveness of a low saturated fat, low cholesterol, weight-reducing diet for the control of hypertriglyceridemia, *Atherosclerosis* **16:**389–403.

Havel, R. J., 1975, Editorial: Hyperlipoproteinemia: Problems in diagnosis and challenges posed by the "type III" disorder, *Ann. Intern. Med.* **82:**273, 274.

Hazzard, W. R., and Bierman, E. L., 1975a, Broad-β disease versus endogenous hypertriglyceridemia: Levels and lipid composition of chylomicrons and very low density lipoproteins during fat-free feeding and alimentary lipemia, *Metabolism* **24:**817–828.

Hazzard, W. R., and Bierman, E. L., 1975b, The spectrum of electrophoretic mobility of very low density lipoproteins: Role of slower migrating species in endogenous hypertriglyceridemia (type IV hyperlipoproteinemia) and broad-β disease (type III), *J. Lab. Clin. Med.* **86:**239–252.

Hazzard, W. R., Goldstein, J. L., Schrott, H. G., Motulsky, A. G., and Bierman, E. L., 1973, Hyperlipidemia in coronary heart disease. III. Evaluation of lipoprotein phenotypes of 156 genetically defined survivors of myocardial infarction, *J. Clin. Invest.* **52:**1569–1577.

Hazzard, W. R., O'Donnell, T. F., and Lee, Y. L., 1975, Broad-β disease (type III hyperlipoproteinemia) in a large kindred: Evidence for a monogenic mechanism, *Ann. Intern. Med.* **82:**141–149.

Jackson, R. L., Sparrow, J. T., Baker, H. N., Morrisett, J. D., Taunton, O. D., and Gotto, A. M., Jr., 1974, The primary structure of apolipoprotein-serine, *J. Biol. Chem.* **249:**5308–5313.

Kane, J. P., Sata, T., Hamilton, R. L., and Havel, R. J., 1975, Apoprotein composition of very low density lipoproteins of human serum, *J. Clin. Invest.* **56:**1622–1634.

Kannel, W. B., Dawber, T. R., Kagan, A., Revotskie, N., and Stokes, J., III, 1961, Factors of risk in the development of coronary heart disease—Six year follow-up experience. The Framingham study, *Ann. Intern. Med.* **55:**33–50.

Kannel, W. B., Castelli, W. P., Gordon, T., and McNamara, P. M., 1971, Serum cholesterol, lipoproteins and the risk of coronary heart disease, *Ann. Intern. Med.* **74:**1–12.

Kaufmann, R. L., Assal, J. Ph., Soeldner, J. S., Wilmshurst, E. G., Lemaire, J. R., Gleason, R. E., and White, P., 1975, Plasma lipid levels in diabetic children. Effect of diet restricted in cholesterol and saturated fats, *Diabetes* **24:**672–679.

Keys, A., 1975, Coronary heart disease—The global picture, *Atherosclerosis* **22:**149–192.

Khachadurian, A. K., Lipson, M., and Kawahara, F. S., 1975, Diagnosis of familial hypercholesterolemia by measurement of sterol synthesis in cultured skin fibroblasts, *Atherosclerosis* **21:**235–244.

Krogh, L., and Wickens, J. T., 1974, Portacaval shunt for hypercholesterolemia, *S. Afr. Med. J.* **48:**(56):2302.

Lees, R. S., and Wilson, D. E., 1971, The treatment of hyperlipidemia, *N. Engl. J. Med.* **284:**186–195.

Levy, R. I., Morganroth, J., and Rifkind, B. M., 1974, Drug therapy. Treatment of hyperlipidemia, *N. Engl. J. Med.* **290:**1295–1301.

Lindner, A., Charra, B., Sherrard, D. J., and Scribner, B. H., 1974, Accelerated atherosclerosis in prolonged maintenance hemodialysis, *N. Engl. J. Med.* **290:**697–701.

Lux, S. E., John, K. M., Ronan, R., and Brewer, H. B., Jr., 1972, Isolation and characterization of the tryptic and cyanogen bromide peptides of ApoLy-Gln II (Apo-II), a plasma high density apolipoprotein, *J. Biol. Chem.* **247:**7519–7527.

Mattson, F. H., Erickson, B. A., and Kligman, A. M., 1972, Effect of dietary cholesterol on serum cholesterol in man, *Amer. J. Clin. Nutr.* **25:**589–594.

Mattson, F. H., Hollenbach, E. J., and Kligman, A. M., 1975, Effect of hydrogenated fat on the plasma cholesterol and triglyceride levels of man, *Amer. J. Clin. Nutr.* **28:**726–731.

McCosh, E. J., Solangi, K., Rivers, J. M., and Goodman, A., 1975, Hypertriglyceridemia in patients with chronic renal insufficiency, *Amer. J. Clin. Nutr.* **28:**1036–1043.

Mishkel, M. A., Nazir, D. J., and Crowther, S., 1975, A longitudinal assessment of lipid ratios in the diagnosis of type III hyperlipoproteinemia, *Clin. Chim. Acta* **58:**121–136.

Mitchell, S., and Levy, R. I., 1974, Portacaval shunt in familial hypercholesterolemia, *Lancet* **2:**1263, 1264.

Morganroth, J., Levy, R. I., and Fredrickson, D. S., 1975, The biochemical, clinical, and genetic features of type III hyperlipoproteinemia, *Ann. Intern. Med.* **82:**158–174.

Morrisett, J. D., Jackson, R. L., and Gotto, A. M., Jr., 1975, Lipoproteins: Structure and function, *Annu. Rev. Biochem.* **44:**183–207.

Nikkilä, E. A., and Aro, A., 1973, Family study of serum lipids and lipoproteins in coronary heart disease, *Lancet* **1:**954–959.

Norum, K. R., Glomset, J. A., Nichols, A. V., Forte, T., Albers, J. J., King, W. C., Mitchell, C. D., Applegate, K. R., Gong, E. L., Cabana, V., and Gjone, E., 1975, Plasma lipoproteins in familial lecithin:cholesterol acyltransferase deficiency: Effects of incubation with lecithin:cholesterol acyltransferase *in vitro*, *Scand. J. Clin. Lab. Invest.* **35** (Suppl. 142):31–55.

Patsch, J. R., Sailer, S., and Braunsteiner, H., 1975, Lipoprotein of the density 1.006–1.020 in the plasma of patients with type III hyperlipoproteinemia in the postabsorptive state, *Eur. J. Clin. Invest.* **5:**45–55.

Pierides, A. M., Alvarez-Ude, F., Kerr, D. N. S., and Skillen, A. W., 1975, Clofibrate-induced muscle damage in patients with chronic renal failure, *Lancet* **2:**1279–1282.

Rose, H. G., Kranz, P., Weinstock, M., Juliano, J., and Haft, J. I., 1973, Inheritance of combined hyperlipoproteinemia: Evidence for a new lipoprotein phenotype, *Amer. J. Med.* **54:**148–160.

Shulman, R. S., Herbert, P. N., Wehrly, K., and Fredrickson, D. S., 1975, The complete amino acid sequence of C-I (ApoLpSer), an apolipoprotein from human very low density lipoproteins, *J. Biol. Chem.* **250**:182–190.

Sigler, G. F., Soutar, A., Gotto, A. M., Jr., and Sparrow, J. T., 1975, The total synthesis of apolipoprotein-C-I, *Circulation* **52** (Suppl. II):II-17.

Sigurdsson, G., Nicoll, A., and Lewis, B., 1975, Conversion of very low density lipoprotein to low density lipoprotein: A metabolic study of apolipoprotein B kinetics in human subjects, *J. Clin. Invest.* **56**:1481–1490.

Simons, L. A., Reichl, D., Myant, N. B., and Mancini, M., 1975, The metabolism of the apoprotein of plasma low density lipoprotein in familial hyperbetalipoproteinemia in the homozygous form, *Atherosclerosis* **21**:283–298.

Slack, J., 1969, Risks of ischemic heart disease in familial hyperlipoproteinemia states, *Lancet* **2**:1380–1382.

Starzl, T. E., Putnam, C. W., Chase, H. P., and Porter, K. A., 1973, Portacaval shunt in hyperlipoproteinemia, *Lancet* **2**:940–944.

Starzl, T. E., Chase, H. P., Putnam, C. W., Nora, J. J., Fennell, R. H., Jr., and Porter, K. A., 1974, Portacaval shunt in hyperlipidemia, *Lancet* **2**:1263.

Stein, E. A., Mieny, C., Spitz, L., Saaron, I., Pettifor, J., Heimann, K. W., Bersohn, I., and Dinner, M., 1975, Portacaval shunt in four patients with homozygous hypercholesterolemia, *Lancet* **1**:832–835.

Stone, N. J., Levy, R. I., Fredrickson, D. S., and Verter, J., 1974, Coronary artery disease in 116 kindred with familial type II hyperlipoproteinemia, *Circulation* **49**:476–488.

Teisberg, P., Gjone, E., and Olaisen, B., 1975, Genetics of LCAT (lecithin:cholesterol acyltransferase) deficiency, *Ann. Hum. Genet. London* **38**:327–331.

Thompson, G. R., Lowenthal, R., and Myant, N. B., 1975, Plasma exchange in the management of homozygous familial hypercholesterolemia, *Lancet* **1**:1208–1211.

Torsvik, H., Fischer, J. E., Feldman, H. A., and Lees, R. S., 1975, Effects of intravenous hyperalimentation on plasma-lipoproteins in severe familial hypercholesterolemia, *Lancet* **1**:601–604.

Wilson, W. S., Hulley, S. B., Burrows, M. I., and Nichaman, M. Z., 1971, Serial lipid and lipoprotein responses to the American Heart Association fat-controlled diet, *Amer. J. Med.* **51**:491–503.

Metabolism of Amino Acids and Organic Acids

Leon E. Rosenberg and Kay Tanaka

7.1. Introduction

Investigations into the metabolism of amino acids and their organic acid catabolites can be seen to have followed a few new and old paths during the interval covered by this chapter. Whereas the 1960's seemed to regale us with a new "aminoacidopathy" or "organic acidemia" monthly, recent years have witnessed a definite slowing in the rate of appearance of such "new" diseases. The field has, we believe, moved off its heady descriptive trail, in which a good nose (literally and figuratively), an alert house staff, and an expensive amino acid analyzer or gas chromatograph assured the investigator of at least a modicum of success. It is now traversing an equally exciting, albeit more demanding, analytical route. This route emphasizes pathophysiology, enzymology, and regulation. It asks "how"

LEON E. ROSENBERG and KAY TANAKA • Yale University, New Haven, Connecticut 06510.

rather than "what." Its tools include cell culture, enzyme characterization, and mass spectrometry, thereby emphasizing its dependence on, and linkage to, the basic biomedical sciences of biochemistry, genetics, and cell biology.

The field has continued to evolve clinically as well as scientifically. It is increasingly concerned with early diagnosis, so as to employ dietary or pharmacological means to limit, where possible, the consequences of the metabolic derangement. It has begun to concern itself with prenatal detection as well as postnatal screening, and we expect contributions from the former to be every bit as great as those from the latter.

Our aim in each of these volumes will be to select a few areas that illustrate these themes. If our criticism is sometimes sharp, we hope it is also fair. If our topic choices are seen as capricious, we hope they are also timely. Interested readers can avail themselves of several recent books (Stanbury *et al.*, 1972; Scriver and Rosenberg, 1973; Nyhan, 1974) or chapters (Rosenberg and Scriver, 1974; Tanaka, 1975) that cover the field comprehensively rather than selectively.

7.2. Hyperammonemia and Urea Cycle Enzymes

7.2.1. Ammonia Formation and Removal

Ammonia, a ubiquitous end product of protein metabolism in mammals, is produced in large amounts during the oxidative deamination of amino acids. If allowed to accumulate, ammonia is highly toxic because it impairs the vital tricarboxylic acid cycle. Thus, mammals have evolved a complex and highly efficient system for ammonia disposal. It may be reutilized in the synthesis of amino acids by reversal of deamination reactions, thereby participating indirectly in the synthesis of purines, pyrimidines, and porphyrins. It condenses with glutamate to form glutamine. It is secreted into the urine. All these mechanisms, however, are quantitatively insignificant when compared to the major pathway of ammonia detoxification, the synthesis of urea. Ureagenesis takes place in the liver via the complex cycle originally predicted and described by Krebs and Henseleit (Fig. 1).

The overall reaction catalyzed by this cycle is simple:

$$2\ NH_3 + CO_2 + 3\ ATP + 3\ H_2O \rightarrow urea + 2\ ADP + AMP + 4\ P_i$$

Its details, however, are complex, as shown by the participation of five enzymes and seven chemical intermediates in two subcellular compart-

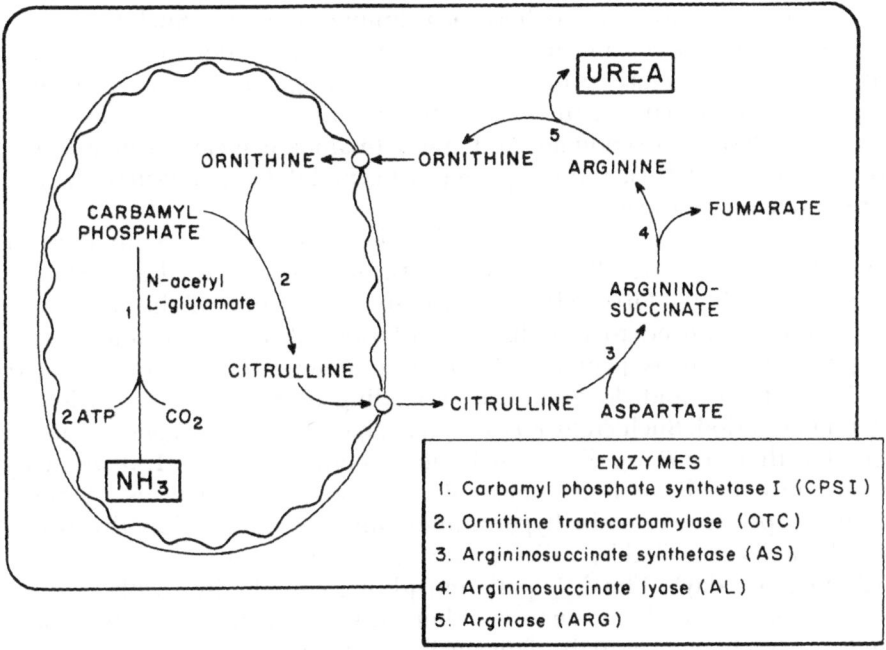

Fig. 1. Krebs-Henseleit urea cycle in liver cell mitochondria and cytoplasm. The five urea cycle enzymes are listed and their sites of action indicated by the numbers. (Reproduced from Gelehrter and Snodgrass, 1974, with permission of author and publisher.)

ments. The cycle is initiated in the mitochondrial matrix, where carbamyl phosphate synthetase I (CPS I) catalyzes the formation of carbamyl phosphate from ammonia, ATP, and bicarbonate. Carbamyl phosphate then condenses with ornithine to form citrulline, this reaction being catalyzed by a second mitochondrial enzyme, ornithine transcarbamylase (OTC). Citrulline diffuses out of the mitochondrion into the cytosol, where urea synthesis is completed by three additional enzymic reactions: the synthesis of argininosuccinate from citrulline and aspartate, the cleavage of argininosuccinate to arginine and fumarate, and the conversion of arginine to urea and ornithine. The latter amino acid reenters the mitochondrion via a specific carrier system, thereby completing the cyclic process.

7.2.2. Ammonia Intoxication

When the system for the removal of ammonia fails in man, ammonia accumulates in tissues and blood, and produces a characteristic encephalopathy highlighted by asterexis, hyperpnea, lethargy, and coma. In adults, hyperammonemia is usually caused by acquired hepatocellular dysfunction secondary to cirrhosis or fulminant hepatitis. Such processes, of course, also occur in children, but three other etiological bases for hyperammonemia are prominent in the young: (1) Reye's syndrome, which will be discussed in detail subsequently; (2) a variety of inborn errors of lysine, propionate, and methylmalonate metabolism (see the review by Hsia, 1974); and (3) specific, inherited defects of each of the five urea cycle enzymes shown in Fig. 1.

The latter group of disorders have been reviewed recently (Scriver and Rosenberg, 1973; Bachmann, 1974), but a few general remarks are appropriate here. First, when the activity of any one of the urea cycle enzymes is reduced to less than 1% of normal, ammonia intoxication appears as soon as protein feeding is initiated, and is almost always followed by a rapid downhill course leading to coma and death in the neonatal period. Such children often have blood ammonia concentrations greater than 1000 μg/dl (normal values being less than 150 μg/dl by commonly used methods). Second, less severe deficiencies of these enzymes produce episodic hyperammonemia and encephalopathy, which can be well controlled by a diet moderately restricted in protein (less than 1.5 g/kg per day). Third, hepatic morphology in children with primary defects of urea cycle enzymes is either entirely normal or demonstrates mild fatty change. Fourth, deficiencies of argininosuccinate synthetase, argininosuccinate lyase, arginase, and (probably) CPS I are each inherited as autosomal recessive traits, whereas OTC deficiency is X-linked (Short *et al.*, 1973; Goldstein *et al.*, 1974; Cathelineau *et al.*, 1974; Ricciuti *et al.*, 1976). It is the latter enzymatic disturbance that we shall focus on.

7.2.3. Biochemical and Clinical Variations in Ornithine Transcarbamylase Deficiency

Females heterozygous for any X-linked trait (e.g., hemophilia, glucose-6-phosphate dehydrogenase deficiency, Duchenne muscular dystrophy) show marked variation in biochemical and clinical phenotype because of random inactivation of one of the two X chromosomes in their cells. Tissues of such females characteristically contain two clones of cells: those in which the normal X chromosome is active, and those in which the X chromosome carrying the mutation is active. Such mosaicism cannot occur in males, of course, since their cells contain only one X chromosome. Thus, biochemical or clinical variation among hemizygous-affected males for X-linked disorders implies that more than one mutation of the gene product in question has occurred, or, in simple terms, that genetic heterogeneity is present. It is now clear that such heterogeneity exists among males with OTC deficiency, and that the observed heterogeneity has clinical significance. Five variants have been well documented (reviewed by Saudubray *et al.*, 1975). One variant is characterized by dramatic hyperammonemia in the first days of life, with coma and death shortly thereafter (Campbell *et al.*, 1973). Such patients have less than 0.5% of normal OTC activity in liver, without significant alteration in pH optimum or apparent K_m's for ornithine and carbamyl phosphate. The second variant was reported by MacLeod *et al.* (1972) in a boy who developed ammonia intoxication at age 5 weeks, died at 4 months, and had 5% of normal OTC activity. This residual activity was not characterized further. A third variant (Saudubray *et al.*, 1975) was noted in a male infant who developed hyperammonemia at age 6 days, but who did well on a protein restricted diet and was thriving at age 15 months. His liver contained 6.5% of normal OTC activity, and this mutant enzyme demonstrated both an altered pH optimum and an increased K_m (reduced affinity) for ornithine. The fourth variant (Levin *et al.*, 1969) was documented in a male who presented with ammonia intoxication at age 9 months, and who also did well thereafter on a low-protein diet. In this child, hepatic OTC activity was reduced to 25% of normal when assayed at pH 7, but was normal when studied at pH 8. In addition, the K_m's for ornithine and carbamyl phosphate were decreased. Finally, to cite an example of the fifth variant, Saudubray *et al.* (1975) reported a male who suddenly developed hyperammonemia and died at age 8 years. Residual OTC activity was 10% of normal, and no aberrations of K_m's for substrates were found. To the biochemical geneticist, such variants imply multiple different mutations of the OTC molecule analogous to the many mutant hemoglobins or G6PD's. To the clinician, such variants mean that OTC deficiency in males may present early or late, may follow a benign or malignant course, and may or may not respond to optimal dietary modification.

7.2.4. Possible Modes of Successful Therapy for Severe Ornithine Transcarbamylase Deficiency

Studies by Campbell *et al.* (1973), Goldstein *et al.* (1974), and Gelehrter and Rosenberg (1975) indicated that males with virtually complete absence of OTC activity (less than 0.5% of normal) could not survive the neonatal period because they could not be given even minimal amounts of essential amino acids without developing lethal hyperammonemia. In such children, exchange transfusion, peritoneal dialysis, or pharmacotherapy seemed futile. Two recent reports, however, revive the possibility that even such severely affected males may be successfully managed. Snyderman *et al.* (1975) described a male infant with virtually complete absence of OTC activity who developed hyperammonemia and profound neurological disturbance in the first days of life. A series of exchange transfusions and peritoneal dialysis, accompanied by adequate caloric intake and ingestion of a special formula containing only the nine essential amino acids plus aspartate and arginine, resulted in clinical improvement and a fall in blood ammonia to less than 200 μg/dl by day 20. He then experienced a short period of well-being, only to succumb on day 54 from *Parapsilosis* pneumonia. Perhaps the fungal infection was an unavoidable complication of the heroic methods needed to sustain life (intravenous catheters, peritoneal dialysis, exchange transfusion, minimal amino acid intake). On the other hand, it is possible that barring such a complication, the boy's life may have been sustained. In either case, this report indicates that neonatal death is not unavoidable in such patients.

Batshaw *et al.* (1975) made a related observation. Based on their work in patients with end-stage renal insufficiency, they proposed that "nitrogen-free" diets could be administered to patients with hyperammonemia by feeding the keto acid analogues of essential amino acids, rather than the amino acids *per se*, thereby taking advantage of reverse transamination to sustain nutrition and limit ammonia formation. They used such a diet in a single 13-year-old girl with hyperammonemia and mental retardation due to partial CPS I deficiency. Her nitrogen balance was sustained on the keto acid–containing diet, and her blood ammonia fell. It now becomes important to test this approach in neonates with severe urea cycle enzyme deficiencies in the hope that such diet therapy, in conjunction with other modalities, may lessen the severity of hyperammonemia and permit normal growth and development.

7.2.5. Pathogenesis of Hyperammonemia in Reye's Syndrome

Since 1963, more than 500 children with Reye's syndrome have been reported (Chaves-Carballo *et al.*, 1975). This entity, characterized by a rapidly progressive encephalopathy and fatty infiltration of the liver and other viscera, follows a fulminant, lethal course in at least 50% of all affected patients. Its exact etiology remains enigmatic, but its temporal association and geographic clustering with outbreaks of infection due to influenza B, varicella-zoster, and other viruses have implicated some kind of host–pathogen (or host–toxin) interaction. The syndrome appears to affect equal numbers of males and females, and those children who do not succumb go on to full recovery. The hepatic histopathology of Reye's syndrome has been studied extensively in biopsy and autopsy material. Its hallmarks include microvesicular steatosis in hepatocytes; swelling, loss of cristae, and rupture of mitochondria; and histochemical evidence for decreased activity of the mitochondrial enzymes succinic dehydrogenase and cytochrome oxidase (Partin *et al.*, 1971; Bove *et al.*, 1975).

In 1969, Huttenlocher *et al.* (1969) reported that hyperammonemia was a regular finding in the acute stages of Reye's syndrome, and this observation has been amply confirmed. It now appears that the encephalopathy observed in these patients is produced in whole or in part by such ammonia accumulation, with its attendant effects on cerebral metabolism. There is, we believe, increasing evidence that implicates the mitochondrial portion of the urea cycle in the pathogenesis of hyperammonemia in Reye's syndrome. First, the plasma amino acid profile in patients with this syndrome is very similar to that of patients with primary, inherited OTC deficiency (Kang and Gerald, 1972; Hilty *et al.*, 1974). In both groups, plasma citrulline is much reduced or absent, whereas the concentrations of several other free amino acids are increased (glutamine, lysine, alanine, tyrosine, and α-aminobutyrate). Second, *in vitro* assays on biopsy or autopsy liver in more than 20 patients with Reye's syndrome have demonstrated a regular reduction in specific activities of CPS I and OTC (Thaler and Hoogenraad, 1974; Thaler *et al.*, 1974; Brown *et al.*, 1974; Sinatra *et al.*, 1975; Tang *et al.*, 1975; Snodgrass and DeLong, 1976), without concomitant reductions in activity of the cytosolic urea cycle enzymes (Snodgrass and DeLong, 1976).

These *in vitro* observations deserve additional comment. As noted in Table I, in which CPS I and OTC activities in liver of Reye's syndrome patients are expressed as the fraction of the control mean in each study, there is marked variation in the degree of enzymatic dysfunction: CPS I activities range from 1 to 116% of control; those for OTC, from 3 to 83% of control. Mean OTC activity (39% of control) among Reye's syndrome patients is slightly less than that for CPS I (54%), but these differences do not appear to be significant. Some of the observed variability must reflect timing of sample availability, i.e., whether tissue was obtained early or late in the course of the disease, and whether by needle biopsy or at autopsy. This view is attested to by the distinct differences in activities noted when the same patient's liver was studied on more than one occasion. In the only two instances in which this was done (Sinatra *et al.*, 1975; Snodgrass and DeLong, 1976), both CPS and OTC activities rose significantly later in the course of the disease.

The qualitative characteristics of OTC in these patients have generated considerable controversy. Thaler *et al.* (1974) reported a girl with Reye's syndrome whose liver had 20% of normal hepatic OTC activity. They found further that the patient's OTC had an 18-fold reduction in affinity for ornithine compared to control OTC and, on this evidence, put forth the rather startling hypothesis that this patient had a genetic variant

Table I. CPS I and OTC Activities in Liver from Patients with Reye's
Syndrome

Reference	Patient No.	Hepatic enzyme activity[a]	
		CPS I	OTC
Thaler and Hoogenraad;	1	—	21
Thaler *et al.* (1974)	2	—	06
Brown *et al.* (1974)	3	80	47
	4	28	16
	5	78	48
	6	42	40
Tang *et al.* (1975)	7	64	10
	8	57	41
Sinatra *et al.* (1975)	9	04	67
	10	82	61
	11	01	03
	12	13	35
	13	82	83
	14	14	31
Snodgrass and DeLong (1976)	15	77	27
	16	77	28
	17	31	72
	18	64	31
	19	116	29
	20	78	70
	21	24	18
	22	70	38
		$\bar{x} = 54$	$\bar{x} = 39$

[a]Values are expressed as percentages of control means. Since control values differed markedly
between studies, each study was treated individually in the calculations of fractional activity
remaining.

of OTC that may have predisposed her to Reye's syndrome. This interesting thesis is marred by two major experimental flaws: First, the K_m for
ornithine was estimated from a double-reciprocal plot constructed from
three nonlinear data points. Second, the K_m's were estimated under less
than optimized assay conditions, in that the OTC was surely not saturated
with the cosubstrate, carbamyl phosphate. Similar assay conditions were
employed in collecting the kinetic data of Sinatra *et al.* (1975), thereby
making their interpretation difficult. On the other hand, Snodgrass and
DeLong (1976) found no abnormalities in K_m for ornithine or carbamyl
phosphate in their study of OTC activity in several Reye's syndrome
patients. It should be emphasized that this study employed assay conditions known to be optimal. Thus, we conclude that there is, as yet, no
convincing evidence for genetic predisposition to Reye's syndrome based
on inherited variation in OTC structure.

Do the observed deficiencies of OTC and CPS I activity interfere with proper functioning of the urea cycle enough to explain the observed hyperammonemia in patients with Reye's syndrome? The data of Snodgrass and DeLong (1976) suggest a qualified affirmative answer to that question. They pointed out that the degree of OTC deficiency noted in their Reye's patients was as great as that observed in females heterozygous for inherited OTC deficiency, who may develop hyperammonemia when stressed with dietary protein increase or infection. They also observed that 24-hr urinary nitrogen excretion in 2 patients with Reye's syndrome was massively increased—to values greater than that reported in patients with massive burns or after major surgery. This important finding suggests that exaggerated proteolysis with marked expansion of the body burden for ammonia removal must be considered, along with enzymatic impairment of urea cycle enzymes, in the pathogenesis of hyperammonemia in this syndrome.

7.3. Inherited Defects of Cobalamin (Vitamin B$_{12}$) Metabolism

7.3.1. Genetic Control of Vitamin Metabolism

The very fact that each of the organic compounds called vitamins must be supplied in the diet is incontrovertible evidence that in the course of evolution, mankind has lost the genetic information required to synthesize these compounds. However, it does not follow therefrom that man's genes play no part in vitamin utilization. On the contrary, it is clear that a number of proteins, and therefore a number of genes, regulate all facets of vitamin metabolism, once ingestion has occurred. These proteins are of two general types: those required for vitamin transport, and those needed for vitamin activation intracellularly. Take vitamin B$_{12}$, or, as it is more appropriately called, cobalamin, as an example. At least a dozen different proteins are required if ingested cobalamins are to function appropriately as coenzymes (Babior, 1975; Rosenberg, 1976): gastric intrinsic factor (IF), a glycoprotein that binds the vitamin in the gastric lumen and carries it to the ileum; specific ileal mucosal receptors, which facilitate intestinal absorption; three serum proteins (transcobalamins I, II, and III), which carry the vitamin in blood; receptor proteins, which facilitate binding and endocytotic internalization of transcobalamin II (TC II)-bound cobalamins by tissue cells (Fig. 2); lysosomal protease(s), which degrade TC II and release free cobalamin to the cytosol; three activating enzymes (two reductases and an adenosyltransferase), which catalyze the

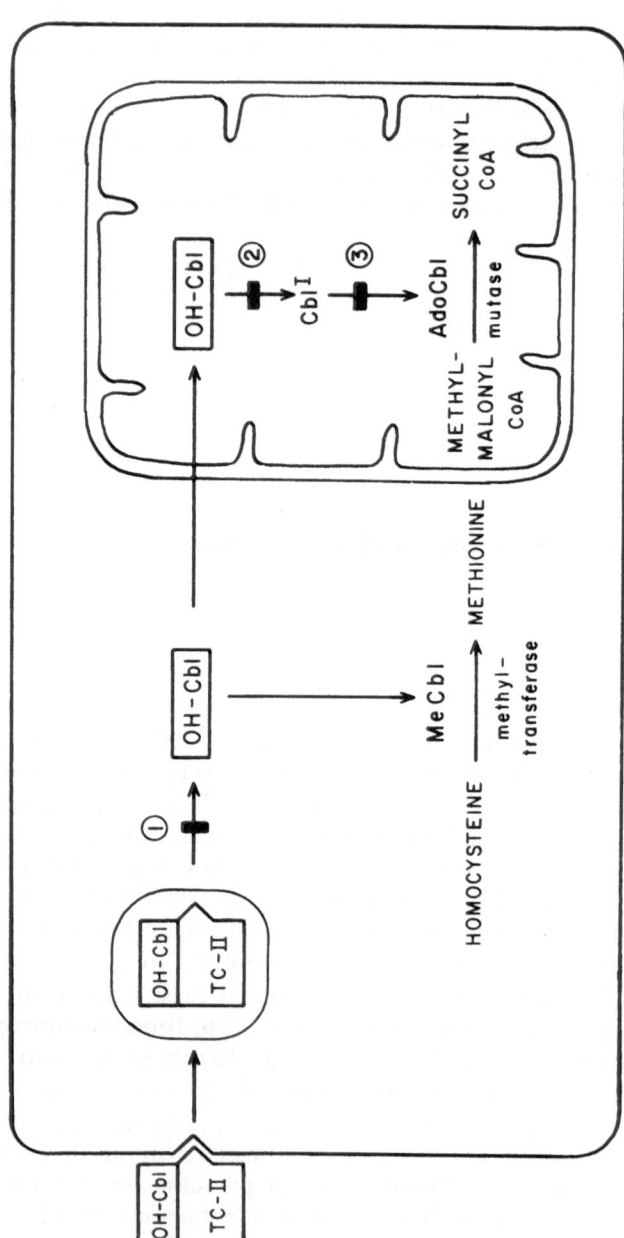

Fig. 2. Proposed pathway of cellular utilization of vitamin B_{12} (cobalamin) in mammals. As discussed in the text, numerous steps are involved: binding of the transcobalamin II (TC II)–vitamin (OH–Cbl) complex to the cell membrane; internalization of the complex; lysosomal degradation of the TC II; transmitochondrial transfer; formation of the two coenzymes, methylcobalamin (MeCbl) and adeno-sylcobalamin (AdoCbl); and binding to their respective apoenzymes, homocystein-methyltetrahydrofolate methyltransferase and methyl-malonyl-CoA mutase. The circled numbers 1–3 denote the probable localization of three known defects in intracellular cobalamin metabolism, as follows: (1) cbl C mutant; (2) cbl A mutant; (3) cbl B mutant. See the text for additional details.

conversion of the vitamin to one of its active coenzyme forms, adeno-sylcobalamin (AdoCbl); and, finally, two apoenzymes (methylmalonyl CoA mutase and homocysteine–methyltetrahydrofolate methyltransferase), which require cobalamin coenzymes for their catalytic activity.

From the foregoing comments, it follows that a wide variety of different mutations could theoretically interfere with cobalamin action. Mutations affecting cobalamin transport could occur in any of several organ systems—the gut, the blood, or tissues such as the liver, muscle, and brain. Mutations could block any one of the intracellular reactions by which the vitamin is converted to its active cobalamin coenzymes (see Fig. 2). Mutations could alter either of the cobalamin-dependent apoenzymes in such a way that they would no longer bind coenzyme avidly, thereby impairing holoenzyme activity. The clinical and chemical manifestations of such mutations could be predicted to vary considerably. Those interfering with intestinal absorption of cobalamins would be expected to produce a disorder identical to that observed in acquired nutritional deficiency of the vitamin. In this event, serum and tissue stores of the vitamin and its coenzymes would be reduced and both cobalamin-dependent holoenzyme activities impaired. At the other extreme, mutations involving a single coenzyme-dependent apoenzyme such as methylmalonyl CoA mutase would alter only that enzymatic function. In this instance, serum and tissue vitamin stores would be normal, as would methyltransferase activity. A third situation, between these extremes, deserves mention. Deficiency of one of the intracellular activating enzymes specific for AdoCbl synthesis would be predicted to lead to normal serum cobalamin content and normal methyltransferase activity, at the same time that tissue stores of AdoCbl and the activity of the AdoCbl-dependent mutase would be impaired.

7.3.2. Enumeration and Characterization of Specific Inherited Defects

As noted in Table II, these theoretical considerations are rapidly being converted to observed phenomena. Eight different human disorders have been traced to specific, inherited defects in cobalamin metabolism (reviewed by Rosenberg, 1976). Three interfere with intestinal absorption and produce a syndrome in children identical to that of pernicious anemia in adults (Donaldson, 1975). Some children with such "juvenile pernicious anemia" lack immunologically identifiable intrinsic factor; others synthesize a mutant IF that lacks binding activity. Still others have an as yet undefined defect in ileal transport of cobalamins. Regard-

Table II. Inherited Defects of Cobalamin (Vitamin B$_{12}$) Metabolism[a]

Metabolic phase affected	Nature of defect	Serum Cbl concentration	Manifestation of defect			Quantitative Cbl requirement in vivo
			Megaloblastic anemia	Methylmalonic-aciduria	Homo-cystinuria	
Intestinal absorption	IF deficiency	low	yes	yes	yes	normal
	Inactive IF	low	yes	NR	NR	normal
	Defective ileal transport	low	yes	NR	NR	normal
Plasma transport	TC I deficiency	low	no	NR	NR	normal
	TC II deficiency	normal	yes	no	no	increased
Tissue utilization	Defective AdoCbl synthesis (cbl A and cbl B)[b]	normal	no	yes	no	increased
	Defective AdoCbl and MeCbl synthesis (cbl C)[b]	normal	variable	yes	yes	increased

[a] The following abbreviations are used: (IF) gastric intrinsic factor; (TC) plasma transcobalamin; (Cbl) cobalamin; (AdoCbl) adenosylcobalamin; (MeCbl) methylcobalamin; (NR) not reported.

[b] The abbreviations cbl A, B, and C refer to different mutations, which are defined further in the text and in Fig. 2.

less of etiology, all such children have low serum cobalamin concentrations, develop megaloblastic anemia, and respond completely to *parenteral* replacement of *physiological* amounts of the vitamin.

Infantile megaloblastic anemia was also the presenting finding in American female siblings (Hakami *et al.*, 1971) and Swiss male siblings (Hitzig *et al.*, 1974) in two unrelated families with a different defect. Each of the affected children also demonstrated leukopenia, thrombopenia, recurrent infections, and failure of normal development. In addition, the Swiss patient had intestinal malabsorption and marked hypogammaglobulinemia involving all immunoglobulin classes. Although their serum cobalamin and folate concentrations were normal, radiochromatographic study of serum transcobalamins revealed complete absence of TC II. A variety of immunological techniques also failed to detect any protein cross-reacting with anti-TC II antiserum in the Swiss patient (Gimpert *et al.*, 1975). No clinical or hematological response was observed when these children were given physiological (1–10 μg/day) doses of vitamin B_{12}, but complete and sustained remissions were produced by parenteral administration of 500–1000 μg/day. These observations lend strong support to the idea that TC II is required for the transport of newly absorbed cobalamin in serum and for the uptake of cobalamins by hematopoietic and other rapidly dividing cells. In the absence of TC II, tissue cobalamin stores can be maintained only by increasing dramatically the concentration of vitamin in the extracellular fluid, thereby permitting cellular entry of cobalamins by passive diffusion. Curiously, when the American patients were allowed to relapse hematologically, they failed to demonstrate methylmalonicaciduria, homocystinuria, or hypomethioninemia (Scott *et al.*, 1972).

In contrast to these prominent effects of TC II deficiency are the results in two brothers with TC I deficiency reported by Carmel and Herbert (1969). Although their serum cobalamin concentrations were reduced much below normal, they were not anemic and appeared to suffer no pathophysiological consequences of the TC I lack. Hence, we can conclude that TC I carries the majority of cobalamin in serum, and that this bound cobalamin is not crucial to cellular functions that require cobalamin coenzymes.

Three other mutations result from primary intracellular defects in cobalamin coenzyme synthesis. The clinical and chemical phenotype in these conditions differs markedly from that of the disorders of cobalamin absorption or extracellular transport discussed above, and focuses on the enzymatic isomerization of L-methylmalonyl CoA to succinyl CoA by the AdoCbl-dependent enzyme methylmalonyl CoA mutase (see Fig. 2). It has long been known that patients with pernicious anemia excrete increased amounts of methylmalonate, because AdoCbl depletion leads to impaired mutase activity. Within the past ten years, however, it has become apparent that methylmalonicacidemia (uria) also results from at least four primary, inherited defects of mutase activity (Rosenberg, 1976). Clinically, three of these entities are very similar. In each, young children develop profound metabolic ketoacidosis in response to protein feeding or increased catabolic stress such as infection. The ketosis and acidosis result from accumulation of methylmalonate, its precursor propionate, and such other by-products of blocked methylmalonate catabolism as lactate, acetoacetate, α-methylacetoacetate, acetone, and butanone (Rosenberg, 1972). These children have normal serum cobalamin concentrations, and exhibit none of the hematological or neurological stigmata of acquired cobalamin deficiency. They differ, however, in their response to pharmacological doses of cobalamins. In some patients, such supplements have absolutely no effect on methylmalonate excretion or protein tolerance; in others, cobalamin supplementation produces a marked fall in methylmalonate excretion. This difference led to a number of *in vitro* studies with liver, leukocytes, and cultured skin fibroblasts, all aimed at identifying the underlying lesion in these children, and at explaining the different therapeutic responses to cobalamin loading. Only the conclusions of this large body of work will be stated here. Some of these children have primary defects of the mutase apoenzyme (Morrow *et al.*, 1975); their cellular metabolism of cobalamins is completely normal (Morrow *et al.*, 1975; Mahoney and Rosenberg 1975; Rosenberg *et al.*, 1975), and they do not respond to cobalamin supplementation *in vivo*. The others have been shown to have a normal mutase apoenzyme and defective AdoCbl synthesis (Mahoney *et al.*, 1975a). The latter group has been further subdivided into two mutant classes (cbl A and cbl B) by studies with intact cultured fibroblasts and extracts thereof (Fig. 2). Although the precise defects in cbl A and cbl B mutants are unclear, it seems very likely that they result from different enzymatic lesions in the mitochondrial pathway by which the cobalamin vitamin is converted to AdoCbl coenzyme.

The third mutation of cobalamin coenzyme synthesis, designated cbl C, differs clinically and chemically from those just mentioned. Homocystinuria and hypomethioninemia are observed along with methylmalonicacidemia. These findings, initially reported in a 6-week-old male who died with developmental failure (Mudd *et al.*, 1969), were interpreted as evidence for defective synthesis of both cobalamin coenzymes, AdoCbl and MeCbl. Three other patients have been described subsequently; none has exhibited ketoacidosis. Two affected brothers were reported by Goodman *et al.* (1970). The older boy, age 14 years, was psychotic, retarded, and had abnormal cerebellar and spinal cord function. At 2 years of age, his younger brother was clinically well. The last-reported patient was a girl who died at age 7 years following a long illness highlighted by megaloblastic anemia and severe mental retardation (Dillon *et al.*, 1974). At autopsy, brain and spinal cord abnormalities typical of those observed in patients with pernicious anemia were noted. Biochemical investigations from several laboratories have confirmed the thesis that the primary lesion in these patients involves defective synthesis of AdoCbl and MeCbl (reviewed by Mudd, 1974, and Rosenberg, 1976). Cultured skin fibroblasts from these patients have proved to be a particularly helpful research resource. They demonstrate markedly reduced amounts of AdoCbl and MeCbl (Linnell *et al.*, 1976), as well as an inability to synthesize these coenzymes from precursor OH–Cbl (Mahoney *et al.*, 1971). These findings suggested a defect in an early step of cobalamin metabolism common to the synthesis of both coenzymes. Rosenberg *et al.* (1975) reported that the plasma membrane of cells from such patients appears to bind cobalamins normally, but that such cells are unable to retain accumulated cobalamins. They also found that cell extracts from such patients contained almost no cobalamin bound to intracellular proteins (presumably the cobalamin-dependent apoenzymes). It seems likely, then, that the primary defect in cbl C mutants involves internalization of the TC II-cobalamin complex lysosomal degradation of TC II or release of cobalamin from the lysosome.

7.3.3. Cobalamin Supplementation as Therapy— Some Caveats

Since the initial description of "B$_{12}$-responsive methylmalonicacidemia" (Rosenberg *et al.*, 1968; Hsia *et al.*, 1970) a number of children have been described whose clinical and chemical findings improve when they are given 500–1000 μg parenteral CN–Cbl or OH–Cbl daily. Thus far, all these responsive patients have been shown to have one of the primary defects of cobalamin coenzyme synthesis discussed above. Several features of such treatment deserve comment. In 1974, the parents of the index patient with responsive methylmalonicacidemia chose to have their son discontinue dietary protein restriction and cobalamin supplements. The boy was then 7 years old and in excellent health, with an I.Q. higher than 100 and good school performance. When seen 1 year later, he was excreting 3–4 g methylmalonate daily (about 1000 times normal), but was otherwise well. He had experienced no episodes of ketosis or acidosis, and had continued to do well in school. Continued follow-up should determine whether discontinuation of treatment in this disease after several years is wise and innocuous.

Although some patients with primary defects in cobalamin metabolism will respond chemically to supplements, this is not true of all such patients. Kaye *et al.* (1974) described 2 children with methylmalonicacidemia whose methylmalonate excretion was unchanged by several days of high-dose cobalamin administration. One of these children is a cbl A mutant, as is the index patient with responsive methylmalonicacidemia; the other is a cbl B mutant. Thus, it appears that further clinical and chemical heterogeneity exists within these mutant classes. This observation also raised the following question: What is an adequate therapeutic trial of cobalamin in patients with methylmalonicacidemia? We know of patients who have responded to 1 mg CN–Cbl daily in one day, and others who have taken as long as 2 weeks. If cobalamin supplements were completely innocuous, it would not matter how long or how much cobalamin was given. Recent experience, however, suggests that this may not be the case. Mahoney *et al.* (1976) reported a male infant with methylmalonicacidemia due to a defect in AdoCbl synthesis (cbl B). He appeared to respond to OH–Cbl supplements (1 mg/day) initially, but then relapsed. When larger doses of the vitamin were then pushed, his condition seemed to deteriorate, and his methylmalonate excretion actually increased. At the time of his death, his serum cobalamin concentration was as high as 3 μg/dl (1000 times normal). Additional studies revealed that OH–Cbl is a potent inhibitor of methylmalonyl CoA mutase activity by competing with AdoCbl for binding to the apoenzyme. Thus, it seems likely that in the face of impaired AdoCbl formation, huge excesses of OH–Cbl may be toxic. The findings in this patient imply that cobalamin supplements cannot be administered with total impunity. Our suggestion would be to use 1–2 mg CN–Cbl or OH–Cbl/day for 14 days. If no beneficial response has been observed by then, none can likely be expected thereafter.

7.3.4. Prenatal Diagnosis and Treatment of Methylmalonicacidemia

In 1970, Morrow *et al.* (1970) correctly predicted an affected fetus in a pregnancy at risk for methylmalonyl CoA mutase apoenzyme deficiency by demonstrating increased methylmalonate content in amniotic fluid and maternal urine at midtrimester. Subsequently it was shown (Mahoney *et al.*, 1975b) that mutase apoenzyme deficiency could be detected by 15 weeks' gestation, using cultured amniotic fluid cell assays. Ampola *et al.* (1975) utilized both these approaches in a most interesting way. They detected a female fetus with defective AdoCbl synthesis (cbl A mutant) in cultured amniocytes at about 16 weeks' gestation. Methylmalonate content of maternal urine and amniotic fluid was increased. When large amounts of CN–Cbl were administered to the mother orally and parenterally, her methylmalonate excretion fell considerably, suggesting that the administered cobalamin was crossing the placenta and was being utilized by the fetus to correct its aberrant AdoCbl synthesis. Following delivery, the infant was shown to respond to cobalamin supplementation, and is doing very well. Although these results show unequivocally that prenatal treatment was biochemically effective here, they do not answer the more fundamental questions relating to the need for such treatment. Are inborn errors of this type harmless to the fetus, as we have always supposed? Do the maternal metabolic capacity and placental circulation effectively protect the fetus with a disorder of diffusible metabolites? Such questions can be answered, we believe, by study of other affected fetuses and at-risk pregnancies, and may open an entirely new area of approach to inborn errors of metabolism.

7.4. Use of Stable Isotopes in the Investigation of Disorders of Amino Acid and Organic Acid Metabolism

7.4.1. Stable Isotopes

The use of isotopes as tracers has been one of the major factors responsible for the rapid progress of biochemical research in the last three decades. The utilization of radioactive isotopes such as carbon-14 (^{14}C) and hydrogen-3 or tritium (^{3}H) has been instrumental in the elucidation of metabolic pathways for many substances, including amino acids and organic acids. It should be noted, however, that with rare exceptions, experimental animals have been employed in the *in vivo* experiments in which radioactive isotopes have been used to explore metabolism in mammals. Radioisotopes such as carbon-14 and hydrogen-3 have had limited *in vivo* use in human investigation, out of concern for the possible deleterious effects of internal radiation with these long-lived isotopes.

Since metabolism in man is not always the same as in other mammals, we cannot always extrapolate to humans the knowledge obtained from animal experiments. Mechanisms of conjugation and detoxification differ considerably from species to species (Williams, 1967). For instance, in man, phenylacetate is excreted largely as phenylacetylglutamine in urine, whereas it is excreted as phenylacetylglycine in rats (Meister, 1965a). For this reason, clinical investigators have long felt the need of safe tracers that can be used in man *in vivo;* this perceived need has been appreciated particularly by investigators of metabolic disorders.

There are nonradioactive (stable) isotopes of carbon, hydrogen, and nitrogen; they are carbon-13 (^{13}C), hydrogen-2 or deuterium (^{2}H), and nitrogen-15 (^{15}N), and they were used as early as 1934 (Caprioli, 1972). The crucial advantages of such stable isotopes for investigative purposes are, as immediately realized, their stability and lack of radioactivity. Their use in human biochemical investigation has, until recently, been almost negligible for two reasons: their limited availability, and technical difficulties in detecting them.

7.4.2. Advances in Instrumentation: Combined Gas Chromatography–Mass Spectrometry and ^{13}C Nuclear Magnetic Resonance

Recent progress in analytical instrumentation has alleviated the latter problem. The use of mass spectrometry (MS), particularly when combined with gas chromatography (GC–MS), and of ^{13}C-nuclear magnetic resonance (^{13}C-NMR) has made it possible to detect these stable isotopes in biological materials with relative ease. With these new techniques, the use of stable isotopes as tracers can provide even more information than that obtained using radioactive isotopes. The production of stable isotopes has also been greatly expanded at the Los Alamos National Scientific Laboratories (Matwiyoff and Ott, 1973). These developments have quickened the interest of clinical investigators in the use of stable isotopes, and pioneering reports began to appear in 1972 and 1973 (Curtius *et al.*, 1972a,b; Bier *et al.*, 1973; Hofmann *et al.*, 1973; Sweetman *et al.*, 1973).

It may be worthwhile to summarize briefly the basic principles of GC–MS and ^{13}C-NMR. Mass spectrometry depends on two phenomena: ionization of molecules to be tested for by some means, such as bombardment with an electron beam (electron impact) or transfer of charge from other ionized substances (chemical ionization); and measurement of the molecular weight of the ions thus produced by electromagnetic detection. Since the energy used for ionization will fragment organic molecules at weak bonds, it is often possible to measure the molecular weight of the intact molecule (M^+), as well as the molecular weights of the fragments (F^+) produced. The molecular structure of the compound may then be elucidated by reassembling this information. When this technique is applied to the analysis of compounds labeled with stable isotopes, the mass of the intact molecule and its fragments will be increased to $M + n_0$, $F_1 + n_1$, and $F_2 + n_2$, respectively, where n_0, n_1, and n_2 denote the number of isotopes incorporated. In this way, it is possible not only to measure the incorporation of isotopes, but also to identify the specific localization of isotopes in the molecule (Biemann, 1962).

It must be emphasized that the compound to be tested by conventional MS must be chemically pure, and this requirement limited its use in biomedical research. This difficulty was solved when GC was successfully combined with MS (Ryhage, 1964). It is now possible to obtain mass spectra of compounds in a complex biological mixture without prepurification. With this method, the sample is injected into the GC part of the system, and when the peak to be tested emerges, its mass spectrum may be taken by simply pressing a button. The sample size may be as small as 0.1– 1 μg. However, the information on intramolecular localization of stable isotopes obtained by GC–MS is neither as specific nor as conclusive as that obtained by ^{13}C-NMR.

Only with the recent advancement of computer technology did ^{13}C-NMR become of practical use. The nuclei of certain atoms such as ^{13}C behave like spinning magnets. If a ^{13}C atom is placed in an external magnetic field, it absorbs radiofrequency energy and produces a signal. Since most of the carbon atoms in an organic molecule have different physical environments due to different neighboring atoms, each produces a signal at a different magnetic field. Thus, a spectrum of signals of all carbon atoms of a given molecule can be obtained by changing the magnetic field. Unlike that of the proton (nucleus of the hydrogen atom), the signal of ^{13}C is weak, and the numbers of ^{13}C atoms in natural compounds are small. Therefore, it was technically difficult to obtain ^{13}C-NMR of natural compounds until recently.

With the use of Fourier-transform and a computer, weak signals from ^{13}C spin resonance can be integrated, so that the ^{13}C-NMR of a compound with a molecular weight up to a few hundred daltons can be obtained in a relatively short time, using several milligrams of pure compound. Thus, signals of essentially all the individual ^{13}C atoms in a molecule can be resolved, and the labeling of each carbon atom can be measured separately, without resorting to the tedious degradation procedures needed when ^{14}C is used as a tracer (Sequin and Scott, 1974). Labeling of a metabolite with ^{13}C can be further assured by the use of a doubly labeled precursor, which will have ^{13}C–^{13}C coupling (London et al., 1976; Tanaka and Armitage, 1976). With this technique, the direct labeling of a metabolite from the precursor may be readily distinguished from that due to the reutilization of tracer atoms.

The requirement for several milligrams of pure compound continues to be a drawback to biomedical application of ^{13}C-NMR. Therefore, GC–MS and ^{13}C-NMR should be seen as complementary methods enhancing each other's versatility of application and precision of information.

7.4.3. Biohazards

The biological safety of stable isotopes is of foremost concern to clinical investigators. ^{13}C is naturally present in a quantity of 1.1% of all carbon atoms; i.e., all the organic compounds in the human body contain this amount of ^{13}C. In human in vivo experiments such as

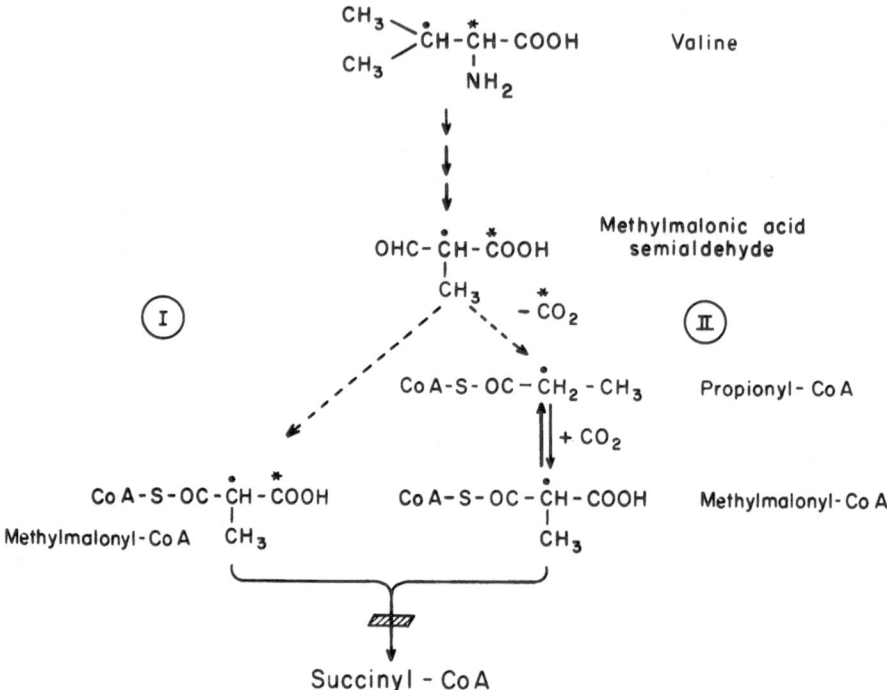

Fig. 3. Possible routes of valine metabolism after formation of methylmalonic acid semi-aldehyde. The α- and β-carbons of valine are marked with* and ●, respectively, to illustrate expected labeling patterns for the two routes.

those described subsequently, ^{13}C-labeled compounds are used in amounts that result, at most, in transient enrichment of ^{13}C to several times the natural abundance in pools of the parent compounds or of their metabolites. Changes in total body ^{13}C are insignificant. It is therefore highly unlikely on theoretical grounds that this isotope would have any adverse biological effects (Matwiyoff and Ott, 1973). In fact, the biological effects of very large doses of ^{13}C-labeled compounds have been little studied. At the Los Alamos Scientific Laboratory, 2 weanling mice were kept for 6 months on a yeast *(Candida utilis)* diet in which 90% of the carbon fed was ^{13}C. During this period, their weight gain was normal and their body ^{13}C content increased to about 60 ^{13}C atoms/100 C atoms. No discernible toxic effects were observed. One of the mice died of accidental asphyxiation during the fourth month (Matwiyoff and Ott, 1973). Later studies have confirmed the nontoxic nature of ^{13}C-labeled compounds (Gregg *et al.,* 1976).

The mass difference between ^2H and ^1H is much greater than that between ^{13}C and ^{12}C. ^2H is present in natural compounds in a quantity of

0.015 ^{2}H atom/100 H atoms. Consequently, there are considerable chemical and biological effects produced by the use of deuterium. It is well known that mammals cannot survive replacement of more than 35% of total body water with heavy water (^{2}H$_2$O). There were noticeable changes in metabolism when 50% ^{2}H$_2$O was given to rats as drinking water for more than 5 days (Thomson, 1960). However, no significant side effects were found in 5 human subjects who were maintained on 0.5% ^{2}H$_2$O enrichment of their body water for 6–8 weeks, except for occasional transient episodes of vertigo, which occurred shortly after administration of the initial priming dose (140–200 g ^{2}H$_2$O) (Taylor et al., 1966). In rats, feeding of 5% ^{2}H$_2$O in drinking water may be considered safe for at least 7 months (Peng et al., 1972).

The amounts of deuterated compounds employed as tracers, however, are much smaller than these extreme conditions. We wish to illustrate the usefulness of studies with stable isotopes by considering three recent investigations.

7.4.4. Recent Investigations with Stable Isotopes

7.4.4.1. [^{13}C]Valine Metabolism in a Patient with Methylmalonicacidemia, Using ^{13}C-NMR— Identification of Propionate as an Obligate Intermediate

As stated earlier in this discussion, there are several known precursors of methylmalonyl CoA: isoleucine, methionine, threonine, cholesterol, odd-chain fatty acids, thymine, and valine. It has been well established that all these precursors, other than valine and thymine, are first converted to propionyl CoA, and then carboxylated to D-methylmalonyl CoA. The exact route by which valine was converted to methylmalonyl CoA was not known until very recently (Tanaka, 1975). There were two contradicting views on the pathway of conversion of methylmalonic acid semialdehyde (MMS) to methylmalonyl CoA (MMCoA). According to one hypothesis, MMS is directly oxidized to MMCoA (see route I, Fig. 3) (Robinson et al., 1957). The second hypothesis proposes that MMS is first decarboxylated to propionate, and then carboxylated to MMCoA (route II) (Kinnory et al., 1955).

The controversy over these specific steps in valine metabolism was rejoined following the discovery of two closely related inborn errors of propionate metabolism—propionicacidemia and methylmalonicacidemia. Ando et al. (1972) administered [U-^{14}C]valine to a patient with methylmalonicacidemia due to defective MMCoA mutase activity, and observed a considerable amount of radioactivity in urinary 3-hydroxypropionic acid, a by-product of propionic acid. From this observation, they proposed that valine is metabolized through MMS to propionic acid (route II). However, their observation could also be explained by route I, since the propionyl CoA carboxylase reaction is reversible. Thus, the question about the pathway of conversion of MMS to methylmalonic acid (MMA) remained unsettled. This matter may have clinical as well as biochemical significance. If, for instance, propionate is an obligate intermediate in the catabolism of valine, the amount of valine fed to patients with propionicacidemia may have to be restricted.

To solve this problem, Tanaka et al. (1975) administered [α-^{13}C]- and [α,β-^{13}C]valine to a patient with methylmalonicacidemia at different times, isolated MMA from multiple urine specimens, and analyzed the MMA specimens by Fourier-transform ^{13}C-NMR to determine the intramolecular labeling with ^{13}C. If MMS metabolism follows route I, the carboxyl carbons would be enriched with ^{13}C after the administration of either compound. In contrast, if it follows route II, the methine ($-CH-$) carbon alone would be enriched after [α,β-^{13}C]valine administration (Fig. 3). The results showed that only the methine carbon was enriched with carbon-13 after [α,β-^{13}C]valine administration; no ^{13}C enrichment was observed at the carboxyl carbons. These results indicate unequivocally that propionate is produced as an obligate intermediate in this patient.

7.4.4.2. Identification of a Minor Pathway of Isoleucine Metabolism

It has been well established that the major catabolic pathway for isoleucine in mammals is that shown as route I in Fig. 4. In this pathway, L-isoleucine is first transaminated to s-2-keto-3-methylvaleric acid, which is subsequently decarboxylated to 2s-methylbutyryl CoA. Three subsequent steps yield propionyl CoA. The labels R and S denote stereospecific configurations, replacing the old D and L nomenclature. In 1959, Stalder identified small amounts of 2-ethylmalonic acid (EMA) in urines from normal man and rats. Since the amounts of EMA increased significantly after rats were loaded with D,L-isoleucine, he proposed that isoleucine may also be metabolized through route II (Fig. 4), taking the steps of 2-ethylacrylate, 2-ethylhydracrylate (2-hydroxymethylbutyrate) to ethylmalonate. This pathway was further investigated by Mamer and Tjoa (1973, 1975), who detected a small amount of ethylhydracrylic acid (EHA) in normal human urine. They also found an increased amount of this compound in a child with an inborn error of isoleucine metabolism at the step of cleavage of 2-methylacetoacetyl CoA (β-ketothiolase reaction).

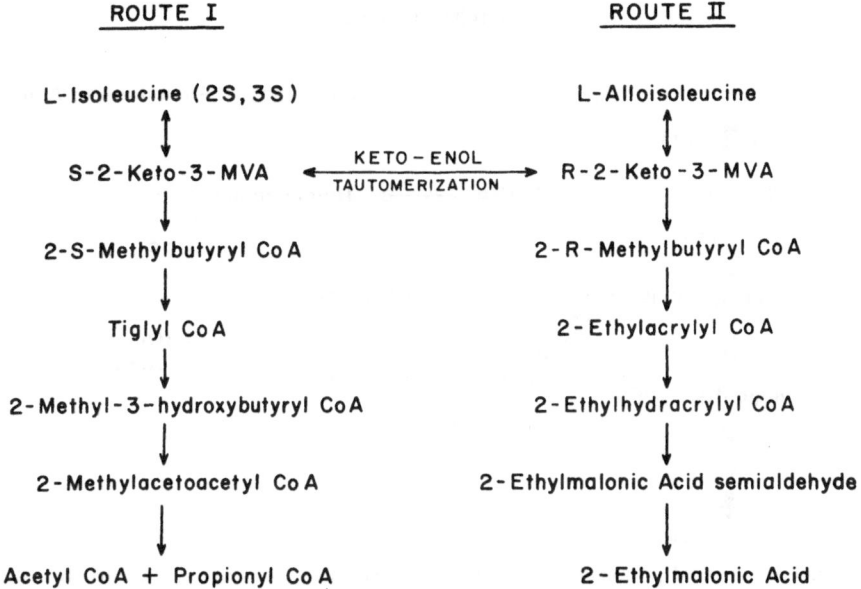

Fig. 4. Pathways of isoleucine metabolism. The evidence for the existence of the minor pathway (route II) is discussed in the text. (MVA) Methylvaleric acid.

They postulated that s-2-ketomethylvaleric acid may be converted in part to the R-form by keto–enol tautomerization, and subsequently metabolized by route II.

To prove this hypothesis, they injected RS*-2-[^{2}H$_3$-methyl]]butyrate (a mixture of the R and s forms) into rats intraperitoneally, and analyzed urinary organic acids by GC–MS. Virtually all urinary EHA (97%) was labeled with ^{2}H, indicating that EHA probably originated from isoleucine. Surprisingly, however, only 11% of urinary EHA was labeled with 2 ^{2}H's, and 86% of the compound had only 1 deuterium. If the [^{2}H$_3$-methyl] group of the precursor had simply remained as the hydroxymethyl group of EHA, as depicted in route II, the resulting EHA would be expected to have 2 ^{2}H atoms. From these findings, they speculated that there was a specific exchange of the second of the original 3 deuterium labels with endogenous ^{1}H, and that this exchange is due to the result of reversible oxidation of EHA to EMA semialdehyde by 3-hydroxyacyl CoA dehydrogenase. The reduction of the aldehyde group back to hydroxymethyl would result in the incorporation of ^{1}H taken up from body water in place of ^{2}H lost in the oxidation. The precursor–product relationship of EHA to EMA could not be obtained, since all the ^{2}H is lost when EHA is oxidized to EMA. If ^{13}C-labeled precursor had been used in lieu of

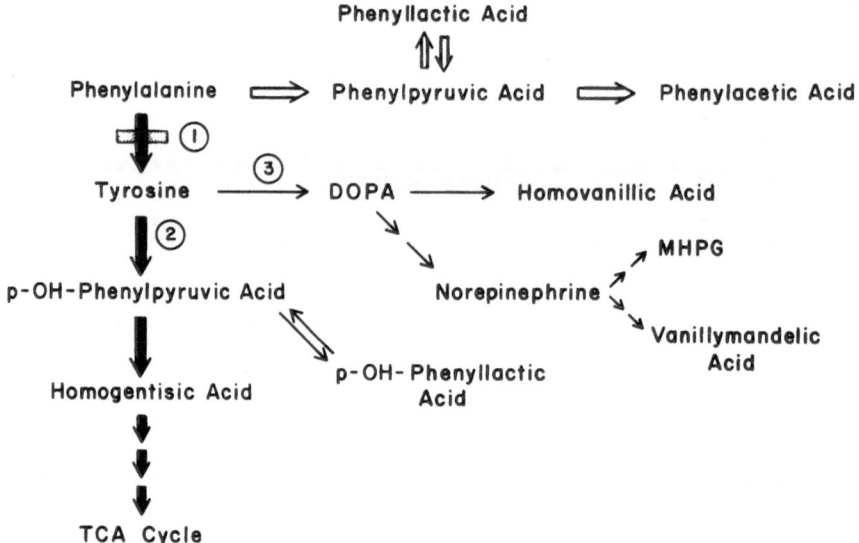

Fig. 5. Pathways of phenylalanine metabolism. Normal pathways are shown by solid arrows; the alternate pathway in phenylketonuria is shown by outline arrows. Abbreviations are as follows: (DOPA) dihydroxyphenylalanine; (MHPG) 3-methoxy-4-hydroxy-phenyleneglycol. The circled numbers 1, 2, and 3 denote reactions catalyzed by phenylalanine hydroxylase, tyrosine transaminase, and tyrosine hydroxylase, respectively.

^{2}H-, the precursor–product definition could have been gained, but the interesting observation on the equilibrium between EHA and EMA semi-aldehyde would have been missed. As these statements illustrate, different types of information may be obtained by use of different isotopes. The physiological role of this minor pathway remains to be elucidated.

7.4.4.3. Use of Deuterated Phenylalanine and Tyrosine in Studies of Phenylketonuria *In Vivo*

Curtius and associates (Curtius *et al.*, 1972b) pioneered in this field. They administered deuterated phenylalanine ([^{2}H]Phe) and tyrosine ([^{2}H]Tyr) orally to patients with phenylketonuria (PKU) and hyperphenyl-lalaninemia, as well as to a normal individual, and analyzed urinary aromatic acids by GC–MS. In the normal subject, such aromatic acids as *p*-hydroxy(OH)phenylpyruvic, *p*-OH-phenyllactic, and *p*-OH-phenylacetic acids, all known to be produced via tyrosine (see Fig. 5), were deuterated. In contrast, there was no incorporation of ^{2}H into these tyrosine metabolites in the urine of either a patient with PKU or a patient with hyper-phenylalaninemia. This labeling pattern is as expected from the known deficiency of phenylalanine hydroxylase activity in patients with

PKU or hyperphenylalaninemia. The data of these investigators were of special interest, however, in that the amounts of p-hydroxylated aromatic acids are known to be *increased* in the urine of patients with PKU (Meister, 1965b). The latter finding has been explained by proposing that Phe, which accumulates intracellularly, acts as a competitive inhibitor of Tyr hydroxylase, the enzyme that catalyzes the conversion of Tyr to dihydroxyphenylalanine (DOPA) (Udenfriend, 1967).

Since inhibition of DOPA synthesis would lead to a depression of synthesis of biogenic amines, Curtius and associates postulated that this inhibition may be a contributing factor to the brain dysfunction seen in patients with PKU. They pursued this problem further by administering deuterated Tyr to patients with PKU and hyperphenylalaninemia (Curtius *et al.*, 1972a). They measured the incorporation of ^{2}H into homovanillic acid (HVA), vanillylmandelic acid (VMA), and 3-methoxy-4-hydroxyphenyleneglycol (MHPG) at a time when the plasma Phe concentration was high, and compared the findings to those obtained when the plasma Phe concentration was low. The ^{2}H content of urinary HVA, VMA, and MHPG was low when the plasma Phe concentration was high, but increased significantly when the plasma Phe concentration was low. These data support the contention that Phe accumulation impairs synthesis of biogenic amines.

Milstein and Kaufman (1975) utilized deuterated Phe differently in the study of Phe metabolism *in vivo*. They administered ^{2}H$_5$-Phe to rats intraperitoneally, and measured the release of deuterium into body water by IR spectrophotometry as an *in vivo* assay for Phe-hydroxylase activity. This method is based on the principle that on conversion of Phe to Tyr by Phe-hydroxylase, the deuterium of the hydroxyl group exchanges with a hydrogen atom (^{1}H) from body water. The amount of deuterium released into body water would thus reflect Phe-hydroxylase activity. The rate of deuterium release was linear for 60–90 min, and was maximal at a dose of about 0.5 g/kg. The method was sensitive enough to detect the higher hydroxylase activity found in male rats compared with that in female rats (Brenneman and Kaufman, 1965). They utilized two known inhibitors of the hydroxylase, p-chlorophenylalanine and methotrexate, to compare their inhibitory effects on the *in vivo* assay with those on *in vitro* measurement of hydroxylase activity. The results obtained with the *in vivo* assay were in excellent agreement with those noted *in vitro*.

This *in vivo* assay method produces a valid estimate of hydroxylase activity only if this reaction is the rate-limiting step in the pathway of Phe metabolism. They tested this hypothesis by comparing the rate of deuterium release from ^{2}H$_5$-Phe to that from ^{2}H$_4$-Tyr; the deuterium release from the latter was twice as great as from the former. They also tested tritium release from ^{3}H$_5$-Phe in rats treated with triamcinolone. In these rats, Tyr-transaminase was induced 6-fold over controls, but the rate of tritium release into the body water was identical to that in controls. These results strongly indicated that Phe hydroxylation is, in fact, the rate-limiting step in the pathway of Phe catabolism. They confirmed, in addition, that the results of this *in vivo* test were unaffected by alteration in the rate of protein synthesis.

This method will be valuable in clinical investigation of PKU patients and heterozygotes, since *in vitro* enzymatic studies of Phe-hydroxylase are limited by the need for liver tissue. Although hydroxylase activity is detectable in pancreas and kidney, such activity is minuscule compared with that in liver (Scriver and Rosenberg, 1973). Currently, the best method available for measuring the hydroxylase activity *in vivo* is the Phe tolerance test, which is relatively insensitive and cannot be used to distinguish between a heterozygote for classic PKU and a homozygote for benign hyperphenylalaninemia. The hydroxylase activity is approximately 15% of normal in the former, whereas it is about 5% of control in the latter. Milstein and Kaufman (1975) emphasized that these two groups may be accurately differentiated by using the new method. They claim that if this method were applied to human investigation, it would be as innocuous as the commonly employed Phe tolerance test, which requires a few small samples of blood (1 ml for one point).

References

Introduction (Section 7.1)

Nyhan, W. L., 1974, *Heritable Disorders of Amino Acid Metabolism. Patterns of Clinical Expression and Genetic Variation,* John Wiley and Sons, New York.

Rosenberg, L. E., and Scriver, C. R., 1974, Disorders of amino acid metabolism, *in: Duncan's Diseases of Metabolism,* Seventh Ed. (P. K. Bondy and L. E. Rosenberg, eds.), pp. 465–654, W. B. Saunders, Philadelphia.

Scriver, C. R., and Rosenberg, L. E., 1973, *Amino Acid Metabolism and Its Disorders,* W. B. Saunders, Philadelphia.

Stanbury, J. B., Wyngaarden, J. B., and Frederickson, D. S., 1972, *The Metabolic Basis of Inherited Disease,* Third Ed., McGraw-Hill, New York.

Tanaka, K., 1975, Disorders of organic acid metabolism, *in: Biology of Brain Dysfunction,* Vol. III (G. Gaull, ed.), pp. 145–214, Plenum Press, New York.

Hyperammonemia and Urea Cycle Enzymes (Section 7.2)

Bachman, C., 1974, Urea cycle, *in: Heritable Disorders of Amino Acid Metabolism. Patterns of Clinical Expression and Genetic Variation* (W. L. Nyhan, ed.), pp. 361–386, John Wiley and Sons, New York.

Batshaw, M., Brusilow, S., and Walser, M., 1975, Treatment of carbamyl phosphate synthetase deficiency with keto analogues of essential amino acids, N. Engl. J. Med. **292:**1085.

Bove, K. E., McAdams, A. J., Partin, J. C., Partin, J. S., Hug, G., and Schubert, W. K., 1975, The hepatic lesion in Reye's Syndrome, Gastroenterology **69:**685.

Brown, T., Hug, G., Bove, K., Brown, H., and Lansky, L., 1974, Reye's syndrome, Lancet **2:**716.

Campbell, A. G. M., Rosenberg, L. E., Snodgrass, P. J., and Nuzum, C. T., 1973, Ornithine transcarbamylase deficiency—A cause of lethal neonatal hyperammonemia in males, N. Engl. J. Med. **288:**1.

Cathelineau, L., Saudubray, J-M, and Polonovski, C., 1974, Heterogenous mutations of the structural gene of human ornithine carbamyltransferase as observed in five personal cases, Enzyme **18:**103.

Chaves-Carballo, E., Gomez, M. R., and Sharbrough, F. W., 1975, Encephalopathy and fatty infiltration of the viscera (Reye-Johnson Syndrome). A 17-year experience, Mayo Clin. Proc. **50:**209.

Gelehrter, T. D., and Rosenberg, L. E., 1975, Ornithine transcarbamylase deficiency. Unsuccessful therapy of neonatal hyperammonemia with N-carbamyl-L-glutamate and L-arginine, N. Engl. J. Med. **292:**351.

Gelehrter, T. D., and Snodgrass, P. J., 1974, Lethal neonatal deficiency of carbamyl phosphate synthetase, N. Engl. J. Med. **290:**430.

Goldstein, A. S., Hoogenraad, N. J., Johnson, J. D., Fukanaga, K., Swierczewski, E., Cann, H. M., and Sunshine, P., 1974, Metabolic and genetic studies of a family with ornithine transcarbamylase deficiency, Pediatr. Res. **8:**5.

Hilty, M. D., Romshe, C. A., and Delamater, P. V., 1974, Reye's syndrome and hyperaminoacidemia, J. Pediatr. **84:**362.

Hsia, Y. E., 1974, Inherited hyperammonemic syndromes, Gastroenterology **67:**347.

Huttenlocher, P. R., Schwartz, A. D., and Klatskin, G., 1969, Reye's syndrome: Ammonia intoxication as a possible factor in the encephalopathy, Pediatrics **43:**443.

Kang, E. A., and Gerald, P. S., 1972, Hyperammonemia and Reye's syndrome, N. Engl. J. Med. **286:**1216.

Levin, B., Dobbs, R. H., Burgess, E. A., and Palmer, T., 1969, Hyperammonaemia. A variant type of deficiency of liver ornithine transcarbamylase, Arch. Dis. Child. **44:**162.

MacLeod, P., Mackenzie, S., and Scriver, C. R., 1972, Partial ornithine carbamyl transferase deficiency: An inborn error of the urea cycle presenting as orotic aciduria in a male infant, Can. Med. Assoc. J. **107:**405.

Partin, J. C., Schubert, W. K., and Partin, J. S., 1971, Mitochondrial ultrastructure in Reye's syndrome (encephalopathy and fatty degeneration of the viscera), N. Engl. J. Med. **285:**1339.

Ricciuti, F. C., Gelehrter, T. D., and Rosenberg, L. E., 1976, X chromosome inactivation in human liver: Confirmation of X-linkage of ornithine transcarbamylase, Amer. J. Hum. Genet. **28:**332.

Saudubray, J. M., Cathelineau, L., Laugier, J. M., Charpentier, C., Lejeune, J. A., and Mozziconacci, P., 1975, Hereditary ornithine transcarbamylase deficiency. Report of two male cases with residual enzymatic activity, *Acta Pae-diatr. Scand.* **64**:464.

Scriver, C. R., and Rosenberg, L. E., 1973, Urea cycle and ammonia, *in: Amino Acid Metabolism and Its Disorders* (C. R. Scriver and L. E. Rosenberg, eds.), pp. 234–249, W. B. Saunders, Philadelphia.

Short, E. M., Conn, H. O., Snodgrass, P. J., Campbell, A. G. M., and Rosenberg, L. E., 1973, Evidence for X-linked dominant inheritance of ornithine transcar-bamylase deficiency, *N. Engl. J. Med.* **288**:7.

Sinatra, F., Yoshida, T., Applebaum, M., Mason, W., Hoogenraad, N. J., and Sunshine, P., 1975, Abnormalities of carbamyl phosphate synthetase and ornithine transcarbamylase in liver of patients with Reye's syndrome, *Pediatr. Res.* **9**:829.

Snodgrass, P. J., and DeLong, G. R., 1976, Urea-cycle enzyme deficiencies and an increased nitrogen load producing hyperammonemia in Reye's syndrome, *N. Engl. J. Med.* **294**:855.

Snyderman, S. E., Sansaricq, C., Phansalkar, S. V., Schacht, R. G., and Norton, P. M., 1975, The therapy of hyperammonemia due to ornithine transcarbamyl-ase deficiency in a male neonate, *Pediatrics* **56**:65.

Tang, T. T., Siegesmund, K. A., Sedmak, G. V., Casper, J. T., Varma, R. R., and McCredie, S. R., 1975, Reye syndrome. A correlated electron-microscopic, viral, and biochemical observation, *J. Amer. Med. Assoc.* **232**:1339.

Thaler, M. M., and Hoogenraad, N. J., 1974, Reye's syndrome, *Lancet* **2**:1203.

Thaler, M. M., Hoogenraad, N. J., and Boswell, M., 1974, Reye's syndrome due to a novel protein-tolerant variation of ornithine–transcarbamylase deficiency, *Lancet* **2**:438.

Inherited Defects of Cobalamin Metabolism (Section 7.3)

Ampola, M. G., Mahoney, M. J., Nakamura, E., and Tanaka, K., 1975, Prenatal therapy of a patient with vitamin B_{12}-responsive methylmalonic acidemia, *N. Engl. J. Med.* **293**:313.

Babior, B. M., ed., 1975, *Cobalamin: Biochemistry and Pathophysiology*, John Wiley and Sons, New York, 477 pp.

Carmel, R., and Herbert, V., 1969, Deficiency of vitamin B_{12}-binding alpha globulin in two brothers, *Blood* **33**:1.

Dillon, M. J., England, J. M., Gompertz, D., Goodey, P. A., Grant, D. B., Hussein, H. A. A., Linnell, J. C., Mathews, D. M., Mudd, S. H., Newns, G. H., Seakins, J. W. T., Uhlendorf, B. W., and Wise, I. J., 1974, Mental retardation, megalo-blastic anemia, methylmalonic aciduria and abnormal homocysteine metabo-lism due to an error in vitamin B_{12} metabolism, *Clin. Sci. Mol. Med.* **47**:43.

Donaldson, R. M., Jr., 1975, Mechanisms of malabsorption of cobalamin, *in: Coba-lamin: Biochemistry and Pathophysiology* (B. M. Babior, ed.), pp. 335–368, John Wiley and Sons, New York.

Gimpert, E., Jakob, M., and Hitzig, W. H., 1975, Vitamin B_{12} transport in blood. I. Congenital deficiency of transcobalamin II, *Blood* **45**:71.

Goodman, S. I., Moe, P. G., Hammond, K. B., Mudd, S. H., and Uhlendorf, B. W., 1970, Homocystinuria with methylmalonic aciduria: Two cases in a sibship, *Biochem. Med.* **4**:500.

Hakami, N., Neiman, P. E., Cannellos, G. P., and Lazerson, J., 1971, Neonatal megaloblastic anemia due to inherited transcobalamin II deficiency in two siblings, *N. Engl. J. Med.* **285**:1163.

Hitzig, W. H., Dohmann, U., Pluss, H. J., and Vischer, D., 1974, Hereditary transcobalamin II deficiency: Clinical findings in a new family, *J. Pediatr.* **85**:622.

Hsia, Y. E., Lilljeqvist, A.-C., and Rosenberg, L. E., 1970, Vitamin B_{12}-dependent methylmalonicaciduria: Amino acid toxicity, long-chain ketonuria and protective effect of vitamin B_{12}, *Pediatrics* **46**:497.

Kaye, C. I., Morrow, G., III, and Nadler, H. L., 1974, *In vitro* "responsive" methylmalonic acidemia: A new variant, *J. Pediatr.* **85**:55.

Linnell, J. C., Matthews, D. M., Mudd, S. H., Uhlendorf, B. W., and Wise, I. J., 1976, Cobalamins in fibroblasts cultured from normal control subjects and patients with methylmalonic aciduria, *Pediatr. Res.* **10**:179.

Mahoney, M. J., Rosenberg, L. E., Mudd, S. H., and Uhlendorf, B. W., 1971, Defective metabolism of vitamin B_{12} in fibroblasts from children with methylmalonicaciduria, *Biochem. Biophys. Res. Commun.* **44**:375.

Mahoney, M. J., and Rosenberg, L. E., 1975, Inborn errors of cobalamin metabolism, *in: Cobalamin, Biochemistry and Pathophysiology,* (B. M. Babior, ed.), pp. 369–402, John Wiley and Sons, New York.

Mahoney, M. J., Hart, A. C., Steen, V. D., and Rosenberg, L. E., 1975a, Methylmalonicacidemia: Biochemical heterogeneity in defects of 5'-deoxyadenosylcobalamin synthesis, *Proc. Nat. Acad. Sci. U.S.A.* **72**:2799.

Mahoney, M. J., Rosenberg, L. E., Waldenstrom, J., Lindblad, B., and Zetterstrom, R., 1975b, Prenatal diagnosis of methylmalonic aciduria, *Acta Paediatr. Scand.* **64**:44.

Mahoney, M. J., Nicholson, J. F., Hart, A. C., Rosenberg, L. E., and Challop, R., 1976, Cobalamin (vitamin B_{12}) toxicity in methylmalonicacidemia, *Pediatr. Res.* (abstract) **10**:368.

Morrow, G., III, Schwartz, R. H., Hallock, J. A., and Barness, L. A., 1970, Prenatal detection of methylmalonic acidemia, *J. Pediatr.* **77**:120.

Morrow, G., III, Mahoney, M. J., Mathews, C., and Lebowitz, J., 1975, Studies of methylmalonyl coenzyme A carbonylmutase activity in methylmalonic acidemia. I. Correlation of clinical, hepatic, and fibroblast data, *Pediatr. Res.* **9**:641.

Mudd, S. H., 1974, Homocystinuria and homocysteine metabolism: Selected aspects, *in: Heritable Disorders of Amino Acid Metabolism. Patterns of Clinical Expression and Genetic Variation* (W. L. Nyhan, ed.), pp. 429–451, John Wiley and Sons, New York.

Mudd, S. H., Levy, H. L., and Abeles, R. H., 1969, A derangement in B_{12} metabolism leading to homocystinemia, cystathioninemia and methylmalonicaciduria, *Biochem. Biophys. Res. Commun.* **35**:121.

Rosenberg, L. E., 1972, Disorders of propionate, methylmalonate, and cobalamin metabolism, *in: The Metabolic Basis of Inherited Disease* (J. B. Stanbury, J. B. Wyngaarden, and D. S. Fredrickson, eds.), Third Ed., pp. 440–458, McGraw-Hill, New York.

Rosenberg, L. E., 1976, Vitamin-responsive inherited metabolic disorders, *in:* *Advances in Human Genetics* (H. Harris and K. Hirschhorn, eds.), Vol. 6, pp. 1–74, Plenum Press, New York.

Rosenberg, L. E., Lilljeqvist, A.-C., and Hsia, Y. E., 1968, Methylmalonic aciduria: Metabolic block localization and vitamin B_{12} dependency, *Science* **162**:805.

Rosenberg, L. E., Patel, L., and Lilljeqvist, A.-C., 1975, Absence of an intracellular cobalamin-binding protein in cultured fibroblasts from patients with defective synthesis of 5′-deoxyadenosylcobalamin and methylcobalamin, *Proc. Nat. Acad. Sci. U.S.A.* **72**:4617.

Scott, C. R., Hakami, N., Chiang Teng, C., and Sagerson, R. N., 1972, Hereditary transcobalamin II deficiency: The role of transcobalamin II in vitamin B_{12}-mediated reactions, *J. Pediatr.* **81**:1106.

Stable Isotopes (Section 7.4)

Ando, T., Rasmussen, K., Nyhan, W. L., and Hull, D., 1972, 3-Hydroxpropionate: Significance of β-oxidation of propionate in patients with propionicacidemia and methylmalonic acidemia, *Proc. Nat. Acad. Sci. U.S.A.* **69**:2807.

Biemann, K., 1962, The mass spectra of isotopically labeled molecules, *in:* *Mass Spectrometry, Organic Chemical Applications*, pp. 204–250, McGraw-Hill, New York.

Bier, D. M., Sherman, W. R., Holland, W. H., and Kipnis, D. M., 1973, The *in vivo* measurement of alanine and glucose turnover with deuterium-labeled metabolites, *in:* *Proceedings of the First International Conference on Stable Isotopes in Chemistry, Biology, and Medicine*, pp. 397–403, U.S. Atomic Energy Commission, Technical Information Center, Springfield, Va.

Brenneman, R. R., and Kaufman, S., 1965, Characteristics of the hepatic phenylalanine-hydroxylating system in newborn rats, *J. Biol. Chem.* **240**:3617.

Caprioli, R. M., 1972, Use of stable isotopes, *in:* *Biochemical Applications of Mass Spectrometry* (G. R. Waller, ed.), pp. 735–776, John Wiley and Sons, New York.

Curtius, H. C., Baerlocher, K., and Völmin, J. A., 1972a, Pathogenesis of phenylketonuria: Inhibition of dopa and catecholamine synthesis in patients with phenylketonuria, *Clin. Chim. Acta* **42**:235.

Curtius, H. C., Völmin, J. A., and Baerlocher, K., 1972b, The use of deuterated phenylalanine for the elucidation of the phenylalanine-tyrosine metabolism, *Clin. Chim. Acta* **37**:277.

Gregg, G., Ott, D., Deaven, L., Spielmann, H., Krowke, R., and Neubert, D., 1976, The search for biological effects of carbon-13 enrichment in developing mammalian systems, *in:* *Proceedings of the Second International Conference on Stable Isotopes*, National Technical Information Service, Springfield, Va. (in press).

Hofmann, A. L., Klein, P. D., Thistle, J. L., Hachey, D. L., Hoffman, N. F., LaRusso, N. F., Thomas, P. J., and Szczepanik, P. A., 1973, Studies on the cause and treatment of gallstones using deuterium labeled bile acids, *in:* *Proceedings of the First International Conference on Stable Isotopes in Chemistry,*

Biology, and Medicine, pp. 369–379, U.S. Atomic Energy Commission, Technical Information Center, Springfield, Va.

Kinnory, D. S., Takeda, Y., and Greenberg, D. M., 1955, Isotope studies on the metabolism of valine, *J. Biol. Chem.* **212**:385.

London, R. E., Kollman, V. H., Mueller, D. D., and Matwiyoff, N. A., 1976, Biosynthetic and biophysical information from carbon-13–carbon-13 multiplets by carbon-13 nuclear magnetic resonance, *in: Proceedings of the Second International Conference on Stable Isotopes,* National Technical Information Service, Springfield, Va. (in press).

Mamer, O. A., and Tjoa, S. S., 1974, 2-Ethylhydracrylic acid: A newly described urinary organic acid, *Clin. Chim. Acta,* **55**:199.

Mamer, O. A., and Tjoa, S. S., 1975, 2-Ethyl-3-deutero-hydracrylic acid, the major urinary metabolite of 2-trideuteromethylbutyric acid by a new metabolic pathway, *Biomed. Mass Spectrom.* **2**:133.

Matwiyoff, N. A., and Ott, D. G., 1973, Stable isotope tracers in the life sciences and medicine, *Science* **181**:1125.

Meister, A., 1965a, Acylation of amino acids, *in: Biochemistry of the Amino Acids,* pp. 441–452, Academic Press, New York.

Meister, A., 1965b, Phenylalanine and tyrosine metabolism, *in: Biochemistry of the Amino Acids,* pp. 1059–1084, Academic Press, New York.

Milstein, S., and Kaufman, S., 1975, Studies on the phenylalanine hydroxylase system *in vivo, J. Biol. Chem.* **250**:4782.

Peng, S. K., Ho, K. J., and Taylor, C. B., 1972, Biologic effects of prolonged exposure to deuterium oxide. A behavioral, metabolic, and morphologic study, *Arch. Pathol.* **94**:81.

Robinson, W. G., Nagle, R., Bachhawat, B. K., Kupiecki, F. P., and Coon, M. J., 1957, Coenzyme A thiol esters of isobutyric, methacrylic and β-hydroxyisobutyric acids as intermediates in the enzymatic degradation of valine, *J. Biol. Chem.* **224**:1.

Ryhage, R., 1964, Use of a mass spectrometer as a detector and analyzer for effluents emerging from high temperature gas liquid chromatography column, *Anal. Chem.* **36**:759.

Scriver, C. R., and Rosenberg, L. E., 1973, Phenylalanine, *in: Amino Acid Metabolism and Its Disorders,* pp. 290–337, W. B. Saunders, Philadelphia.

Séquin, U., and Scott, I. A., 1974, Carbon-13 as a label in biosynthetic studies, *Science* **186**:101.

Stalder, K., 1959, Über das Vorkommen von Äthylmalonsäure im Harn, *Z. Physiol. Chem.* **314**:204.

Sweetman, L., Nyhan, W. L., Klein, P. D., and Szczepanik, P. A., 1973, Glycine 1,2-^{13}C in the investigation of children with inborn errors of metabolism, *in: Proceedings of the First International Conference on Stable Isotopes in Chemistry, Biology, and Medicine,* pp. 404–409, U.S. Atomic Energy Commission, Technical Information Center, Springfield, Va.

Tanaka, K., 1975, Disorders of organic acid metabolism, *in: Biology of Brain Dysfunction,* Vol. III (G. Gaull, ed.), pp. 145–214, Plenum Press, New York.

Tanaka, K., and Armitage, I. M., 1976, Investigation of ^{13}C-valine metabolism in methylmalonic acidemia using nuclear magnetic resonance: Identification of propionate as an obligate intermediate, *in: Proceedings of the Second International Conference on Stable Isotopes,* National Technical Information Service, Springfield, Va. (in press).

Tanaka, K., Armitage, I. M., Ramsdell, H. S., Hsia, Y. E., Lipsky, S. R., and Rosenberg, L. E., 1975, [^{13}C]Valine metabolism in methylmalonicacidemia using nuclear magnetic resonance: Propionate as an obligate intermediate, *Proc. Nat. Acad. Sci. U.S.A.* **72:**3692.

Taylor, C. B., Mikkelson, R., Anderson, J. A., and Forman, D. T., 1966, Human serum cholesterol synthesis measured with the deuterium label, *Arch. Pathol.* **81:**213.

Thomson, J. F., 1960, Physiological effects of D_2O in mammals, *Ann. N.Y. Acad. Sci.* **84:**736.

Udenfriend, S., 1967, The primary enzymatic defect in phenylketonuria and how it may influence the central nervous system, *in: Proceedings of a Conference on Phenylketonuria and Allied Metabolic Diseases* (J. A. Anderson and K. F. Swaiman, eds.), U.S. Department of Health, Education, and Welfare, Washington, D.C., pp. 1–8.

Williams, R. T., 1967, Comparative patterns of drug metabolism, *Fed. Proc. Fed. Amer. Soc. Exp. Biol.* **26:**1029.

Disorders of Purine and Pyrimidine Metabolism

J. Edwin Seegmiller

8.1. Introduction

During the past year, a number of developments have increased substantially our understanding of the coordinated relationship of human
purine and pyrimidine metabolism and the role of specific aberrations of
metabolism in this area in causation of human disease. However, in order
to understand and appreciate the significance of these developments,
background information is required. Since the subject has not previously
been reviewed in this series, the considerable material relating clinical and
biochemical correlations needs to be presented. A comprehensive description with specific citations of all major contributions of even the recent
years is not possible within the space limitations of this chapter. Therefore, the information will be summarized largely by referencing more

J. EDWIN SEEGMILLER • The University of California, La Jolla, California.

comprehensive reviews and more recent reports, rather than crediting, in all cases, the original citations of the various observations.

The primary objective has been to bring the clinician and the investigator in metabolic diseases up to date on the current state of our knowledge. Particular emphasis is given to the areas of research that need yet to be undertaken, and to the evolution of our concepts of the mechanism of development of disease, rather than to a recitation of all work in the field.

8.1.1. Role of Gout and Hyperuricemia in Development of New Medical Concepts

Human disorders of purine metabolism have provided an important chapter in the historical development of our knowledge of medicine. The first recognized disorder, gouty arthritis, very early became the focus for a continuing fruitful cooperation of the chemist, and, more recently, the biochemist, with the physician in investigations leading to development of many new medical concepts (Seegmiller, 1974; Wyngaarden and Kelley, 1972).

8.1.1.1. Pathology Produced by Sparingly Soluble Substances

The interest of the chemist in gouty arthritis began in 1776 with the isolation by the Swedish chemist Scheele of uric acid from a concretion of the urinary tract. In 1798, the British chemist Wollaston isolated the same substance from a gouty tophus that he is purported to have removed from his own ear. A half-century later, an elevated concentration of uric acid was demonstrated in the serum of gouty patients by the British physician Alfred Baring Garrod. In subsequent work, he formulated the essential concept of the pathology in gout being produced by crystalline deposits of sparingly soluble substances. This concept was lost for a time as an explanation of the pathological mechanism of the acute attack of gout, but additional evidence of its validity has been obtained during the past 15 years (Seegmiller *et al.*, 1963; McCarty, 1974). We now recognize the major pathological changes of gout as a consequence of the deposition of crystals of monosodium urate monohydrate in and about the joints and in the parenchymal portion of the kidney from supersaturated plasma, while at the lower pH of urine, crystals of free uric acid can accumulate as calculi in the kidney and bladder. This early recognition of the role of uric acid in the pathogenesis of gout led to the further exploration of correlates of chemical components in serum with pathological states—an exploration that still continues today.

8.1.1.2. Concept of Genetic Heterogeneity in Causation of Disease

In recent years, detailed studies of the causes of hyperuricemia responsible for the supersaturation of urate in serum of gouty patients have provided concrete evidence of a variety of mechanisms. Some patients show predominantly a diminished renal excretion of uric acid, while others show primarily an excessive synthesis of uric acid. Some patients show evidence of both processes (Seegmiller *et al.*, 1963). Further evidence of genetic heterogeneity in the causes of hyperuricemia has come with the identification during the past decade of a number of different enzyme defects responsible for hyperuricemia and gout, reviewed by Becker and Seegmiller (1974) and Kelley and Wyngaarden (1974). Genetic heterogeneity has also been found from one family to another in the types of mutational defects within a single gene responsible for impairment of an enzyme activity (Kelley *et al.*, 1969).

8.1.2. Insight into Cellular and Physiological Mechanisms Revealed by Mutations

The highly specific nature of the metabolic lesion produced by most of the abnormal gene products serves as a beacon for illuminating in a unique manner complex metabolic interrelationships in the intact organism that might otherwise be impossible to deduce. The bacterial geneticists have used this approach to develop at will specific mutations that are of value in revealing the biochemical basis for ever more complex biological phenomena. Only in recent years have we begun to use similar approaches to study the mammalian cell. For similar studies of human cellular processes, we have been almost completely dependent on spontaneous mutations presenting clinically as human disease for obtaining our human mutations until very recently (DeMars and Held, 1972; Sato *et al.*, 1972; Lever *et al.*, 1974; Nuki *et al.*, 1974). The specific human enzyme defects identified from spontaneous human mutations have already provided many detailed insights into normal cellular and physiological mechanisms made apparent by the perturbation created by the mutation.

8.1.2.1. Regulation of Purine Synthesis

Of special value has been the insight gained into the normal regulation of the rate of purine biosynthesis. Mutations in two different human genes have been particularly informative. A gross deficiency of the enzyme hypoxanthine–guanine phosphoribosyltransferase (HPRT), an

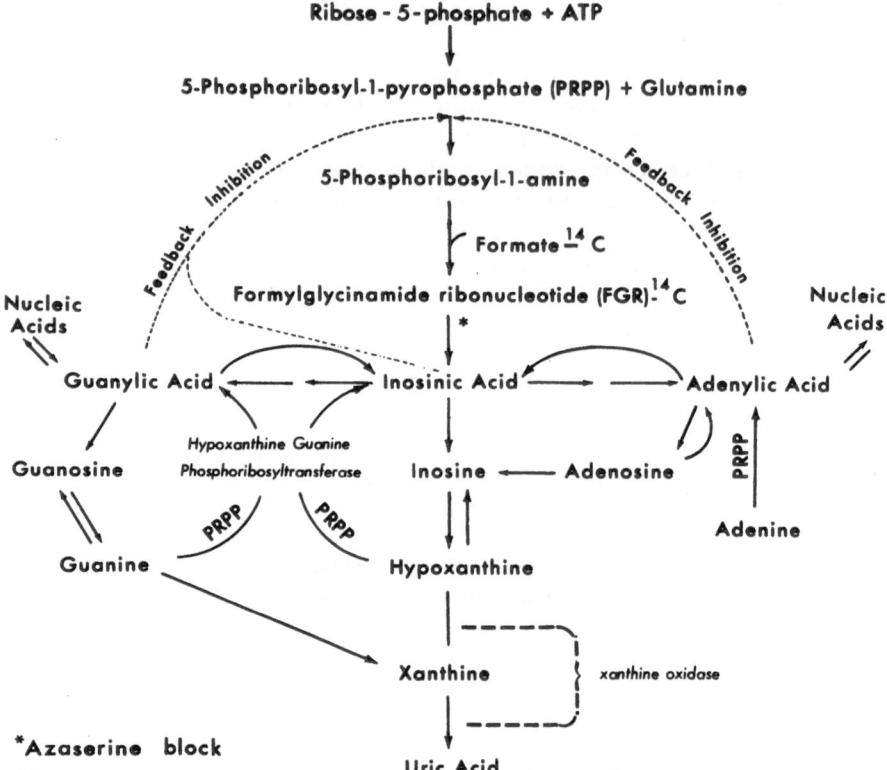

Fig. 1. Regulation of purine synthesis and site of the enzyme defect in the Lesch-Nyhan syndrome. Although purine nucleotides inhibit the presumed rate-limiting enzyme phosphoribosylpyrophosphate (PRPP) glutamine amidotransferase, the excessive rate of purine synthesis in the Lesch-Nyhan syndrome is apparently driven by the accumulation of PRPP, a substrate for the missing enzyme hypoxanthine-guanine phosphoribosyltransferase as well as for the rate-limiting amidotransferase. (Reproduced from Seegmiller *et al.*, 1967, with permission of the publishers. Copyright 1976 by the American Association for the Advancement of Science.)

X-linked defect responsible for the Lesch-Nyhan syndrome and its variants (Seegmiller *et al.*, 1967) (Fig. 1), is accompanied by a 4–8 fold increase in the rate of purine biosynthesis. The cause of this increased synthetic rate has been traced to the intracellular accumulation of a substrate for the missing enzyme HPRT; this substrate, phosphoribosylpyrophosphate (PP-ribose-P) (Rosenbloom *et al.*, 1968), enhances the rate of the presumed rate-limiting enzyme in two different ways: (1) It exerts an allosteric activation of the rate-limiting enzyme, PP-ribose-P glutamine amidotransferase (see below), by converting it to an active monomeric form, thus reversing the action of the purine nucleotides in producing an inactive

dimer form of the enzyme, as shown in Fig. 2 (Holmes *et al.*, 1973a,b).
(2) That PP-ribose-P is normally present in rate-limiting concentrations, substantially lower than required for maximal enzyme activity at substrate saturation, provides the second mechanism, by which increases in intracellular concentration of PP-ribose-P increase the rate of purine synthesis (Wood and Seegmiller, 1973; Fox, I. H., and Kelley, 1974a).

Confirmation of this concept was provided by the discovery of a mutation in a different gene that is also responsible for an increased concentration of intracellular PP-ribose-P associated with purine overproduction in gouty arthritis in additional gouty families (Henderson *et al.*, 1968; Hershko *et al.*, 1968). A diminished inhibition of purine synthesis in response to preformed purine compounds in cells cultured from 2 gouty patients suggested the presence of an abnormal regulatory enzyme (PP-ribose-P glutamine amidotransferase) that is less responsive than normal to feedback inhibitors (Henderson *et al.*, 1968). However, in both patients (Becker *et al.*, 1974b; Becker and Seegmiller, 1974, 1975), and in a family from Israel (Sperling *et al.*, 1974a), the increased PP-ribose-P was traced to an increased rate of its synthesis from overactivity of the enzyme PP-ribose-P synthetase. Correlations of the rate of purine synthesis with changes in the intracellular concentration of PP-ribose-P induced by a variety of pharmacological agents both *in vitro* (Boyle *et al.*, 1972; Kelley *et al.*, 1970a; Fox, I. H., and Kelley, 1973) and *in vivo* (Kelly *et al.*, 1970b; Kelley, 1975a,b) provide additional evidence of the important role of intra-

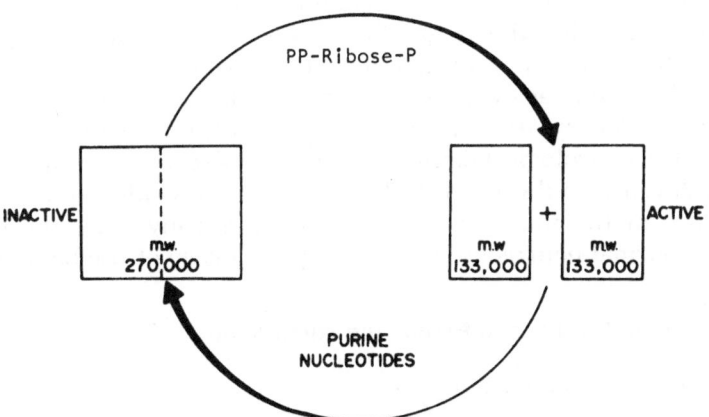

Fig. 2. Molecular mechanism of regulation of the rate of purine biosynthesis. The activity of the enzyme phosphoribosylpyrophosphate glutamine amidotransferase is regulated by its conversion to a relatively inactive dimer by purine nucleotides and its reversal to an active monomer by phosphoribosylpyrophosphate (PP-ribose-P). (Reproduced from Holmes *et al.*, 1974b, with permission of the publishers.)

cellular PP-ribose-P concentration as a determinant of the rate of purine biosynthesis.

8.1.2.2. Physiological Consequences of Failure To Repair DNA Damaged by Ultraviolet (UV) Light

Mutations in the purine and pyrimidine metabolizing systems have revealed additional cellular and physiological mechanisms involving these compounds. Exposure of cells to UV light results in a dimerization of adjacent thymine bases of DNA that are normally repaired by excision and replacement catalyzed by a series of repair enzymes. In the recessively inherited disease xeroderma pigmentosum (XP), the repair mechanism is defective (Cleaver, 1968). Hybridization of XP fibroblasts from different families has revealed four complementation groups (A, B, C, and D) that repair the defect, and a fifth that produces no such complementing repair (Robbins *et al.*, 1974; Pedrini *et al.*, 1974). The failure to correct these UV-induced changes in DNA in patients with XP results in an increased sensitivity to sunlight and multiple cutaneous neoplasms in exposed areas of the skin.

8.1.2.3. Role of Purine and Pyrimidine Nucleotide Metabolism in Brain Function

Some indication of the essential role of purine and pyrimidine nucleotide metabolism in brain function is provided by the mental retardation accompanying the virtual loss of the two enzymes orotate phosphoribosyltransferase and orotate decarboxylase in the autosomal recessive disorder orotic aciduria (see the recent summaries by Smith *et al.*, 1972; Seegmiller, 1974; and Levine *et al.*, 1974; see also Section 8.4.1). Likewise, the neurological damage and compulsive self-mutilating behavior of children with the Lesch-Nyhan syndrome provide evidence of the importance of the purine reutilization pathways involving the enzyme HPRT in normal neurological function, particularly of the basal ganglia.

8.1.2.4. Role of Purine and Pyrimidine Nucleotide Metabolism in Normal Development and Function of the Hematological System

Organ systems with a rapid cellular proliferation inherently require a constant large supply of purine and pyrimidine nucleotides to meet the needs for new synthesis of the nucleic acids DNA and RNA. In fact, considerable evidence has accumulated of the need of such rapidly proliferating tissues for a supplemental source of purine compounds supplied by the liver and transported by erythrocytes as an additional function not commonly recognized (Pritchard *et al.*, 1970; Lerner and Lowy, 1974; Lowy and Lerner, 1974). Such a carrier role of the erythrocyte is also implicit in the relatively rapid turnover of purine compounds of mature erythrocytes coupled with their inability to synthesize purine compounds *de novo* (Lowy and Lerner, 1974; Lerner and Lowy, 1974). The rapid uptake by the normal kidney of purine compounds generated within the liver (Lowy and Lerner, 1974) suggests a possible role of this system in the renal failure accompanying severe liver dysfunction in the "hepatorenal" syndrome. No measurements of intracellular nucleotides or of plasma purine compounds have yet been made. The liver may provide, in addition, pyrimidine compounds for nourishment of other organs, including brain, as summarized by Levine *et al.* (1974).

The consistent association of orotic aciduria with a megaloblastic anemia and its occasional association with the Lesch-Nyhan syndrome provide evidence of the importance of these enzymes of pyrimidine and of purine metabolism in the normal functioning and development of these systems as well. The importance of the enzyme HPRT in the normal proliferation of stem cell precusors of the hematopoetic system is shown by a curious characteristic of females heterozygous for the X-linked deficiency of HPRT. A consequence of the random inactivation of one of the two X chromosomes at an early stage in the development of female zygote (see the summaries by Seegmiller, 1974; and Kelley and Wyngaarden, 1972) is the presence of both normal and mutant cell populations in the somatic cells of heterozygote females. Such mosaicism is readily demonstrated in fibroblasts cultured from heterozygote females, but their red cells and leukocytes show only normal cells in families with severe enzyme deficiency (Rosenbloom *et al.*, 1967; Nyhan *et al.*, 1970). These observations suggest an enhanced differential rate of proliferation for the normal hematopoetic stem cell, as compared with the mutant. This selective advantage is not seen in families with less severe enzyme defects (Emmerson *et al.*, 1972).

8.1.2.5. Role of Purine Nucleoside Interconversion and Pyrimidine Metabolism in the Immune Response

A completely unanticipated role for enzymes of purine interconversion was revealed by the discovery by Giblett *et al.* (1972) of adenosine deaminase deficiency in 2 patients with combined immunodeficiency disease. The subsequent identification by Giblett *et al.* (1975a) of a patient with isolated T-cell dysfunction associated with a gross deficiency of purine nucleoside phosphorylase has provided additional evidence for the concept. In addition, a low-activity allele of uridine monophosphate kinase was found in 2 children with frequent infections (Giblett *et al.*, 1974) (see Section 8.4.3).

8.1.2.6. Purine and Pyrimidine Biosynthesis as a Major Function of Carbon Dioxide Required by Mammalian Cells *In Vitro*

New perspective on the relative importance of carbon dioxide fixation in the metabolism of a variety of mammalian cells has come from recent studies of Scheffler (1974). The absolute requirement of several cell lines for carbon dioxide for growth can be met by addition of the purine hypoxanthine and the pyrimidine uridine to the medium, suggesting that the major role of carbon dioxide as a nutrient in these cell lines may be its incorporation into the purine and pyrimidine rings. As expected, hypoxanthine was unable to replace carbon dioxide in HPRT-deficient human fibroblasts.

8.1.2.7. Use of Purine and Pyrimidine Mutants in Somatic Cell Genetics

Mammalian cell lines deficient in the enzyme HPRT have been very useful in cell hybridization studies. Azaguanine can be used to allow selective survival of mutant cells deficient in the enzyme HPRT and therefore unable to convert azaguanine to its toxic nucleotide form. Conversely, the HPRT-deficient cells can be selectively killed by inhibiting purine synthesis *de novo* with either aminopterin of "HAT" medium (Sato *et al.*, 1972) or azaserine and providing hypoxanthine in the medium, thereby making cell survival dependent on the presence of HPRT for utilization of the hypoxanthine (Seegmiller *et al.*, 1969). The greater requirement of the HPRT-deficient cells for exogenous carbon dioxide suggests the use of low carbon dioxide concentrations as an alternate to "HAT" medium in selection against HPRT-deficient cells (Scheffler, 1974).

In an analogous manner, the thymidine analogue bromodeoxyuridine (BUdR) has been used to select for cells deficient in thymidine kinase. In addition, the lethal effects of exposure to light of cells that have incorporated BUdR forms the basis of a general system for selection of a variety of auxotrophic mutants analogous to the use of penicillin in selection of bacterial mutants. The selection is based on the failure of auxotrophic mutants to grow in the presence of minimal growth medium. They therefore fail to incorporate the BUdR, thereby escaping its lethal action, and are subsequently "rescued" by growth on enriched medium.

8.2. Abnormalities of Purine Metabolism

8.2.1. Adenine Phosphoribosyltransferase Deficiency

The heterozygous state for adenine phosphoribosyltransferase (APRT) deficiency was first observed as an autosomal dominantly inherited trait in erythrocytes of 4 persons over three generations with enzyme activities ranging from 21 to 37% of normal (Kelley *et al.*, 1968). The defect has since been found in additional families, including some families with gout, but no disease state has yet been found as a consistent accompaniment of the partial deficiency (Fox, I. H., *et al.*, 1973; Fox I. H., and Kelley 1974c; Emmerson *et al.*, 1974; Delbarre *et al.*, 1974a,b). Srivastava *et al.* (1972) found a frequency for the trait of 1 per 100 individuals screened in a small series.

The clinical consequence of homozygosity for the enzyme defect has only recently been observed in a 4-year old girl who presented with calculi of the urinary tract. Her first episode of dysuria 6 months earlier was relieved spontaneously by her expulsion of a microcalculus (Cartier *et al.*, 1974). The second required retrograde intervention under anesthesia, with the removal via the urethra of 26 calculi weighing a total of 460 mg. In both cases, chemical examination of the calculi with the murexide test indicated that these were uric acid stones. Although her serum urate was only 6 mg/dl, she was admitted for more detailed study of her purine metabolism. Ion-exchange chromatography of the calculi revealed the presence of around 5–10% uric acid, with a second component that was identical with 2,8-dioxyadenine by UV absorption spectrum at pH's of 2, 7, and 12; by migration on electrophoresis in borate buffer, pH 9.0; by IR absorption spectra; and by X-ray diffraction pattern of the crystalline material. Her 24-hr urine contained normal quantities of uric acid (Cartier and Hamet, personal communication), but 40 mg adenine, as compared with around 1.5 mg in the 24-hr urine of a normal person.

The activity of APRT was grossly deficient. Her erythrocyte hemolysate showed an activity less than 0.01% of normal, while the activity of her HPRT was in the normal range. Unfortunately, no cell cultures could be obtained. Both parents and her maternal grandfather showed APRT activities of their erythrocyte lysates in the range 30–46% of normal, thus providing good evidence of the recessive inheritance of this disorder.

From cell hybridization studies of a similar mutation in animal cells, Tischfield and Ruddle (1974) concluded that the APRT locus is on chromosome 16. This location suggests the need for studies of possible linkage between APRT and alpha haptoglobin (McKusick, 1975).

The absence of obvious neurological, hematological, or other gross pathology in this child suggests that adenine reutilization may be of less importance in normal physiological function of cells than is the reutilization of hypoxanthine or guanine. However, before this conclusion can be definitely established, the possibility of significant amounts of residual APRT activity being present in other body cells must be ruled out.

8.2.2. Hypoxanthine–Guanine Phosphoribosyltransferase (HPRT) Deficiency

HPRT deficiency continues to be a consistent accompaniment of the Lesch-Nyhan syndrome and its variants. Several reviews have appeared (de Bruyn, 1976; Seegmiller, 1974; Kelley, 1974; Kelley and Wyngaarden, 1972, 1974). The primary mutation appears to be in the structural gene coding for HPRT, as immunologically cross-reacting material has been reported by several investigators. Capecchi *et al.* (1974) and Arnold and Kelley (1974) found evidence of an accelerated destruction of mutant HPRT enzyme in mouse fibroblasts carrying this enzyme deficiency, with evidence that the abnormal gene product is present in substantially reduced amounts. Similar studies have not yet been done on human mutant cells. Bakay *et al.* (1975) found evidence of restoration of human HPRT activity after fusion of HPRT-deficient human and mouse cell lines.

The purine overproduction is also consistently associated with an increased intracellular concentration of PP-ribose-P. The range of clinical presentation in general tends to reflect the severity of the enzyme deficit, although some exceptions have been found (Emmerson and Thompson, 1973). Children with even the most severe enzyme defect appear normal at birth, but the enzyme defect and characteristic biochemical changes are present. In many infants, careful questioning of the mothers reveals that the first indication of any abnormality is the occasional presence of reddish-orange "sand" noted in the diapers, which is undoubtedly crystals of uric acid from its excessive production. In the past, no significance has been attached to this finding by either the parent or the physician, but it obviously deserves greater attention. Obstruction of the urinary tract, particularly during periods of dehydration or passage of calculi, is an additional consequence of the excessive uric acid production, and may lead to early impairment of renal function. Neurological symptoms first appear around 6 months of age with inability to hold up the head, followed by development of spasticty and hypereflexia and choreoathetosis. The appearance of self-mutilation by biting of lips, tongue, and fingers is extremely variable in time of onset and severity. In occasional patients, it has been first noted with the appearance of the lower incisors; in others, it has been as late as 14 years of age. In occasional patients, it may even be sporadic in appearance.

Treatment consists of a high fluid intake, allopurinol to diminish uric acid production and to control hyperuricemia, and diazepam (Valium) to diminish spasticity. Beneficial effects of hydroxytryptophan in controlling self-mutilating behavior were reported by Mizuno and Yugari (1974). Rockson *et al.* (1974) reported an increased activity of dopamine-β-hydroxylase, suggesting an increased adrenergic activity, as well as a curious absence of the pressor response to cold. These observations, if confirmed, suggest the possibility of a relative imbalance between catecholamines and serotonin, which is the metabolic product formed from hydroxytryptophan in brain (Fernstrom, 1974). These concepts suggest new avenues of exploration for possible approaches to treatment of the neurological and behavior problems of these children.

Since no fully effective treatment of the neurological dysfunction has been found, its preventive control through prenatal diagnosis of pregnancies at risk for carrying a affected child is warranted. In our own laboratory, we have now monitored 17 pregnancies at risk for this disease, and have found 6 affected fetuses, in each case sufficiently early that the parents' desire to terminate the pregnancy could be met (Boyle *et al.*, 1970; Van Heeswijk *et al.*, 1972). Since the disease is X-linked, female relatives at risk for the disease should be notified of the need to monitor their pregnancies if they are to avoid the chance of producing an affected male. Heterozygous carriers can be identified by demonstrating the normal and mutant cells by biochemical tests of cultured skin fibroblasts or of hair roots (Rosenbloom *et al.*, 1968; Francke *et al.*, 1973).

With this development, the identification of all affected males becomes of crucial importance. A simple screening test is the determination of the ratio of uric acid to creatinine in a casual urine specimen (Kaufman *et al.*, 1968), with confirmation by assay for the enzyme in a heparinized blood sample.

The HPRT locus has been identified on the midportion of the long arm of the X-chromosome (McKusick, 1975) within mapping distance of the more distally located glucose-6-phosphate dehydrogenase (Francke *et al.*, 1974), with the α-galactosidase and phosphoglycerate kinase loci residing in the adjacent regions toward the centromere. This same relative relationship is confirmed by the X-ray fragmentation method for mapping genes (Goss and Harris, 1975).

The nature of the primary mutation varies from one family to another. In some instances, the mutation has affected primarily the affinity constant K_m for one of the substrates (McDonald and Kelley, 1974; Benke et al., 1973a). As a consequence, very sophisticated kinetic analysis has been required in some cases to demonstrate the enzyme deficit (Fox, I. H., et al., 1975).

Associated with the enzyme defect is an increased activity of APRT in erythrocytes, but not in fibroblasts or other cell types. A stabilization of the APRT by the high erythrocyte content of PP-ribose-P against attrition with time provides one possible explanation (Seegmiller, 1974). Increases in activity of a variety of other enzymes have also been observed in association with HPRT deficiency. An increased activity of PP-ribose-P synthetase was reported by Reem (1975), but this finding is at variance with previous work of other investigators (Rosenbloom et al., 1968; Becker et al., 1973b).

A defect in intracellular transport of hypoxanthine (and guanine) was described in HPRT-deficient cells (Benke et al., 1973b), and HPRT was reported in normal erythrocyte cell membranes (de Bruyn and Oei, 1974). However, considerable evidence argues against HPRT serving a transport function in the mammalian cell (Berlin and Oliver, 1975).

8.2.3. Adenosine Deaminase Deficiency

A gross deficiency of adenosine deaminase (ADA) was first discovered during screening for isoenzyme patterns of ADA as genetic markers by Giblett et al. (1972). No red cell ADA activity was detectable in 2 young unrelated females with combined immunodeficiency disease. Intermediate activity of ADA in the erythrocytes of their parents with consanguinity in one family supported a recessive mode of inheritance. Additional patients were soon found (Ochs et al., 1973; Dissing and Knudsen, 1972; Yount et al., 1974). The available data were recently summarized (Meuwissen and Pollara, 1974; Meuwissen et al., 1975a,b; Bergsma, 1975) from two recent conferences on immunodeficiency disease.

8.2.3.1. Range of Clinical Presentation

The clinical presentation in both children suggested a severe T-lymphocyte dysfunction associated with varying degrees of B-lymphocyte dysfunction (Giblett et al., 1972). One child, 22 months of age, had a history of recurrent respiratory infections and candidiasis, and marked lymphopenia of 50–500 lymphocytes/mm³ from neonatal life. She showed no delayed hypersensitivity response to Candida, mumps, or streptokinase–streptodornase, and could not be sensitized to dinitrochlorobenzene. The response of her lymphocytes to the phytohemagglutinin and pokeweed mitogens, as well as to allogeneic cells, was very poor. Plasma immunoglobulins declined from normal or elevated levels during the first 9 months to very low levels, particularly of IgG and IgM, and secretory IgA was undetectable in saliva. Despite her blood group O, she failed to develop anti-A and anti-B. Only a minimal response was produced by injection of diphtheria, pertussis, tetanus (DPT), and typhoid vaccine, and her Schick test remained positive. She did show antibodies to herpes and adenoviruses. Following a transplant of fetal thymus and liver, which was without therapeutic benefit, she nevertheless developed a strong titer of cytotoxic antibodies against a panel of human lymphocytes.

The second child, age 3½ years, was purportedly healthy during the first 2 years of life. However, her immunological status had been studied in detail because of the death from immunological deficiency of a female sibling. Despite a moderate lymphopenia of 800–1250/mm^3 and up to 25% eosinophils at 2 weeks of life, she had no significant clinical symptoms until the onset, at 24 months of age, of a series of mild upper respiratory infections, which rapidly became worse. At age 30 months, she showed hepatosplenomegaly and a progressive deterioration of her pulmonary system. At age 40 months, a variety of bronchial flora including *Candida* were cultured, and she showed signs of severe airway obstruction. Her leukocyte count ranged from 4400 to 9900/mm^3, with 680–4160 lymphocytes/mm^3 and 5–25% eosinophils. Platelets, hemoglobin, and karyotype were all normal, but her lymphocytes responded only minimally to phytohemagglutinin and allogeneic cells. As with the previous patient, she showed no delayed hypersensitivity to *Candida* or streptokinase–streptodornase, and could not be sensitized to dinitrochlorobenzene. Her serum showed no anti-A or anti-B, despite blood group O. Antibody response to DPT was minimal, and Schick test remained positive. She had nevertheless formed antibodies against some common viruses and bacteria. Immunoglobulin levels ranged as follows: IgG, 1700–1200 mg; IgM, 1312–145 mg; IgA, 98–56 mg; and IgE, 23 µg/100 ml plasma.

A fatal combined immunodeficiency disease with many similarities to the human disorder was described by McGuire *et al.* (1974) in foals of Arabian horses. This holds forth the possibility of an experimental animal for more detailed study, and ADA should be examined.

In a series of 23 patients with combined immunodeficiency disease, severe ADA deficiency was found in 12 (Meuwissen *et al.*, 1975b; Cohen, 1975). Many clinical symptoms in the groups with and without ADA deficiency were very similar in frequency, and included chronic diarrhea and malabsorption, chronic pneumonia, and noninfectious skin lesions.

Infection with opportunistic pathogens and recurrent otitis media were noted in both groups, but were somewhat more frequent in the ADA-deficient patients. All patients with ADA deficiency showed candidiasis and failure to thrive, while only 50% of the patients with normal ADA had these problems. Most ADA-deficient patients showed impairment of cell-mediated immunity suggestive of fairly severe impairment of T-cell function (Cohen and Lightbody, 1975), with variable degrees of impairment of humoral immunity and B-cell function (Wara and Ammann, 1975). Correlations have not yet been made between severity of clinical disease and quantities of residual (if any) ADA activity in fibroblasts or lymphoblasts, but genetic heterogeneity is to be expected as a major factor to account for the range of clinical expression (Giblett *et al.*, 1975b).

The identification of ADA deficiency in association with combined immunodeficiency disease in more than two dozen patients, and the absence of gross ADA deficiency in over 54,000 individuals of the general population (Spencer *et al.*, 1968; Dissing and Knudsen, 1970; Hopkinson *et al.*, 1969; Meuwissen *et al.*, 1975b), argue strongly for a possible etiological relationship. The presence of gross ADA deficiency in erythrocytes of a 12-year-old native of the !Kung tribe of the Kalahari desert of South Africa in the absence of any clinical evidence of immunodeficiency has been puzzling (Giblett *et al.*, 1975b). Although only 2–3% of normal ADA activity was found in erythrocytes, normal ADA activity was eventually found in his lymphocytes (Meuwissen *et al.*, 1975b).

8.2.3.2. Radiographic Changes

Children with ADA deficiency also show characteristic radiographic lesions of diagnostic value, summarized by Wolfson and Cross (1975). In addition to the osteoporosis, characteristic lung pattern, and small or absent thymus, tonsils, and adenoids seen in all patients with combined immunodeficiency disease, 9 of 12 patients with ADA deficiency showed one or more of the following bone abnormalities:

1. Cupping concavity and flaring of anterior rib ends at the costochondral junction.
2. Broad, vertically short pelvis, relatively square ilia, and short, bluntly ending ischia.
3. Alteration of contour and articulation of transverse processes and posterior ribs.
4. Platyspondylisis (slight decrease in height of thoracic and lumbar vertebrae).
5. Abnormally thick growth arrest lines.

Some of these changes resemble those of infantile achondroplasia.

8.2.3.3. Genetics

Although initial reports of a genetic linkage of the ADA and the HLA loci suggested a possible small chromosomal deletion of both loci (Giblett *et al.*, 1972), the frequency of occurrence of ADA deficiency makes it very unlikely (Giblett *et al.*, 1975b). Furthermore, the subsequent demonstration of the locus of erythrocyte ADA on chromosome 20 and the HLA locus on chromosome 6 makes this possibility most unlikely (McKusick, 1975). A recessive mode of inheritance as a silent allele (Chen *et al.*, 1974; Giblett *et al.*, 1975b) was shown in all family studies. Scott *et al.* (1974) found that the activity of erythrocyte ADA decreased to a mean value approximately one-half of controls in 9 of 17 individuals in three generations who were at risk for being heterozygous for ADA deficiency. These authors concluded that within a high-risk family, heterozygotes may be identified with 90% confidence.

8.2.3.4. Enzymology of Adenosine Deaminase

ADA was purified 32,000-fold (Rossi *et al.*, 1975) from erythrocytes by affinity chromatography. Less highly purified preparations showed K_m values of 30 μM (Osborne and Spencer, 1973) and 25 μM (Agarwal *et al.*, 1975). In human tissues, ADAs of both low and high molecular weights were found (Akedo *et al.*, 1970, 1972; van der Weyden and Kelley, 1974; van der Weyden *et al.*, 1974). The smaller one, with estimates of molecular weight ranging from 30,000 to 47,000, is converted by incubation with an enzyme found in lung or liver to a larger aggregate with greater thermal stability of mol.wt. 230,000 (Akedo *et al.*, 1972; Hirschhorn, 1975b). The larger can be disaggregated to the smaller molecular species by incubation with guanidine, with partial recovery of enzyme activity after dialysis.

Three electrophoretic isoenzyme patterns of erythrocyte ADA reflecting two alleles were found by Spencer *et al.* (1968), and a third rare allele with a substantially reduced activity was reported by Hopkinson *et al.* (1969). The different isoenzyme patterns of ADA revealed in tissues of various organs on electrophoresis were initially interpreted as evidence for as many as four or five loci for ADA. However, Hirschhorn (1975a,b) showed absence of ADA activity of an affected patient not only in erythrocytes, but also in spleen, muscle, intestine, heart, and liver. Furthermore, incubation of ADA from a normal lymphoblast line or erythrocytes with various tissues of ADA-deficient patients produced the additional isoenzyme patterns characteristic of each of the organs. Evidently, ADA synthesis is controlled by a single structural gene coding for an enzyme of erythrocytes and lymphocytes of molecular weight around 35,000–

47,000. A posttranscriptional modification then increases the molecular weight or alters the charge to produce the various isoenzyme patterns of erythrocytes, lymphocytes, and the various organs. Van der Weyden and Kelley (1974) and van der Weyden *et al.* (1974) found 0.5% of normal ADA activity in the spleen of a child who died with ADA deficiency and severe combined immunodeficiency disease. Sedimentation analysis showed that the diminished activity resided in an intermediate-molecular-weight species, with absence of activity in the high- and low-molecular-weight fractions found as additional peaks in normal human spleen. They concluded that the defect may occur at a step after translation of ADA messenger RNA into protein, and probably does not result from a genetic deletion.

8.2.3.5. Changes with Mitogenic Stimulation

In addition to the three electrophoretic bands of the low-molecular-weight forms of ADA, lymphocytes show 35% of the total activity in the form of a tissue-specific ADA of substantially higher molecular weight. This proportion decreases to 8% on stimulation with phytohemagglutinin. Stimulation with concanavalin A, a presumed T-cell mitogen, produced a similar decrease, while stimulation with pokeweed mitogen, a presumed B-cell mitogen, produced no change in tissue isoenzymes. That the high-molecular-weight form of the enzyme is of lower activity but greater stability, while the lower-molecular-weight form shows a higher activity but a decreased stability, provides a possible mechanism for the cell to obtain a greater activity of enzyme without altering its rate of synthesis of the protein (Hirschhorn, 1975a; Hirschhorn and Levytska, 1974).

8.2.3.6. Proposed Pathogenetic Mechanisms

The association of ADA deficiency with impairment of the immune response was most unexpected. However, in retrospect, it need not have been. In a number of hereditary diseases, the organ system most severely affected by a mutation-induced deficiency is the organ in which the enzyme is normally most abundant, as exemplified by the high HPRT activity in brain, particularly the basal ganglia (Kelley and Wyngaarden, 1972; Seegmiller, 1974). In six mammalian species, ADA is normally most abundant in the spleen and duodenum (Brady and Donovan, 1965). Furthermore, an increase in the ADA activity of cells and lymph draining a sheep lymph node was noted by Hall (1963) to accompany both plasma cell and antibody production in response to antigenic stimulus. In normal human lymphocytes, as well as in cultured lymphoblastoid cell lines,

Coleman and Hutton (1975) found, with some few exceptions, a general correlation between ADA activity, terminal deoxynucleotidyl transferase, and the presence of surface markers of T-cells. Therefore, one might deduce that ADA deficiency could very well impair the function of the lymphatic system. Affected children develop a severe lymphopenia, and those lymphocytes present show only a very weak response to phytohemagglutinin and other mitogenic stimuli.

The mechanism by which the ADA deficiency produces impairment in the lymphatic system has not been elucidated, but several theories have been proposed. Since adenosine and AMP are effective in inhibiting RNA, protein, and DNA synthesis (Hirschhorn *et al.,* 1970), the modulation of ADA enzyme activity observed could represent a mechanism either for removing the potentially toxic metabolite adenosine or for providing an efficient conversion to a form convenient for salvage of purines required for proliferative processes (Hirschhorn, 1975a).

Although an accumulation of adenosine in ADA-deficient cells has not yet been demonstrated, it has been considered as a possible mechanism involved in the disease. An increase in intracellular cyclic adenylic acid (cAMP) was noted from adenosine administration (Hadden, 1975), but has not yet been demonstrated in ADA-deficient cells.

The demonstration of a toxic action of adenosine requires special growth media. The relatively high content of ADA in fetal calf serum and normal human serum used in cell cultures leads to a very rapid deamination of adenosine, within minutes or hours (Green, 1975). Horse serum contains virtually no ADA, and its use permitted a study of the toxicity of adenosine. At concentrations of 10^{-4}–10^{-6} M, it killed a variety of cell lines, and at lower concentrations inhibited their growth (Green and Chan, 1973). This growth inhibition could be fully overcome by pyrimidine, but not by purine compounds (Green and Chan, 1973; Ishii and Green, 1973), suggesting a possible inhibition of pyrimidine synthesis by adenosine. Confirmation for this concept was found by demonstration of a reduced incorporation of ^{14}C-aspartic acid into uridine nucleotides and the appearance of labeled orotic acid in the medium. Further evidence of the pyrimidine starvation was the lowered intracellular concentration of pyrimidine nucleotides found by high-pressure liquid chromatography. Since adenosine, but not inosine or hypoxanthine, produces a marked lowering of intracellular PP-ribose-P, and cells relatively deficient in adenosine kinase are more resistant to the toxic action of adenosine, the effect is thought to be mediated through an adenine nucleotide, possibly ADP, acting to inhibit the activity of PP-ribose-P synthetase (Green, 1975). The diminished intracellular concentration of PP-ribose-P could decrease the rate of pyrimidine synthesis at two different metabolic sites. PP-ribose-P reportedly activates carbamyl phosphate synthetase activity (Tatibana and

Shigesada, 1972), as well as serving as a substrate for the enzyme orotate phosphoriboysltransferase, an obligatory step in pyrimidine nucleotide synthesis.

Attractive as this theory appears, considerable evidence has accumulted indicating that additional processes may be disturbed by adenosine toxicity (Snyder, personal communication). Furthermore, its relevance to ADA deficiency remains to be proved.

8.2.3.7. Therapy

If pyrimdine starvation were the principal mechanism involved in the immunodeficiency of ADA deficiency, its therapy should be quite simple. The pyrimidine nucleoside uridine has already been shown to provide complete replacement therapy for the pyrimidine starvation of orotic aciduria. Attempts to treat the immunodeficiency of ADA deficiency with uridine have not appeared promising (Goldblum, personal communication). Furthermore, no evidence of impaired pyrimidine synthesis in affected children has yet been obtained. Uridine was ineffective in restoring response to PHA (Parkman et al., 1975).

The enzyme deficiency of ADA is also expressed in cultured cells, thus making prenatal diagnosis feasible. Chen et al. (1975) reported activities of 1 and 10% of normal in skin fibroblasts cultured from 2 children with ADA deficiency demonstrated in their erythrocytes. These values could well be spuriously higher than the true values, since the fibroblasts were cultured in medium containing 20% fetal calf serum, from which ADA could very well have found its way into the cells. These authors found the specific activity of ADA in normal cultured amniotic cells to be very similar to the activity in fibroblasts. Hirschhorn et al. (1975) identified an affected fetus in utero, thus demonstrating the capability of prenatal diagnosis. Although the pregnancy was not terminated, it allowed definitive plans to be made for care of the child from birth. In addition, two heterozygous fetuses were identified prenatally (Seegmiller et al., 1976).

Treatment of ADA deficiency is still evolving (Hong, 1975). As in other types of immunodeficiency disease, transplantation of bone marrow (Parkman et al., 1975) or thymus from a suitably matched donor, or even 9-month fetal liver, to convert the patient to a chimera is effective if the patient and donor are sufficiently well matched to prevent development of a rejection reaction to the host (Keightly et al., 1975). The improvement observed in the response of ADA-deficient lymphocytes to mitogens on the addition of ADA to the medium suggests the possible therapeutic value of transfusions of irradiated whole normal blood (Polmar et al., 1975; Goldblum, personal communication). Initial studies appear promising in some cases.

8.2.4. Mutations in Phosphoribosylpyrophosphate Synthetase

The enzyme PP-ribose-P synthetase catalyzes the synthesis of PP-ribose-P from ATP and ribose-5-phosphate, and shows a dependence on inorganic phosphate and magnesium. Schubert *et al.* (1975) found multiple states of aggregation of a 31,000 mol.wt. subunit in the native forms of the bacterial enzyme, with the predominant mol.wt. 150,000–200,000 consisting of five or six subunits. Disaggregation occurred on removal of inorganic phosphate, and was prevented by oxidation of one of the four cysteine residues (Roberts *et al.*, 1975). The mammalian enzyme shows a subunit of mol.wt. of 34,500, with aggregations from 60,000 to 1,200,000 mol.wt. (Fox, I. H., and Kelley, 1974a). It is inhibited by ADP, GDP, and 2,3-diphosphoglycerate. Activity is greatly increased by inorganic phosphate (Fox and Kelley, 1974a; Sciaky *et al.*, 1974), and seems limited by availability of ribose-5-phosphate in the intact cell (Becker and Seegmiller, 1975).

8.2.4.1. Increased Activity of Phosphoribosylpyrophosphate Synthetase

Production of PP-ribose-P at an increased rate has been proposed as the mechanism for the purine overproduction responsible for development of gouty arthritis in the six different types of enzyme abnormalities shown in Table I. The clinical presentation in each demonstrated case was severe gouty arthritis, with a tendency to greater than usual difficulty with renal calculi (Becker and Seegmiller, 1974).

Clinical examples of each of the three types of excessive PP-ribose-P production have been found. However, in type I glycogen storage disease, and to an even greater extent in increased glutathione reductase activity (see Section 8.2.6), the mechanism remains to be proved. In each family, a different type of mutation was present in the same enzyme, thus again revealing genetic heterogeneity. In one family, this disorder appeared to result from a dominantly inherited mutation in a structural gene leading to a specific enzyme activity 2–3 times higher than normal, with normal enzyme kinetic and inhibitory constants, and thus represents a new type of mammalian mutation (Becker *et al.*, 1973a,b, 1974b, 1975b).

In a second family, the high activity resulted from a markedly decreased responsiveness to normal physiologically active nucleotide inhibitors, ADP and GDP, of PP-ribose-P synthetase (Sperling *et al.*, 1974a; Zoref *et al.*, 1975). In a third family, the increased activity resulted from an increased affinity of the mutant enzyme for the substrate ribose-5-phosphate (Becker and Seegmiller, 1974, 1975).

Table I. Proposed Enzymatic Mechanisms Responsible for Excessive Uric Acid Synthesis in Man

Mechanism	Enzyme abnormality	Status of association
Increased PP-ribose-P production	Increased PP-ribose-P synthetase activity:	
	1. Diminished response to feedback inhibition	Demonstrated
	2. Increased specific activity of enzyme	Demonstrated
	3. Higher affinity for a substrate (ribose-5-P)	Demonstrated
	4. Increased concentration of a substrate (ribose 5-P)	Demonstrated
	Glucose-6-phosphatase deficiency (Type 1 glycogenosis)	Unconfirmed
	Increased glutathione reductase activity	Unconfirmed
Decreased PP-ribose-P utilization	Severe HPRT deficiency (Lesch-Nyhan syndrome)	Demonstrated
	Partial HPRT deficiency	Demonstrated
Altered feedback inhibition	PP-ribose-P amidotransferase relatively insensitive to feedback inhibition	Uncomfirmed
	Adenosine Kinase deficiency[a]	Unconfirmed

[a]Described in 3T6 mouse fibroblast cells; human correlate not yet identified.

8.2.4.2. Decreased Activity of Phosphoribosylpyrophosphate Synthetase

A partial deficiency of PP-ribose-P synthetase was reported in 4 patients with hereditary nonspherocytic hemolytic anemia in three families associated with basophilic stippling and increased red cell glutathione and nucleotide content, presumably adenine nucleotides (Valentine *et al.*, 1972). Eventually, these authors identified the increased nucleotide content as being composed of pyrimidine nucleotides, and the primary defect was a gross deficiency of pyrimidine-5'-nucleotidase (Valentine *et al.*, 1974), which is described in Section 8.4.2. However, a gross but inconstant deficiency of PP-ribose-P synthetase was found in the erythrocytes of an infant with mental retardation reported by Wada *et al.* (1974).

8.2.5. Hereditary Xanthinuria from Xanthine Oxidase Deficiency

The majority of patients with hereditary xanthinuria show no symptoms of the disorder, and are therefore unaware of its presence unless an especially curious physician attempts to find the cause of their very low serum urate concentrations (Seegmiller, 1974). However, these patients carry a very high risk of developing renal calculi composed of xanthine, which have been observed in about one-third of the known patients. In addition, 2 of the 18 known cases have shown clinical evidence of myalgias, particularly after moderate exercise. Muscle biopsies of both patients demonstrated intracellular crystals composed of xanthine and hypoxanthine (Parker *et al.*, 1970).

The diagnosis is made by demonstration of a serum urate concentration of less than 1 mg/dl and urinary uric acid excretion of less than 50 mg in a 24-hr collection. The possible occurrence of variants of xanthinuria with excretion of quantities of uric acid somewhat greater than 50 mg/day along with increased quantities of oxypurines in the urine should be considered. The diagnosis of xanthinuria is confirmed with the demonstration of xanthine as the major purine component of urine, along with lesser amounts of hypoxanthine. A variety of analytical methods are available (Seegmiller, 1974).

The heterozygous state is not detectable. The possibility of the heterozygosity being revealed by hepatic failure was suggested by Rapado *et al.* (1975). The brother of one known xanthinuric showed no evidence of the disease when first seen, but was a known alcholic. His serum urate initially was in the normal range, but after developing severe liver cirrhosis with ascites and hepatic encephalopathy, he had a persistent hypouricemia (0.85 mg/dl), and his 24-hr urine contained 50 mg uric acid, along with 269 mg xanthine and 68 mg hypoxanthine, suggesting the possibility that hepatic insufficiency may have unmasked a partial defect of xanthine oxidase in a heterozygote. Rapado *et al.* (1975) suggested examining urine for xanthinuria in all patients with hypouricemia and hepatic disease, and looking among members of such a patient's family for asymptomatic xanthinurics.

The drug allopurinol not only is an inhibitor of xanthine oxidase, but also is metabolized by this enzyme to its oxidized form, oxipurinol. This drug has therefore been used to study possible residual xanthine oxidase activity *in vivo* (Holmes *et al.*, 1974a; Simmonds *et al.*, 1974, 1975). Of the 5 patients to whom allopurinol was administered, 2 failed to show any conversion to oxipurinol; however, a secondary effect of allopurinol on pyrimidine metabolism was observed. All 3 patients in whom it was measured showed an increased excretion of orotic acid and orotidine in the urine in response to allopurinol administration (Simmonds *et al.*, 1974, 1975). Allopurinol administration produced no change in total purine excretion in all 5 patients.

The observation of Holmes *et al.* (1974a) of failure of allopurinol to alter erythrocyte PP-ribose-P content suggests the possibility that the enzyme HPRT is virtually saturated with hypoxanthine and xanthine *in vivo* in the xanthinuric patient. In 1 of the 5 patients, allopurinol produced an increase in xanthine excretion, suggesting the possibility of a residual xanthine oxidase activity being functionally active *in vivo*. Watts *et al.* (1971a,b) reported identification of xanthine and hypoxanthine crystals in muscles of gout patients treated with allopurinol. However, patients were asymptomatic, and the observation has been challenged (Hitchings, 1971).

8.2.6. Evidence of Influence of Carbohydrate Metabolism on Purine Metabolism

The association of uric acid overproduction with glycogen storage disease type I (glucose-6-phophatase deficiency) shown in Table I provides convincing evidence of the close relationship of carbohydrate and purine metabolism (Seegmiller, 1974; Wyngaarden and Kelley, 1972). It suggests the possibility that an increased intracellular glucose-6-phosphate content in the liver could enhance the oxidation of glucose-6-phosphate to ribose-5-phosphate. The increase in the oxidative pathway of glucose could thereby give rise to an increased formation of PP-ribose-P as a cause of purine overproduction in this disease. Erythrocyte content of PP-ribose-P is not abnormal in this disease, but neither do erythrocytes normally show glucose-6-phosphatase activity. These considerations have led to the suggestion that the enhanced rate of purine synthesis occurs primarily in the liver, the organ in which the enzyme deficiency is demonstrable. With recent reports of beneficial effects of portocaval shunt in treatment of this disease, the possibility of obtaining liver for more detailed analysis of PP-ribose-P content and rate of formation may be tested.

An increased activity of glutathione reductase in erythrocytes of gouty patients was reported by Long (1967), with the suggestion that this enzyme abnormality might also stimulate the oxidative pathway of glucose and thereby increase PP-ribose-P generation and purine synthesis. No evidence was presented of an increased rate of purine synthesis in his patients. Furthermore, Beutler (1969) presented evidence of activation of glutathione reductase by riboflavin administration, thus raising questions of the accuracy of all previous measurements of this enzyme.

An increase in PP-ribose-P formation by rat liver was shown by Henderson (personal communication) to accompany the administration *in vivo* of methylene blue, as well as of a variety of hormones such as ACTH and growth hormone. These observations suggest that increased activity of the oxidative pathway of glucose may be a general regulatory process for rapidly controlling the rate of purine synthesis *de novo*.

Becker and Seegmiller (1975) observed a patient with gout who showed an excessive rate of PP-ribose-P synthesis in the absence of any demonstrable abnormality of PP-ribose-P synthetase, but associated with an increased intracellular concentration of ribose-5-phosphate, suggesting the possibility of a primary defect at an earlier stage in the regulation of the oxidative pathway of glucose. Becker (1975) found a consistent correlation of increased content of PP-ribose-P in fibroblasts cultured *in vitro* with an increased rate of uric acid generation *in vivo* in all 7 patients studied, while their erythrocyte content of PP-ribose-P showed no consistent correlation.

Hereditary fructose intolerance—a disorder of metabolism characterized by a grossly deficient phosphofructoaldolase—was associated with hyperuricemia in 6 children described by Perheentupa and Raivio (1967). A rapid fructose infusion produces a hyperuricemia associated with an enhanced rate of purine synthesis *de novo* (Raivio *et al.*, 1975) in both normal and gouty subjects. An abnormal increase in serum urate concentration of certain gouty patients in response to fructose infusion was observed by Müller and Frank (1974).

8.3. Abnormalities in Serum Urate Concentration

8.3.1. Hyperuricemia

Hyperuricemia is being found with an increasing number of clinical abnormalities in addition to gouty arthritis, and has been reviewed in detail (Newcombe, 1975; Klinenberg, 1975). The most prevalent cause is the administration of a wide range of pharmacological agents (Kelley, 1975a), including salicylates at doses less than 3 gr./day and most antihypertensive drugs except the spironolactones. In a prospective study, Fessel (1972; Fessel *et al.*, 1973) observed a tendency for hyperuricemic patients to develop diabetes mellitus. Herman *et al.* (1974) reported a significantly lower serum urate in patients with known diabetes. However, hyperuricemia is known to accompany the ketoacidosis of diabetes as well as that of starvation. Hyperuricemia also accompanied the ketoaciduria of one child with branched-chain ketoaciduria (maple syrup urine disease) described by Schulman *et al.* (1970), and is an example of a primary defect in amino acid metabolism associated with hyperuricemia. The hyperuricemia associated with obesity is substantially diminished by weight reduction. Other associated disorders include hypertension, polycystic kidney (Newcombe, 1973), myocardial infarction, and Down's syndrome, with a recent report of gout in such a patient (Cayla *et al.*, 1974). Avascular necrosis of the hip associated with hyperuricemia and a tendency to excessive alcohol consumption was also described (Hunder *et al.*, 1968; Mielants *et al.*, 1975).

The possibility of an excessive rate of purine synthesis being associated with a deficiency of adenosine kinase has been raised by the excretion of excessive amounts of purines into the medium in a cultured mammalian cell line grossly deficient in this enzyme (see Table I), as reported by Chan et al. (1973). This defect, however, has not yet been identified in patients with gout or any other human disorder. Gout was also recently described in a patient with Bartter's syndrome (Meyer et al., 1975).

A variety of neurological disorders has been found associated with hyperuricemia in addition to the Lesch-Nyhan syndrome, and are summarized in recent reviews (Kelley and Wyngaarden, 1972; Seegmiller, 1974; Newcombe, 1975). These disorders include ataxia, weakness, deafness, and renal insufficiency with varying degrees of disability reported by Rosenberg et al. (1970) in 5 of 22 family members. Gout was associated with benign symmetrical lipomatosis of Lanoid Bensaud, and was found in a 30-year-old woman who presented with muscle cramps, pes cavis deformity, oligomenorrhea, and extensor plantar reflexes (Greene et al., 1970). She also showed an excessive rate of incorporation of glycine-1-^{14}C into urinary uric acid. Two additional patients described by Müller and Frank (1974) showed an excessive incorporation of glycine-U-^{14}C into urinary uric acid, and an enhanced increase in serum urate concentration in response to fructose infusion. A child with autistic behavior and mental retardation, but with normal HPRT activity, showed a markedly excessive rate of purine synthesis (Nyhan et al., 1969). A young girl with encephalopathy, self-mutilation, and excessive uric acid production, but no hyperuricemia, was also described (Hooft et al., 1968). A 15-year-old boy with a history of renal calculi from age 2 years with excessive uric acid synthesis presented with an idiopathic tremor of the right arm (Becker and Seegmiller, unpublished observation). A hyperuricemic child with uncontrollable seizures showed a dramatic clinical improvement with control of the seizures by allopurinol therapy (Coleman, 1971; Coleman et al., 1974). In none of the patients described above has the primary enzyme defect been identified. However, new methods for assessing purine metabolism in human cells in vitro have been developed by Henderson et al. (1974a,b), and only with identification of additional patients can we be certain that the association of the clinical disorder with hyperuricemia is a valid one.

8.3.2. Effects of Hyperuricemia on Renal Function

Berger and Yü (1975) concluded from a prospective study of 524 gouty patients that hyperuricemia per se had no adverse effects on renal function. Deterioration of renal function in the gouty subject was associated primarily with aging, renal vascular disease, renal calculi with pylonephritis, or independently occurring nephropathy. Diminished renal function was ascribable to gout alone in very few patients. However, the higher incidence of renal dysfunction in patients with overproduction of uric acid (Kelley et al., 1969; Greene, 1972) from partial HPRT deficiency provides strong evidence for the toxic effects of large loads of uric acid on the kidney. Renal damage is associated initially with an enhanced renal clearance of uric acid with respect to creatinine (Berger and Yü, 1975).

8.3.3. Clinical Disorders Associated with Hypouricemia

Hypouricemia results from, in addition to the well-known uricosuric drugs, a variety of other drugs. These include doses of salicylates greater than 4 g/day and radioopaque dyes used in radiographic studies of the kidney. Hepatic failure can also be associated with a hypouricemia in occasional patients (see Section 8.3.2).

A primary defect in renal tubular reabsorption of uric acid analogous to the tubular defect present normally in the Dalmatian dog was described recently by Greene et al. (1972) and Simkin et al. (1974). Tubular abnormalities of Fanconi's syndrome can also produce a hypouricemia distinguishable from that of xanthinuria by the excretion of normal quantities of uric acid in the 24-hr urine, and distinguished from the Dalmatian dog syndrome in its being associated with amino aciduria. Sperling et al. (1974b) described a patient with hypouricemia, hypercalciuria, and decreased bone density.

A diminished synthesis of uric acid in a mentally retarded child with microcephaly and a gross defect in folic acid metabolism consisting of a deficiency of forminotransferase was described by Arakawa et al. (1972). The urine of affected patients shows a positive ferric chloride test due to the excretion of large amounts of formimino glutamic acid, which is not altered by administration of folic acid (Niederwieser et al., 1974).

8.3.4. Convenient Clinical Method for Evaluation of Uric Acid Production

The classification of patients into overexcretors and normal excretors of uric acid becomes especially important as an initial method for identifying patients who could be candidates for known enzyme defects. It is also of practical value in aiding the physician in selecting the best drug for management of his particular patient. This selection is of special importance when one considers the lifetime commitment being made to drug treatment. The test is most conveniently performed immediately after the diagnosis of gouty arthritis has been made and the patient has been started on colchicine to control the acute symptoms. He is usually well motivated at that time to follow the purine-free diet and avoid alcohol and drugs for a period of 6 days. During the last 3 days of the diet, 24-hr urine collections are made, each in a separate bottle containing 3 ml toluene as a preservative. Urine collections are stored at room temperature until dilution for analysis for uric acid and creatinine content. The urine is warmed to dissolve any crystalline deposits that may be present before removal of an aliquot for analysis and measurement of the total volume. The mean 24-hr excretion of uric acid in the normal adult male is 528 mg, with the upper range of normal being 600 mg. This test is not reliable as an index of purine overproduction in patients with significant degrees of renal dysfunction. Patients with substantial renal dysfunction, as well as those excreting excessive quantities of uric acid (greater than 600 mg/24 hr), should be on allopurinol. This drug not only diminishes uric acid content of serum and urine by blocking its formation, thus reducing the load of uric acid passing through the kidney, but also provides a specific therapeutic action in substantially correcting the excessive purine production. Only in patients with HPRT deficiency does the diminution in total purine production fail to occur in response to allopurinol (Kelley et al., 1969). Patients excreting less than 600 mg/24 hr with a normal renal function presumably have a diminished renal excretion of uric acid. Therefore, the uricosuric drug probenecid provides specific corrective therapy. Indications for allopurinol, in addition to renal dysfunction or excessive uric acid production, are a history of renal calculi composed of uric acid or intolerance of a uricosuric drug.

8.4. Abnormalities of Pyrimidine Metabolism

Abnormalities of pyrimidine metabolism have been reviewed recently by Levine et al. (1974), Gröbner and Zöllner (1975), Seegmiller (1974), and Smith et al. (1972).

8.4.1. Orotic Aciduria

Excretion of increased quantities of orotic acid in the urine can result from a variety of primary genetic defects. These defects include a primary aberration of pyrimidine metabolism, and a variety of primary defects in the urea cycle enzymes, producing hyperammonemia. It can also result from the action of a variety of pharmacological agents.

8.4.1.1. Hereditary Orotic Aciduria

This enzyme abnormality, causing mental retardation, impaired growth, and megaloblastic anemia, is unusual in its involvement of gross deficiencies of two sequential enzymes, orotate phosphoribosyltransferase (OPRT) and orotidine-5-phosphate decarboxylase (ODC) (see Fig. 3).

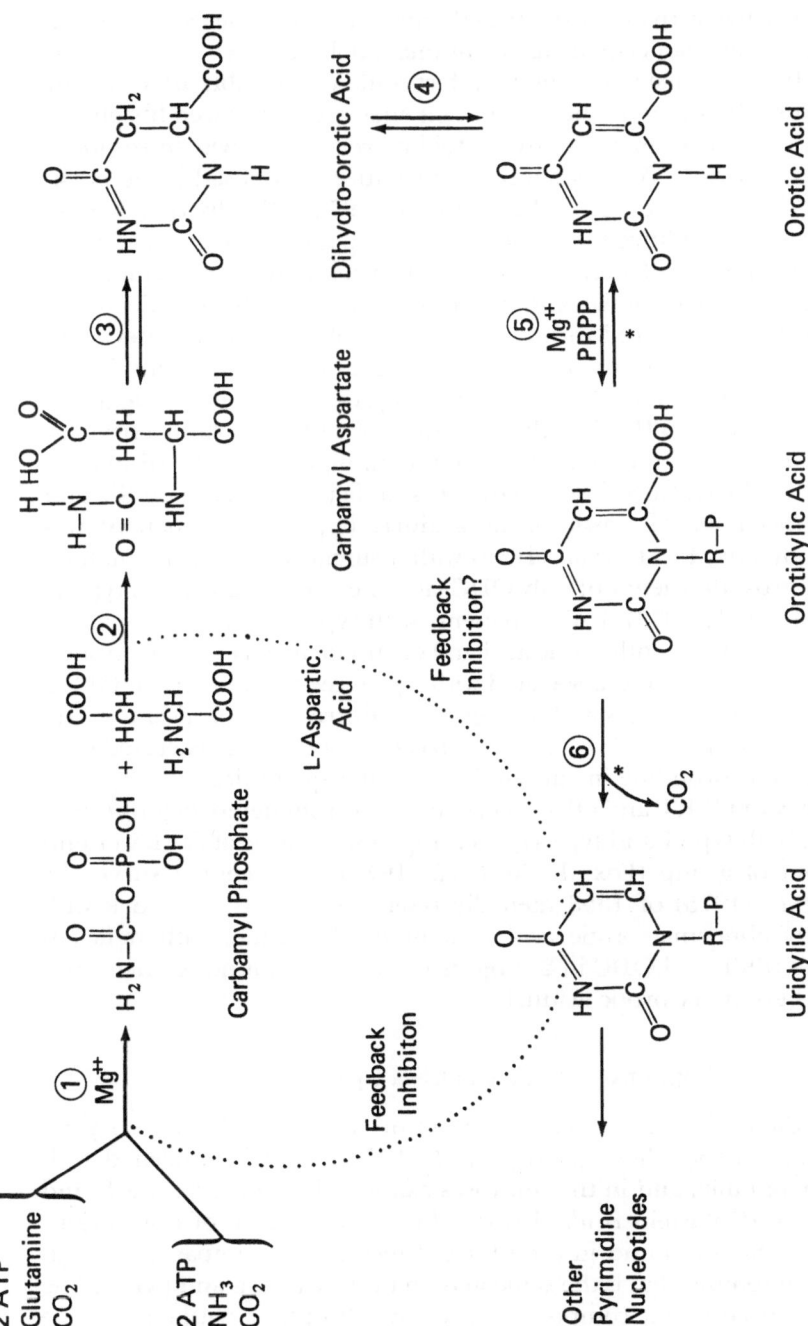

Fig. 3. Pyrimidine biosynthesis pathway with feedback control mechanisms. Enzymes 5 and 6 are grossly deficient in hereditary orotic aciduria. (R) Ribose; (P) phosphate. (Reproduced from Seegmiller, 1969, with permission of the publisher.) * Enzymes deficient in hereditary orotic aciduria.

However, the two activities are purified together from a variety of tissues, suggesting their association as a bifunctional complex (Reyes and Guganig, 1975), so that a hereditary defect could conceivably affect one or both activities. In addition, the two mutant enzymes in cultured fibroblasts show a curious and dramatic 10- to 100-fold increase in activity in response to a variety of drugs. Among several explanations proposed is the possible action of a regulator gene (Krooth *et al.*, 1974). Worthy *et al.* (1974) treated fibroblasts cultured from oroticaciduric patients with azauridine to increase the amount of mutant enzymes sufficiently to allow demonstration of greater thermolability and different electrophoretic mobility of the mutant ODC as compared with that of normal fibroblasts. An intermediate thermolability was found in one heterozygous cell strain of fibroblasts, but normal values were found in two others. These data suggest a mutation in a gene affecting the structure of either or both enzymes, rather than action of a regulatory gene mutation, as the cause of hereditary orotic aciduria. In addition to the gross deficiency of both OPRT and ODC characteristic of classic orotic aciduria (type I), one patient was described by Fox, R. M. *et al.* (1969) with a similar clinical presentation, but with a gross deficiency of only ODC, and therefore classified as type II (Fox, R. M. *et al.*, 1973). Unlike patients with type I disease, this patient excreted in the urine both orotic acid and orotidine in excessive quantities. Therapy with uridine was associated with a progressive decrease in OPRT activity of his erythrocytes and a progressive decrease in orotidine excretion (Fox, R. M. *et al.*, 1973). The heterozygous mother also excreted both orotic acid and orotidine in substantially smaller quantities.

Activity of OPRT and ODC in erythrocytes from heterozygous family members, both type I and type II, overlapped with those at the lower end of the control group (Fox, R. M. *et al.*, 1973). A screening survey by Rogers *et al.* (1975) of 1358 mentally retarded subjects showed 9 with persistently abnormal orotic acid content of the urine, with deficient activity of OPRT and ODC in 2 subjects in the range found for heterozygotes for hereditary orotic aciduria.

8.4.1.2. Orotic Aciduria from Defects in Urea Synthesis

Hereditary deficiencies have been found in each of the five enzymes involved in urea synthesis (Levine *et al.*, 1974). Each is associated with hyperammonemia, and in the few cases examined, orotic acid was found in the urine (Goldstein *et al.*, 1974). The possible cause of this curious association may be found in a postulated incomplete compartmentalization of a compound that is the same in both urea synthesis and pyrimidine synthesis. This unstable compound, carbamyl phosphate synthetase, is the first intermediate in the synthesis of both urea and pyrimidines (see Fig. 3), and is produced from ATP, bicarbonate, and glutamine or ammonia by the enzyme carbamyl phosphate synthetase, which is of two different origins. One is present in liver mitochondria, utilizes ammonia, requires acetyl glutamate, and is involved in urea synthesis. The other enzyme, which is found in the soluble portion of both hepatic and nonhepatic tissues, requires glutamine for maximal activity, but also reacts with ammonia and is concerned with pyrimidine nucleotide synthesis. The first two enzymes involved in pyrimidine nucleotide synthesis, cytoplasmic carbamyl phosphate synthetase and aspartate transcarbamylase, are induced together as an associated complex of mol.wt. 600,000 in human lymphocytes in response to phytohemagglutinin stimulation (Ito and Uchino, 1973). The activity of aspartate transcarbamylase was around 100 times that of carbamyl phosphate synthetase, so the rate of pyrimidine synthesis is probably determined by the amount of carbamyl phosphate available for reaction. The close association of the two enzymes presumably aids in stabilizing the unstable carbamyl phosphate and in channeling it into pyrimidine nucleotide synthesis. The activity of carbamyl phosphate synthetase is regulated by a variety of compounds. The glutamine-requiring enzyme of liver is inhibited by UMP-UDP (Fig. 3). UTP synthesis is stimulated by purine nucleotides, particularly inosinic acid, with greatest activation by exposure to PP-ribose-P (Tatibana and Shigesada, 1972), but is inhibited by adenosine (see Section 8.2.3.6) (Green and Chan, 1973). The marked decrease in orotic acid excretion of patients with hereditary orotic aciduria on treatment with uridine provides evidence of the operation of such a mechanism of feedback inhibition *in vivo*. In a similar manner, provision of preformed pyrimidines in the form of oral RNA decreased the orotic acid excretion of patients receiving allopurinol (Zöllner and Gröbner, 1971).

Although carbamyl phosphate of mitochondrial origin was initially thought to remain compartmentalized, evidence has recently been found suggesting that it can spill over into the cytoplasm and stimulate pyrimidine biosynthesis under certain conditions of accumulation. The excretion in the urine of orotic acid, uridine, and other pyrimidine compounds in patients with hyperammonemia from any one of a number of primary defects in the enzymes of urea synthesis, such as deficiency of ornithine transcarbamylase, is presumably on this basis. Goldstein *et al.* (1974) showed a correlation in the urinary excretion of orotic acid and the blood ammonia concentration in a patient with congenital hyperammonemia due to ornithine transcarbamylase deficiency. Dhondt and Farriaux (1975) used orotic acid excretion after a protein load to identify carriers for this disorder, which shows an X-linked dominant pattern of inheritance (Short *et al.*, 1973). Since the enzyme normally resides in the mitochondria, the possibility of this disorder being transmitted only through females as a mitochondrial defect must be considered. It might show an X-linked dominant pattern of inheritance, if it were indeed coded in the DNA of mitochondria. However, the number of genes that could be coded in the amount of DNA in mitochondria is severely limited, and considerable evidence is accumulating for a nuclear coding for a number of enzymes that are found in the mitochondria. Hyperammonemia in infants receiving total parental nutrition ("hyperalimentation") is also accompanied by an orotic aciduria (Levine *et al.*, 1974), presumably as a result of a concomitant inhibition of some step in urea synthesis.

8.4.1.3. Pharmacologically Induced Orotic Aciduria

The drug azauridine produces an inhibition of orotic acid decarboxylase, with a resulting orotic aciduria (Fallon *et al.*, 1961). A mild orotic aciduria and orotidinuria, accompanied by an increased activity of OPRT and ODC of erythrocytes is a secondary effect of therapy with the drug allopurinol (Fox, R. M. *et al.*, 1970; Kelley and Beardmore, 1970; Fox, R. M. *et al.*, 1971; Kelley *et al.*, 1971). No evidence has yet been found of any deleterious effect in the human from the mild orotic aciduria produced by allopurinol. Cultured cells show an increase in activity of both OPRT and ODC by addition to the culture medium of allopurinol, 6-azauridine, 5-azaorotic acid, or barbituric acid, which appears to result from simultaneous inhibition and stabilization of OPRT and ODC by the nucleotide formed from these substances or their metabolites (Fox, R. M. *et al.*, 1971; Brown *et al.*, 1972; Krooth *et al.*, 1974; Becker *et al.*, 1974a). Becker *et al.* (1974a, 1975a) showed the conversion of a single low-molecular-weight species (41,000) of ODC to a larger, more stable form with mol. wt. 108,000 on addition of oxipurinol to cultured human lymphoblasts. Gröbner and Kelley (1975) showed the presence of three molecular species of OPRT–ODC enzyme activity in human erythrocytes of mol.wt. 55,000, 80,000, and 113,000. The form with the lowest molecular weight is most abundant, but is least stable to storage at 4°C. It is converted to the more stable form of high molecular weight by incubation of hemolysates *in vitro* with ribonucleotides of either allopurinol or oxipurinol, the latter being the more effective agent. These authors suggest the possibility that the increased activity of OPRT and ODC noted in erythrocyte lysates after allopurinol administration may result from a similar conversion to a more stable form of the enzyme with resistance to destruction during preparation of the cell lysate greater than that of the low-molecular-weight species.

8.4.2. Pyrimidine 5'-Nucleotidase Deficiency

8.4.2.1. Presentation

A gross deficiency of the enzyme pyrimidine 5'-nucleotidase was found by Valentine *et al.* (1974) in a total of 6 patients with congenital

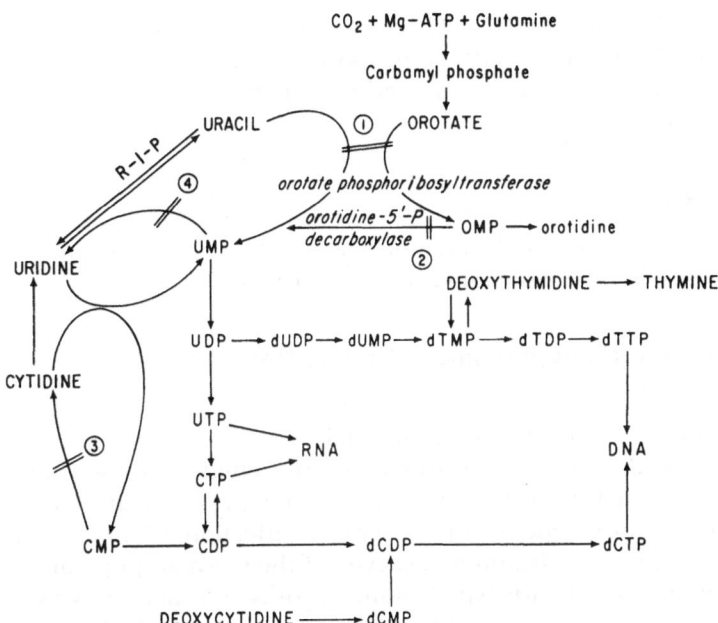

Fig. 4. Pyrimidine nucleotide interconversions. Enzymes 1 and 2 exist as a complex and are grossly deficient in orotic aciduria. Phosphatase activities 3 and 4 are catalyzed by a single enzyme, pyrimidine-5′-nucleotidase, which is grossly deficient in the form of hereditary hemolytic anemia described by Valentine et al. (1974).

nonspherocytic hemolytic anemia. Increased basophilic stippling was a prominent feature of the disease in all patients (Valentine et al. 1972). This condition was first attributed to a modest decrease in the activity of the enzyme PP-ribose-P synthetase to around 20–30% of normal (see Section 8.2.4.2). A marked accumulation of pyrimidine nucleotides was found in erythrocytes, and spectrophotometric methods for its diagnosis were outlined in Valentine et al. (1974).

8.4.2.2. Biochemical Features

The total nucleotide content of erythrocytes of affected patients was increased 3–4.4 fold over normal. Of the total intracellular nocleotides of erythrocytes, 78–83% were pyrimidine nucleotides, with around 50% cytidine nucleotides. The amount of pyrimidine 5′-nucleotidase activity ranged from 3 to 14% of normal with either uridylic or cytidylic acid as substrate (Fig. 4). An unexplained feature of the disease was a 37–100% increase in the glutathione content of erythrocytes of affected patients. Comparable biochemical studies on other cell types, such as leukocytes, platelets, or cultured skin fibroblasts or lymphoblasts, remain to be done.

Biochemical characteristics of the normal enzyme were described by

Paglia and Valentine, (1975). This enzyme is very sensitive to inhibition by lead, and Paglia *et al.* (1975) proposed its inhibition as part of the mechanism of hemolytic anemia induced by a relatively low level of lead intoxication.

8.4.2.3. Genetics

Initial data on family members are compatible with an autosomal recessive mode of transmission of the deficiency.

8.4.3. Uridine Monophosphate Kinase Relative Deficiency

Giblett *et al.* (1974) found an allele (type 2) of uridine monophosphate kinase that in homozygous form in 3 children showed an activity 29–34% of that found in homozygotes for type 1. Of the 3 children, 2 gave a history of frequent respiratory tract infections. The same two most common alleles were found in a survey of the German population, but in the 1 patient found with type 2 homozygosity, no mention was made of any correlation with increased tendencies to infections (Kuhn *et al.*, 1975).

8.4.4. Carbamyl Phosphate Synthetase Deficiency

A gross deficiency of the enzyme carbamyl phosphate synthetase produced remarkable degrees of hyperammonemia, hyperglycinemia, and low serum urea, accompanied by vomiting, lethargy, mental retardation, and other neurological dysfunction similar to that found in ketotic hyperglycinemia with propionic acidemia. It was a lethal disorder in a patient with severe cerebral damage described by Gelehrter and Snodgrass (1974). The enzyme deficiency was traced, in their patient, to the carbamyl phosphate synthetase associated with mitochondria—and was therefore involved as the first step in urea synthesis—rather than to pyrimidine synthesis. Orotic aciduria would therefore not be an expected accompaniment of the hyperammonemia of this condition.

8.4.5. β-Aminoisobutyric Acid Excretion

A defect in the degradative pathway of thymidine (Fig. 5) has been proposed to account for the excretion of β-aminoisobutyric acid (BAIB) in the urine inherited as a recessive trait in certain families. The condition is entirely harmless, and has been used as a genetic marker (Yanai *et al.*, 1969). BAIB excretion was increased on loading with thymidine, but no studies of the enzyme activity in affected persons have yet been made.

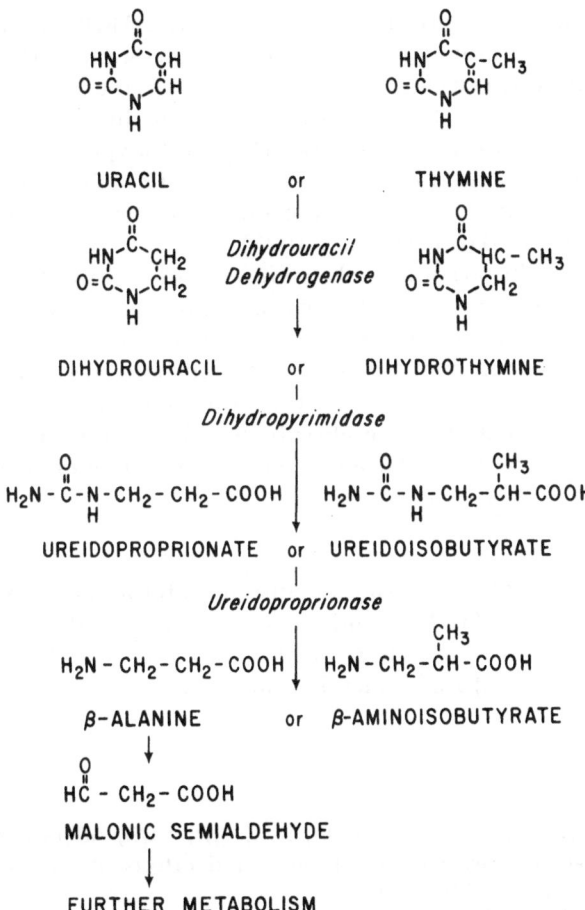

Fig. 5. Pathway for degradation of pyrimidine nucleotides.

8.5. Regulatory Role of Cylic Purine Nucleotides

8.5.1. Cyclic 3′,5′-Adenosine Monophosphate

In recent years, evidence from many biological systems has accumulated establishing a role for cAMP in regulation of a great many variations in cell response, including those mediated by various hormones (Pastan, 1975). In general, increased concentrations of cAMP are correlated with development of differentiated functions and a diminished rate of cell growth, but in special circumstances, cAMP can also enhance some aspects of cell proliferation. In general, the intracellular concentration of GMP tends to vary inversely with the concentration of cAMP, and produces an opposite effect of stimulation of cell proliferation. Some of the phenotypic changes in cultured cells associated with a malignant transformation are reversed by cAMP. A deficiency of receptors for the cAMP signal in the kidney has been proposed in type II pseudohypoparathyroidism to account for the associated increased excretion of cAMP in the urine. The excretion of cAMP was increased even further by administration of parathyroid extract (Drezner et al., 1973).

Mouse lymphosarcoma cells deficient in adenylate cyclase, the enzyme responsible for cAMP formation, were selected in vitro by treatment with isoproteronol (Bourne et al., 1975). From the same parent mouse lymphoma cell line, a subline deficient both in cAMP-dependent histone phosphokinase activity and in the binding of cAMP to the enzyme's regulatory subunit was also obtained by its resistance to dibutyryl cAMP (Daniel et al., 1973). Gross deficiencies of these enzymes have not yet been identified in vivo.

ACKNOWLEDGMENTS

Work reported herein from the author's laboratory was supported in part by United States Public Health Service grants AM-05646, AM-13622, and GM-17702 and by grants from the National Foundation, the Kroe Foundation, and the Josiah Macy Foundation.

References

Agarwal, R. P., Sagar, S. M., and Parks, R. E., Jr., 1975, Adenosine deaminase from human erythrocytes: Purification and effects of adenosine analogs, Biochem. Pharmacol. 24:693–701.

Akedo, H., Nishihara, H., Shinkai, K., and Komatsu, K., 1970, Adenosine deaminases of two different molecular sizes in human tissues, Biochim. Biophys. Acta 212:189–191.

Akedo, H., Nishihara, H., Shinkai, K., Komatsu, K., and Ishikawa, S., 1972, Multiple forms of human adenosine deaminase. I. Purification and characterization of two molecular species, Biochim. Biophys. Acta 276:257–271.

Arakawa, T., Yoshida, T., Konno, T., and Honda, Y., 1972, Defect of incorporation of glycine-1-^{14}C into urinary uric acid in formiminotransferase deficiency syndrome, Tohoku J. Exp. Med. 106:213–218.

Arnold, W. J., and Kelley, W. N., 1974, Hypoxanthine–guanine phosphoribosyltransferase (HGPRT) deficiency: Immunologic studies on the mutant enzyme, Adv. Exp. Med. Biol. 41A:177–185.

Bakay, B., Nyhan, W. L., Croce, C. M., and Koprowski, H., 1975, Reversion in expression of hypoxanthine–guanine phosphoribosyltransferase following cell hybridization, J. Cell Sci. 17:567–578.

Becker, M. A., 1975, Gout with purine overproduction: Patterns of fibroblast phosphoribosylpyrophosphate and ribose-5-phosphate concentration and generation, *Arthritis Rheum.* **18**:385 (abstract).

Becker, M. A., and Seegmiller, J. E., 1974, Genetic aspects of gout, *Annu. Rev. Med.* **25**:15–28.

Becker, M. A., and Seegmiller, J. E., 1975, Recent advances in the identification of enzyme abnormalities underlying excessive purine synthesis in man, *Arthritis Rheum.* **18**(Suppl.):687–693.

Becker, M. A., Kostel, P. J., Meyer, L. J., and Seegmiller, J. E., 1973a, Human phosphoribosylpyrophosphate synthetase: Increased enzyme specific activity in a family with gout and excessive purine synthesis, *Proc. Nat. Acad. Sci. U.S.A.* **70**:2749–2752.

Becker, M. A., Meyer, L. J., and Seegmiller, J. E., 1973b, Gout with purine overproduction due to increased phosphoribosylpyrophosphate synthetase activity, *Amer. J. Med.* **55**:232–242.

Becker, M. A., Argubright, K. F., Fox, R. M., and Seegmiller, J. E., 1974a, Oxipurinol-associated inhibition of pyrimidine synthesis in human lymphoblasts, *Mol. Pharmacol.* **10**:657–668.

Becker, M. A., Meyer, L. J., Kostel, P. J., and Seegmiller, J. E., 1974b, Increased PP-ribose-P synthetase activity: A genetic abnormality leading to excessive purine production and gout, *Adv. Exp. Med. Biol.* **41A**:307–315.

Becker, M. A., Argubright, K. F., and Seegmiller, J. E., 1975a, Effects of oxipurinol on pyrimidine nucleotide synthesis in human lymphoblasts, *Arthritis Rheum.* **18**(Suppl.):871–876.

Becker, M. A., Kostel, P. J., and Meyer, L. J., 1975b, Human phosphoribosylpyrophosphate synthetase. Comparison of purified normal and mutant enzymes, *J. Biol. Chem.* **250**:6822–6830.

Benke, P. J., Hebert, A., and Herrick, N., 1973a, *In vitro* effects of magnesium ions on mutant cells from patients with the Lesch-Nyhan syndrome, *New Engl. J. Med.* **289**:446–450.

Benke, P. J., Herrick, N., and Hebert, A., 1973b, Transport of hypoxanthine in fibroblasts with normal and mutant hypoxanthine–guanine phosphoribosyltransferase, *Biochem. Med.* **8**:309–323.

Berger, L., and Yü, T.-F., 1975, Renal function in gout. IV. An analysis of 524 gouty subjects including long-term follow-up studies, *Amer. J. Med.* **59**:605–613.

Bergsma, D. (editor), 1975, *Immunodeficiency in Man and Animals,* (Birth Defects, Vol. 11, No. 1), Sinauer Associates, Sunderland, Massachusetts.

Berlin, R. D., and Oliver, J. M., 1975, Membrane transport of purine and pyrimidine bases and nucleosides in animal cells, *Int. Rev. Cytol.* **42**:287–336, (G. H. Bourne and J. F. Danielli, eds.), Academic Press, New York.

Beutler, E., 1969, Glutathione reductase: Stimulation in normal subjects by riboflavin supplementation, *Science* **165**:613–615.

Bourne, H. R., Coffino, P., and Tomkins, G. M., 1975, Selection of a variant lymphoma cell deficient in adenylate cyclase, *Science* **187**:750–752.

Boyle, J. A., Raivio, K. O., Astrin, K. H., Schulman, J. D., Graf, M. L., Seegmiller,

J. E., and Jacobsen, C. B., 1970, Lesch-Nyhan syndrome: Preventive control by prenatal diagnosis, *Science* **169**:688–689.

Boyle, J. A., Raivio, K. O., Becker, M. A., and Seegmiller, J. E., 1972, Effects of nicotinic acid on human fibroblast purine biosynthesis, *Biochim. Biophys. Acta* **269**: 179–183.

Brady, T. G., and O'Donovan, C. I., 1965, A study of the tissue distribution of adenosine deaminase in six mammal species, *Comp. Biochem. Physiol.* **14**:101–120.

Brown, G. K., Fox, R. M., and O'Sullivan, W. J., 1972, Alteration of quaternary structural behaviour of an hepatic orotate phosphoribosyltransferase–orotidine-5-phosphate decarboxylase complex in rats following allopurinol therapy, *Biochem. Pharmacol.* **21**:2469–2477.

Capecchi, M. R., Capecchi, N. E., Hughes, S. H., and Wahl, G. M., 1974, Selective degradation of abnormal proteins in mammalian tissue culture cells, *Proc. Nat. Acad. Sci. U.S.A.* **71**:4732–4736.

Cartier, M. P., Hamet, M., and Hamburger, J., 1974, Une nouvelle Maladie métabolique le déficit complete en adenine-phosphoribosyltransférase avec lithiase de 2,8-dihydroxyadénine, *C. R. Acad. Sci. Paris* **279**:883–886.

Cayla, J., Rondier, J., Auscher, C., Perreau, C., and de Gery, A., 1974, Goutte et mongolisme. A propos d'une observation, *Rev. Rheum. Mal Osteoartic* **41**:203–207.

Chan, T.-S., Ishii, K., Long, C., and Green, H., 1973, Purine excretion by mammalian cells deficient in adenosine kinase, *J. Cell. Physiol.* **81**:315–322.

Chen, S.-H., Scott, C. R., and Giblett, E. R., 1974, Adenosine deaminase: Demonstration of a "silent" gene associated with combined immunodeficiency disease, *Amer. J. Hum. Genet.* **26**:103–107.

Chen, S.-H., Scott, C. R., and Swedberg, K. R., 1975, Heterogeneity for adenosine deaminase deficiency: Expression of the enzyme in cultured skin fibroblasts and amniotic fluid cells, *Amer. J. Hum. Genet.* **27**:46–52.

Cleaver, J. E., 1968, Defective repair replication of DNA in xeroderma pigmentosum, *Nature London,* **218**:652–656.

Cohen, F., 1975, Clinical features, in: *Combined Immunodeficiency Disease and Adenosine Deaminase Deficiency. A Molecular Defect* (H. J. Meuwissen, R. J. Pickering, B. Pollara, and I. H. Porter, eds.), pp. 245 and 246, Academic Press, New York.

Cohen, F., and Lightbody, J. J., 1975, Effector phase abnormalities of cell mediated immunity in family members of a child with hereditary T-cell immunodeficiency and absent adenosine deaminase, in: *Combined Immunodeficiency Disease and Adenosine Deaminase Deficiency. A Molecular Defect* (H. J. Meuwissen, R. J. Pickering, B. Pollara, and I. H. Porter, eds.), pp. 201–212, Academic Press, New York.

Coleman, M., 1971, Reversal of organic brain syndrome with seizures and hyperuricosuria subsequent to allopurinol therapy, *Trans. Amer. Neurol. Assoc.* **96**:113–117.

Coleman, M. S., and Hutton, J. J., 1975, Terminal deoxynucleotidyl transferase and adenosine deaminase in human lymphoblastoid cell lines, *Expt. Cell Res.* **94**:440–442.

Coleman, M., Landgrebe, M., and Landgrebe, A., 1974, Progressive seizures with hyperuricosuria reversed by allopurinol, *Arch. Neurol.* **31:**238–242.

Daniel, V., Bourne, H. R., and Tomkins, G. M., 1973, Altered metabolism and endogenous cyclic AMP in cultured cells deficient in cyclic AMP–binding proteins, *Nature London New Biol.* **244:**167–169.

de Bruyn, C. H. M. M., 1976, Hypoxanthine–guanine phosphoribosyltransferase deficiency, *Hum. Genet.* **31:**127–150

de Bruyn, C. H. M. M., and Oei, T. L., 1974, Purine metabolism in intact erythrocytes from controls and HG-PRT deficient individuals, *Adv. Exp. Med. Biol.* **41A:**223–227.

Delbarre, F., Auscher, C., Amor, B., and de Gery, A., 1974a, Gout with adenine phosphoribosyl transferase deficiency, *Adv. Exp. Med. Biol.* **41A:**333–339.

Delbarre, F., Auscher, C., Amor, B., de Gery, A., Cartier, P., and Hamet, M., 1974b, Gout with adenine phosphoribosyl transferase deficiency, *Biomedicine* **21:**82–85.

DeMars, R., and Held, K. R., 1972, The spontaneous azaguanine-resistant mutants of diploid human fibroblasts, *Humangenetik* **16:**87–110.

Dhondt, J.-L., and Farriaux, J.-P., 1975, Essai de dépistage des conductrices pour le déficit en ornithine-carbamyl-transférase par le dosage urinaire de l'acide orotique a propos d'une étude familiale, *Ann. Genet. Paris* **18:**197–202.

Dissing, J., and Knudsen, J. B., 1970, Human erythrocyte adenosine deaminase polymorphism in Denmark, *Hum. Hered.* **20:**178–181.

Dissing, J., and Knudsen, B., 1972, Adenosine-deaminase deficiency and combined immunodeficiency syndrome, *Lancet* **2:**1316.

Drezner, M., Neelon, F. A., and Lebovitz, H. E., 1973, Pseudohypoparathyroidism type II: A possible defect in the reception of the cyclic AMP signal, *New Engl. J. Med.* **289:**1056–1060.

Emmerson, B. T., and Thompson, L., 1973, The spectrum of hypoxanthine–guanine phosphoribosyltransferase deficiency, *Q. J. Med.* **42:**423–440.

Emmerson, B. T., Thompson, C. J., and Wallace, D. C., 1972, Partial deficiency of hypoxanthine–guanine phosphoribosyltransferase: Intermediate enzyme deficiency in heterozygote red cells, *Ann. Intern. Med.* **76:**285–287.

Emmerson, B. T., Gordon, R. B., and Thompson, L., 1974, Adenine phosphoribosyltransferase deficiency in a female with gout, *Adv. Exp. Med. Biol.* **41A:**327–331.

Fallon, H. J., Frei, E., III, Block, J., and Seegmiller, J. E., 1961, The uricosuria and orotic aciduria induced by 6-azauridine, *J. Clin. Invest.* **40:**1906–1914.

Fernstrom, J. D., 1974, Modification of brain serotonin by the diet, *Ann. Rev. Med.* **25:**1–8.

Fessel, W. J., 1972, Hyperuricemia in health and disease, *Semin. Arthritis Rheum.* **1:**275–299.

Fessel, W. J., Siegelaub, A. B., and Johnson, E. S., 1973, Correlates and consequences of asymptomatic hyperuricemia, *Arch. Intern. Med.* **132:**44–54.

Fox, I. H., and Kelley, W. N., 1974a, Human phosphoribosylpyrophosphate (PP-ribose-P) synthetase: Properties and regulation, *Adv. Exp. Med. Biol.* **41A:**79–86.

Fox, I. H., and Kelley, W. N., 1974b, Pharmacological alterations of intracellular phosphoribosylpyrophosphate (PP-ribose-P) in human tissues. *Adv. Exp. Med. Biol.* **41A:**93–99.

Fox, I. H., and Kelley, W. N., 1974c, Adenine phosphoribosyltransferase deficiency: Report of a second family, *Adv. Exp. Med. Biol.* **41A:**319–326.

Fox, I. H., Meade, J. C., and Kelley, W. N., 1973, Adenine phosphoribosyltransferase deficiency in man. Report of a second family, *Amer. J. Med.* **55:**614–620.

Fox, I. H., Dwosh, I. L., Marchant, P. J., Lacroix, S., Moore, M. R., Omura, S., and Wyhofsky, V., 1975, Hypoxanthine–guanine phosphoribosyltransferase. Characterization of a mutant in a patient with gout, *J. Clin. Inv.* **56:**1239–1249.

Fox, R. M., O'Sullivan, W. J., and Firkin, B. G., 1969, Orotic aciduria. Differing enzyme patterns, *Amer. J. Med.* **47:**332–336.

Fox, R. M., Royse-Smith, D., and O'Sullivan, W. J., 1970, Orotidinuria induced by allopurinol, *Science* **168:**861–862.

Fox, R. M., Wood, M. H., and O'Sullivan, W. J., 1971, Studies on the coordinate activity and lability of orotidylate phosphoribosyltransferase and decarboxylase in human erythrocytes, and the effects of allopurinol administration, *J. Clin. Invest.* **50:**1050–1060.

Fox, R. M., Wood, M. H., Royse-Smith, D., and O'Sullivan, W. J., 1973, Hereditary orotic aciduria: Types I and II, *Amer. J. Med.* **55:**791–798.

Francke, U., Bakay, B., and Nyhan, W. L., 1973, Detection of heterozygous carriers of the Lesch-Nyhan syndrome by electrophoresis of hair root lysates, *J. Pediatr.* **82:**472–478.

Francke, U., Bakay, B., Connor, J. D., Coldwell, J. G., and Nyhan, W. L., 1974, Linkage relationships of X-linked enzymes glucose-6-phosphate dehydrogenase and hypoxanthine guanine phosphoribosyltransferase: Recombination in female offspring of compound heterozygotes, *Amer. J. Hum. Genet.* **26:**512–522.

Gelehrter, T. D., and Snodgrass, P. J., 1974, Lethal neonatal deficiency of carbamyl phosphate synthetase, *New Engl. J. Med.* **290:**430–433.

Giblett, E. R., Anderson, J. E. Cohen, F., Pollara, B., and Meuwissen, H. J., 1972, Adenosine-deaminase deficiency in two patients with severely impaired cellular immunity, *Lancet* **2:**1067–1069.

Giblett, E. R., Anderson, J. E., Chen, S.-H., Teng, Y.-S., and Cohen, F., 1974, Uridine monophosphate kinase: A new genetic polymorphism with possible clinical implications, *Amer. J. Hum. Genet.* **26:**627–635.

Giblett, E. R., Ammann, A. J., Wara, D. W., Sandman, R., and Diamond, L. K., 1975a, Nucleoside-phosphorylase deficiency in a child with severely defective T-cell immunity and normal B-cell immunity, *Lancet* **1:**1010–1013.

Giblett, E. R., Scott, C. R., and Chen, S.-H., 1975b, Adenosine deaminase: Genetic aspects, *in: Combined Immunodeficiency Disease and Adenosine Deaminase Deficiency. A Molecular Defect* (H. J. Meuwissen, R. J. Pickering, B. Pollara, and I. H. Porter, eds.), pp. 103–110, Academic Press, New York.

Goldstein, A. S., Hoogenraad, N. J., Johnson, J. D., Fukanaga, K., Swierczewski, E., Cann, H. M., and Sunshine, P., 1974, Metabolic and genetic studies of a family with ornithine transcarbamylase deficiency, *Pediatr. Res.* **8:**5–12.

Goss, S. J., and Harris, H., 1975, New method for mapping genes in human chromosomes, *Nature London* **255:**680–684.

Green, H., 1975, Pyrimidine starvation induced by adenosine in cultured cells and its bearing on the lymphocyte deficiency disease associated with absence of adenosine deaminase, *in: Combined Immunodeficiency Disease and Adenosine Deaminase Deficiency. A Molecular Defect* (H. J. Meuwissen, R. J. Pickering, B. Pollara, and I. H. Porter, eds.), pp. 141–155, Academic Press, New York.

Green, H., and Chan, T.-S., 1973, Pyrimidine starvation induced by adenosine in fibroblasts and lymphoid cells: Role of adenosine deaminase, *Science* **182**:836, 837.

Greene, M. L., 1972, Clinical features of patients with the "partial" deficiency of the X-linked uricaciduria enzyme, *Arch. Intern. Med.* **130**:193–198.

Greene, M. L. Glueck, C. J., Fujimoto, W. Y., and Seegmiller, J. E., 1970, Benign symmetric lipomatosis (Launois-Bensaude adenolipomatosis) with gout and hyperlipoproteinemia, *Amer. J. Med.* **48**:239–246.

Greene, M. L., Marcus, R., Aurbach, G. D., Kazam, E. S., and Seegmiller, J. E., 1972, Hypouricemia due to isolated renal tubular defect. Dalmatian dog mutation in man, *Amer. J. Med.* **53**:361–367.

Gröbner, W., and Kelley, W. N., 1975, Effect of allopurinol and its metabolic derivatives in the configuration of human orotate phosphoribosyltransferase and orotidine 5'-phosphate decarboxylase, *Biochem. Pharmacol.* **24**:379–384.

Gröbner, W., and Zöllner, N., 1975, Störungen des menschlichen Pyrimidinstoffwechsels, *Muench. Med. Wochenschr.* **117**:1453–1456.

Hadden, J. W., 1975, Cyclic nucleotides and lymphocyte metabolism, function, and development, *in: Combined Immunodeficiency Disease and Adenosine Deaminase Deficiency* (H. J. Meuwissen, R. J. Pickering, B. Pollara, and I. H. Porter, eds.), pp. 173–186, Academic Press, New York.

Hall, J. G., 1963, Adenosine deaminase activity in lymphoid cells during antibody production, *Aust. J. Exp. Biol. Med. Sci.* **41**:93–97.

Henderson, J. F., Rosenbloom, F. M., Kelley, W. N., and Seegmiller, J. E., 1968, Variations in purine metabolism of cultured skin fibroblasts from patients with gout, *J. Clin. Invest.* **47**:1511–1516.

Henderson, J. F., Fraser, J. H., and McCoy, E. E., 1974a, Methods for the study of purine metabolism in human cells *in vitro, Clin. Biochem.* **7**:339–358.

Henderson, J. F., McCoy, E. E., and Fraser, J. H., 1974b, Purine nucleotide synthesis, interconversion and catabolism in human leukocytes, *Adv. Exp. Med. Biol.* **41A**:113–116.

Herman, J. B., Medalie, J. H., and Goldbourt, J., 1974, Diabetes and uric acid—A relationship investigated by the epidemiological method, *Adv. Exp. Med. Biol.* **41B**:483–484.

Hershko, A., Hershko, C., and Mager, J., 1968, Increased formation of 5-phosphoribosyl-1-pyrophosphate in red blood cells of some gouty patients, *Isr. Med. J.* **4**:939–944.

Hirschhorn, R., 1975a, Adenosine deaminase deficiency: Genetic and metabolic implications, *in: Combined Immunodeficiency Disease and Adenosine Deaminase Deficiency. A Molecular Defect,* (H. J. Meuwissen, R. J. Pickering, B. Pollara, and I. H. Porter, eds.), pp. 121–128, Academic Press, New York.

Hirschhorn, R., 1975b, Conversion of human erythrocyte–adenosine deaminase activity to different tissue-specific isozymes. Evidence for a common catalytic unit, *J. Clin. Invest.* **55**:661–667.

Hirschhorn, R., and Levytska, V., 1974, Alterations in isozymes of adenosine deaminase during stimulation of human peripheral blood lymphocytes, *Cell. Immun.* **12:**387–395.

Hirschhorn, R., Grossman, J., and Weissmann, G., 1970, Effect of cyclic 3',5'-adenosine monophosphate and theophylline on lymphocyte transformation, *Proc. Soc. Exp. Biol. Med.* **133:**1361–1365.

Hirschhorn, R., Beratis, N., Rosen, F. S., Parkman, R. Stern, R., and Polmar, S., 1975, Adenosine-deaminase deficiency in a child diagnosed prenatally, *Lancet* **1:**73–75.

Hitchings, G. H., 1971, Crystals in skeletal muscle, *Br. Med. J.* **4:**555–556.

Holmes, E. W., Wyngaarden, J. B., and Kelley, W. N., 1973, Human glutamine phosphoribosylpyrophosphate amidotransferase. Two molecular forms interconvertible by purine ribonucleotides and phosphoribosylpyrophosphate, *J. Biol. Chem.* **248:**6035–6040.

Holmes, E. W., Jr., Mason, D. H., Jr., Goldstein, L. I., Blount, R. E., Jr., and Kelley, W. N., 1974a, Xanthine oxidase deficiency: Studies of a previously unreported case, *Clin. Chem.* **20:**1076–1079.

Holmes, E. W., Jr., Wyngaarden, J. B., and Kelley, W. N., 1974b, Human glutamine phosphoribosylpyrophosphate (PP-ribose-P) amidotransferase: Kinetic, regulation, and configurational changes, *Adv. Exp. Med. Biol.* **41A:**43–53.

Hong, R., 1975, Summary of therapy in ADA deficient patients. *in: Combined Immunodeficiency Disease and Adenosine Deaminase Deficiency. A Molecular Defect* (H. J., Meuwissen, R. J. Pickering, B. Pollara, and I. H. Porter, eds.), pp. 293–299, Academic Press, New York.

Hooft, C., Van Nevel, C., and De Schaepdryver, A. F., 1968, Hyperuricosuric encephalopathy without hyperuricaemia, *Arch. Dis. Child.* **43:**734–737.

Hopkinson, D. A., Cook, P. J. L., and Harris, H., 1969, Further data on the adenosine deaminase (ADA) polymorphism and a report of a new phenotype, *Ann. Hum. Genet.* **32:**361–367.

Hunder, G. G., Worthington, J. W., and Bickel, W. H., 1968, Avascular necrosis of the femoral head in a patient with gout, *J. Amer. Med. Assoc.* **203:**47–49.

Ishii, K., and Green, H., 1973, Lethality of adenosine for cultured mammalian cells by interference with pyrimidine biosynthesis, *J. Cell Sci.* **13:**429–439.

Ito, K., and Uchino, H., 1973, Control of pyrimidine biosynthesis in human lymphocytes: Simultaneous increase in activities of glutamine-utilizing carbamyl phosphate synthetase and aspartate transcarbamylase in phytochemagglutinin-stimulated human peripheral lymphocytes and their enzyme co-purification, *J. Biol. Chem.* **248:**389–392.

Kaufman, J. M., Greene, M. L., and Seegmiller, J. E., 1968, Urine uric acid to creatinine ratio. A screening test for inherited disorders of purine metabolism, *J. Pediatr.* **73:**583–592.

Keightly, R. G., Lawton, A. R., Yu, L. Y. F., and Cooper, M. D., 1975, Correction of combined immunodeficiency by fetal liver transplantation in a patient with adenosine deaminase deficiency, *in: Combined Immunodeficiency Disease and Adenosine Deaminase Deficiency. A Molecular Defect* (H. J. Meuwissen, R. J. Pickering, B. Pollara, and I. H. Porter, eds.), pp. 213–217, Academic Press, New York.

Kelley, W. N., 1974, Pathophysiology of purine metabolism in man, *Enzyme* **18**:161–175.

Kelley, W. N., 1975a, Effects of drugs on uric acid in man, *Annu. Rev. Pharmacol.* **15**:327–350.

Kelley, W. N., 1975b, Pharmacologic approach to the maintenance of urate homeostasis, *Nephron* **14**:99–115.

Kelley, W. N., and Beardmore, T. D., 1970, Allopurinol: Alteration in pyrimidine metabolism in man, *Science* **169**:388–390.

Kelley, W. N., and Wyngaarden, J. B., 1972, The Lesch-Nyhan syndrome, *in: The Metabolic Basis of Inherited Disease*, Third Ed. (J. B. Stanbury, J. B. Wyngaarden, and D. S. Fredrickson, eds.), pp. 969–991, McGraw-Hill, New York.

Kelley, W. N., and Wyngaarden, J. B., 1974, Enzymology of gout, *Adv. Enzymol.* **41**:1–33.

Kelley, W. N., Levy, R. I., Rosenbloom, F. M., Henderson, J. F., and Seegmiller, J. E., 1968, Adenine phosphoribosyltransferase deficiency: A previously undescribed genetic defect in man, *J. Clin. Invest.* **47**:2281–2289.

Kelley, W. N., Greene, M. L., Rosenbloom, F. M., Henderson, J. F., and Seegmiller, J. E., 1969, Hypoxanthine-guanine phosphoribosyltransferase deficiency in gout. A review, *Ann. Intern. Med.* **70**:155–206.

Kelley W. N., Fox, I. H., and Wyngaarden, J. B., 1970a, Regulation of purine biosynthesis in cultured human cells. I. Effects of orotic acid, *Biochim. Biophys. Acta* **215**:512–516.

Kelley, W. N., Greene, M. L., Fox, I. H., Rosenbloom, F. M., Levy, R. I., and Seegmiller, J. E., 1970b, Effects of orotic acid on purine and lipoprotein metabolism in man, *Metabolism* **19**:1025–1035.

Kelley, W. N., Beardmore, T. D., Fox, I. H., and Meade, J. C., 1971, Effect of allopurinol and oxipurinol on pyrimidine synthesis in cultured human fibroblasts, *Biochem. Parmacol.* **20**:1471–1478.

Klinenberg, J. R. (ed.), 1975, Proceedings of the second conference on gout and purine metabolism, *Arthritis Rheum.* **18**(Suppl.):659–888.

Krooth, R. S., Lam, G. F. M., and Kiang, S. Y. C., 1974, Oxipurinol and orotic aciduria: Effect on the orotidine-5′-monophosphate decarboxylase activity of cultured human fibroblasts, *Cell* **3**:55–57.

Kuhn, B., Bissbort, S., Kompf, J., and Ritter, H., 1975, Red cell uridine-5-monophosphate kinase (UMPK). Formal genetics, linkage analysis and population genetics from southwestern Germany, *Humangenetik* **28**:255–258.

Lerner, M. H., and Lowy, B. A., 1974, The formation of adenosine in rabbit liver and its possible role as a direct precursor of erythrocyte adenine nucleotides, *J. Biol. Chem.* **249**:959–966.

Lever, J. E., Nuki, G., and Seegmiller, J. E., 1974, Expression of purine overproduction in a series of 8-azaguanine-resistant diploid human lymphoblast lines, *Proc. Nat. Acad. Sci. U.S.A.* **71**:2679–2683.

Levine, R. L., Hoogenraad, N. J., and Kretchmer, N., 1974, A review: Biological and clinical aspects of pyrimidine metabolism, *Pediatr. Res.* **8**:724–734.

Long, W. K., 1967, Glutathione reductase in red blood cells: Variant associated with gout, *Science* **155**:712–713.

Lowy, B. A., and Lerner, M. H., 1974, A role of liver adenosine in the renewal of the adenine nucleotides of human and rabbit erythrocytes, *Adv. Exp. Med. Biol.* **41A:**129–139.

McCarty, D. J., 1974, Crystal deposition joint disease, *Annu. Rev. Med.* **25:**279–288.

McDonald, J. A., and Kelley, W. N., 1974, Hypoxanthine–guanine phosphoribosyltransferase deficiency: Altered kinetic properties of a specific mutant form of the enzyme, *Adv. Exp. Med. Biol.* **41A:**167–175.

McGuire, T. C. Poppie, M. J., and Banks, K. L., 1974, Combined (B- and T-lymphocyte) immunodeficiency: A fatal genetic disease in Arabian foals, *J. Amer. Vet. Med. Assoc.* **164:**70–76.

McKusick, V. A., 1975, *Mendelian Inheritance in Man, Catalogs of Autosomal Dominant, Autosomal Recessive, and X-Linked Phenotypes,* Fourth Ed., The Johns Hopkins University Press, Baltimore.

Meuwissen, H. J., and Pollara, B., 1974, Adenosine deaminase deficiency: The first inborn error of metabolism noted in immunodeficiency disease, *J. Pediatr.* **84:**315–316.

Meuwissen, H. J., Pickering, R. J., Pollara, B., and Porter, I. H. (ed.), 1975a, *Combined Immunodeficiency Disease and Adenosine Deaminase Deficiency. A Molecular Defect, Proceedings,* Academic Press, New York.

Meuwissen, H. J., Pollara, B., and Pickering, R. J., 1975b, Combined immunodeficiency disease associated with adenosine deaminase deficiency, *J. Pediatr.* **86:**169–181.

Meyer, W. J., III, Gill, J. R., Jr., and Bartter, F. C., 1975, Gout as a complication of Bartter's syndrome. A possible role for alkalosis in the decreased clearance of uric acid, *Ann. Intern. Med.* **83:**56–59.

Mielants, H., Veys, E. M., de Bussere, A., and Van der Jeught, J., 1975, Relations entre la nécrose avasculaire et le métagolisme des lipides et des purines. Corrélations entre les tauz d'acide urique, des lipides et des lipoprotéines dans la goutte et la nécrose avasculaire, *Rev. Rhum. Mal. Osteo-Articulaires* **42:**505–511.

Mizuno, T.-I., and Yugari, Y., 1974, Letter to Editor: Self-mutilation in Lesch-Nyhan syndrome, *Lancet* **1:**761.

Müller, M. M., and Frank, O., 1974, Lipid and purine metabolism in benign symmetric lipomatosis, *Adv. Exp. Med. Biol.* **41B:** 509–516.

Newcombe, D. S., 1973, Gouty arthritis and polycystic kidney disease, *Ann. Intern. Med.* **79:**605.

Newcombe, D. S., 1975, *Inherited Biochemical Disorders and Uric Acid Metabolism,* First Ed., University Park Press, Baltimore.

Niederwieser, A., Giliberti, P., Matasović, A., Pluznik, S., Steinmann, B., and Baerlocher, K., 1974, Folic acid non-dependent formimimoglutamic aciduria in two siblings, *Clin. Chim. Acta* **54:**293–316.

Nuki, G., Lever, J., and Seegmiller, J. E., 1974, Biochemical characteristics of 8-azaguanine resistant human lymphoblast mutants selected *in vitro, Adv. Exp. Med. Biol.* **41A:**255–267.

Nyhan, W. L., James, J. A., Teberg, A. J., Sweetman, L., and Nelson, L. G., 1969, A new disorder of purine metabolism with behavioral manifestations, *J. Pediat.* **74:**20–27.

Nyhan, W. L., Bakay, B., Connor, J. D., Marks, J. F., and Keele, D. K., 1970, Hemizygous expression of glucose-6-phosphate dehydrogenase in erythrocytes of heterozygotes for the Lesch-Nyhan syndrome, *Proc. Nat. Acad. Sci. U.S.A.* **65:**214–218.

Ochs, H. D., Yount, J. E., Giblett, E. R., Chen, S. H., Scott, C. R., and Wedgwood, R. J., 1973, Adenosine-deaminase deficiency and severe combined immuno-deficiency syndrome, *Lancet* **1:**1393, 1394.

Osborne, W. R. A., and Spencer, N., 1973, Partial purification and properties of the common inherited forms of adenosine deaminase from human erythro-cytes, *Biochem. J.* **133:**117–123.

Paglia, D. E., and Valentine, W. N., 1975, Characteristics of a pyrimidine-specific 5'-nucleotidase in human erythrocytes, *J. Biol. Chem.* **250:**7973–7979.

Paglia, D. E., Valentine, W. N., and Dahlgren, J. G., 1975, Effects of low-level lead exposure on pyrimidine 5'-nucleotidase and other erythrocyte enzymes: Possible role of pyrimidine 5'- nucleotidase in the pathogenesis of lead-induced anemia, *J. Clin. Invest.* **56:**1164–1169.

Parker, R., Snedden, W., and Watts, R. W. E., 1970, The quantitative determina-tion of hypoxanthine and xanthine ("oxypurines") in skeletal muscle from two patients with congenital xanthine oxidase deficiency (xanthinuria), *Biochem. J.* **116:**317, 318.

Parkman, R., Gelfand, E. W., Rosen, F. S., Sanderson, A., and Hirschhorn, R., 1975, Severe combined immunodeficiency and adenosine deaminase defi-ciency, *N. Engl. J. Med.* **292:**714–719.

Pastan, I., 1975, Regulation of cellular growth, *Adv. Metab. Disord.* **8:**7–16.

Pedrini, A. M., Dalpra, L., Ciarrocchi, G., Noy, G. C. F. P., Spadari, S., Nuzzo, F., and Falaschi, A., 1974, Levels of some enzymes acting on DNA in xeroderma pigmentosum, *Nucleic Acids Res.* **1:**193–202.

Perheentupa, J., and Raivio, K. O., 1967, Fructose-induced hyperuricaemia, *Lancet* **2:**528–531.

Polmar, S. H., Wetzler, E. M., Stern, R. C., and Hirschhorn, R., 1975, Restoration of *in-vitro* lymphocyte responses with exogenous adenosine deaminase in a patient with severe combined immunodeficiency, *Lancet* **2:**743–746.

Pritchard, J. B., Chavez-Peon, F., and Berlin, R. D., 1970, Purines: Supply by liver to tissues, *Amer. J. Physiol.* **219:**1263–1267.

Raivio, K. O. Becker, M. A., Meyer, L. J., Greene, M. L., Nuki, G., and Seegmiller, J. E., 1975, Stimulation of human purine synthesis de novo by fructose infusion, *Metabolism* **24:**861–869.

Rapado, A., Mendoza, H. J. C., Castrillo, J. M., Frutos, M., and Delatte, L. C., 1975, Xanthinuria as a cause of hypouricaemia in liver disease, *Br. Med. J.* **2:**560.

Reem, G. H., 1975, Phosphoribosylpyrophosphate overproduction, a new meta-bolic abnormality in the Lesch Nyhan syndrome, *Science* **190:**1098, 1099.

Reyes, P., and Guganig, M. E., 1975, Studies on a pyrimidine phosphoribosyltrans-ferase from murine leukemia P1534J. Partial purification, substrate specific-ity, and evidence for its existence as a bifunctional complex with orotidine 5'-phosphate decarboxylase, *J. Biol. Chem.* **250:**5097–5108.

Robbins, J. H., Kracmer, K. H., Lutzner, M. A., Festoff, B. W., and Coon, H. G., 1974, Xeroderma pigmentosum. An inherited disease with sun sensitivity, multiple cutaneous neoplasms, and abnormal DNA repair, *Ann. Intern. Med.* **80:**221–248.

Roberts, M. F., Switzer, R. L., and Schubert, K. R., 1975, Inactivation of *Salmonella* phosphoribosylpyrophosphate synthetase by oxidation of a specific sulfhydryl group with potassium permanganate, *J. Biol. Chem.* **250:**5364–5369.

Rockson, S., Stone, R., van der Weyden, M., and Kelley, W. N., 1974, Lesch-Nyhan syndrome: Evidence for abnormal adrenergic function, *Science* **186:**934, 935.

Rogers, L. E., Nicolaisen, A. K., and Holt, J. G., 1975, Hereditary orotic aciduria: Results of a screening survey, *J. Lab. Clin. Med.* **85:**287–291.

Rosenberg, A. L., Bergstrom, L., Troost, B. T., and Bartholomew, B. A., 1970, Hyperuricemia and neurologic deficits, a family study, *New Engl. J. Med.* **282:**992–997.

Rosenbloom, F. M., Kelley, W. N., Henderson, J. F., and Seegmiller, J. E., 1967, Lyon Hypothesis and X-linked disease, *Lancet* **2:**305–306.

Rosenbloom, F. M., Henderson, J. F., Caldwell, I. C., Kelley, W. N., and Seegmiller, J. E., 1968, Biochemical bases of accelerated purine biosynthesis *de novo* in human fibroblasts lacking hypoxanthine–guanine phosphoribosyltransferase, *J. Biol. Chem.* **243:**1166–1173.

Rossi, C. A., Lucacchini, A., Montali, U., and Ronca, G., 1975, A general method of purification of adenosine deaminase by affinity chromatography, *Int. J. Pept. Protein Res.* **7:**81–89.

Sato, K., Slesinski, R. S., and Littlefield, J. W., 1972, Chemical mutagenesis at the phosphoribosyltransferase locus in cultured human lymphoblasts, *Proc. Nat. Acad. Sci. U.S.A.* **69:**1244–1248.

Scheffler, I. E., 1974, Conditional lethal mutants of Chinese hamster cells: Mutants requiring exogenous carbon dioxide for growth, *J. Cell Physiol.* **83:**219–230.

Schubert, K. R., Switzer, R. L., and Shelton, E., 1975, Studies of the quaternary structure and the chemical properties of phosphoribosylpyrophosphate synthetase from *Salmonella typhimurium, J. Biol. Chem.* **250:**7492–7500.

Schulman, J. D., Lustberg, T. J., Kennedy, J. L., Museles, M., and Seegmiller, J. E., 1970, A new variant of maple syrup urine disease (branched chain ketoaciduria). Clinical and Biochemical evaluation, *Amer. J. Med.* **49:**118–124.

Sciaky, N., Razin, B., Gazit, B., and Mager, J., 1974, Regulatory aspects of the synthesis of 5-phosphoribosyl-1-pyrophosphate in human red blood cells, *Adv. Exp. Med. Biol.* **41A:**87–92.

Scott, C. R., Chen, S.-H., and Giblett, E. R., 1974, Detection of the carrier state in combined immunodeficiency diseases associated with adenosine deaminase deficiency, *J. Clin. Invest.* **53:**1194–1196.

Seegmiller, J. E., 1969, Diseases of purine and pyrimidine metabolism, *in: Duncan's Diseases of Metabolism,* Sixth Ed. (P. K. Bondy and L. E. Rosenberg, eds.), p. 516, W. B. Saunders Co., Philadelphia.

Seegmiller, J. E., 1974, Diseases of purine and pyrimidine metabolism, *in: Duncan's Diseases of Metabolism, Genetics and Metabolism,* Seventh Ed. (P. K. Bondy and L. E. Rosenberg, eds.), pp. 655–774, W. B. Saunders Co., Philadelphia.

Seegmiller, J. E., Laster, L., and Howell, R. R., 1963, Biochemistry of uric acid and its relation to gout, *New Engl. J. Med.* **268:**712–716, 764–773, 821–827.

Seegmiller, J. E., Rosenbloom, F. M., and Kelley, W. N., 1967, Enzyme defect associated with a sex-linked human neurological disorder and excessive purine synthesis, *Science* **155:**1682–1684.

Seegmiller, J. E., Siniscalco, M., Klinger, H. P., Eagle, H., Koprowski, H., and Fujimoto, W. Y., 1969, Intergenomic complementation of two X-linked genes by hybridization of mutant human fibroblasts, *Trans. Assoc. Amer. Physicians* **82:**239–247.

Seegmiller, J. E., Scott, D., and Snyder, F. F., 1976, Prenatal detection of adenosine deaminase deficiency (in preparation).

Short, E. M., Conn, H. O., Snodgrass, P. J., Campbell, A. G. M., and Rosenberg, L. E., 1973, Evidence for X-linked dominant inheritance of ornithine transcarbamylase deficiency, *New Engl. J. Med.* **288:**7–12.

Simkin, P. A., Skeith, M. D., and Healey, L. A., 1974, Suppression of uric acid secretion in a patient with renal hypouricemia, *Adv. Exp. Med. Biol.* **41B:**723–728.

Simmonds, H. A., Levin, B., and Cameron, J. S., 1974, Variations in allopurinol metabolism by xanthinuric subjects, *Clin. Sci. Mol. Med.* **47:**173–178.

Simmonds, H. A., Levin, B., and Cameron, J. S., 1975, Variations in allopurinol metabolism by xanthinuric subjects, *Clin. Sci. Mol. Med.* **49:**81, 82.

Smith, L. H., Huguley, C. M., Jr., and Bain, J. A., 1972, Hereditary orotic aciduria, *in: Metabolic Basis of Inherited Disease,* Third Ed. (J. B. Stanbury, J. B. Wyngaarden, and D. S. Fredrickson, eds.), pp. 1003–1029, McGraw-Hill, New York.

Spencer, N., Hopkinson, D. A., and Harris, H., 1968, Adenosine deaminase polymorphism in man, *Ann. Hum. Genet.* **32:**9–14.

Sperling, O., Persky-Brosh, S., Boer, P., and de Vries, A., 1974a, Mutant phosphoribosylpyrophosphate synthetase in two gouty siblings with excessive purine production, *Adv. Exp. Med. Biol.* **41A:**299–305.

Sperling, O., Weinberger, A., Oliver, I., Liberman, U. A., and de Vries, A., 1974b, Hypouricemia, hypercalcuria and decreased bone density. A new hereditary syndrome, *Adv. Exp. Med. Biol.* **41B:**717–721.

Srivastava, S. K., Villacorte, D., and Beutler, E., 1972, Correlation between adenylate metabolizing enzymes and adenine nucleotide levels of erythrocytes during blood storage in various media, *Transfusion* **12:**190–197.

Tatibana, M., and Shigesada, K., 1972, Two carbamyl phosphate synthetases of mammals: Specific roles in control of pyrimidine and urea biosynthesis, *Adv. Enzyme Regul.* **10:**249–271.

Tischfield, J. A., and Ruddle, F. H., 1974, Assignment of the gene for adenine phosphoribosyltransferase to human chromosome 16 by mouse–human somatic cell hybridization, *Proc. Nat. Acad. Sci. U.S.A.* **71:**45–49.

Valentine, W. N., Anderson, H. M., Paglia, D. E., Jaffé, E. R., Konrad, P. N., and Harris, S. R., 1972, Studies on human erythrocyte nucleotide metabolism. II. Nonspherocytic hemolytic anemia, high red cell ATP, and ribosephosphate pyrophosphokinase (RPK, E. C. 2.7.6.1) deficiency, *Blood* **39:**674–684.

Valentine, W. N., Fink, K., Paglia, D. E., Harris, S. R., and Adams, W. S., 1974, Hereditary hemolytic anemia with human erythrocyte pyrimidine 5'-nucleotidase deficiency, *J. Clin. Invest.* **54:**866–879.

van der Weyden, M. B., and Kelley, W. N., 1974, Adenosine deaminase deficiency in severe combined immunodeficiency: Evidence for a posttranslational defect, *J. Clin. Invest.* **53:**81A–82A.

van der Weyden, M. B., Buckley, R. H., and Kelley, W. N., 1974, Molecular form of adenosine deaminase in severe combined immunodeficiency, *Biochem. Biophys. Res. Commun.* **57:**590–595.

Van Heeswijk, P. J., Blank, C. H., Seegmiller, J. E., and Jacobson, C. B., 1972, Preventive control of the Lesch-Nyhan syndrome, *Obstet. Gynecol.* **40:**109–113.

Wada, Y., Nishimura, Y., Tanabu, M., Yoshimura, Y., Iinuma, K., Yoshida, T., and Arakawa, T., 1974, Hypouricemic mentally retarded infant with a defect of 5-phosphoribosyl-1-pyrophosphate synthetase of erythrocytes, *Tohoku J. Exp. Med.* **113:**149–157.

Wara, D. W., and Ammann, A. J., 1975, Laboratory data, *in: Combined Immunodeficiency Disease and Adenosine Deaminase Deficiency. A Molecular Defect* (H. J. Meuwissen, R. J. Pickering, B. Pollara, and I. H. Porter, eds.), pp. 247–253, Academic Press, New York.

Watts, R. W. E., Scott, J. T., Chalmers, R. A., Bitensky, L., and Chayen, J., 1971a, Microscopic studies on skeletal muscle in gout patients treated with allopurinol, *Q. J. Med.* **40:**1–14.

Watts, R. W. E., Snedden, W., and Parker, R. A., 1971b, A quantitative study of skeletal muscle purines and pyrazolo-[3,4-d]pyrimidines in gout patients treated with allopurinol, *Clin. Sci.* **41:**153–158.

Wolfson, J. J., and Cross, V. F., 1975, The radiographic findings in forty-nine patients with combined immunodeficiency, *in: Combined Immunodeficiency Disease and Adenosine Deaminase Deficiency. A Molecular Defect* (H.J. Meuwissen, R. J. Pickering, B. Pollara, and I. H. Porter, eds.), pp. 255–274, Academic Press, New York.

Wood, A. W., and Seegmiller, J. E., 1973, Properties of 5-phosphoribosyl-1-pyrophosphate amidotransferase from human lymphoblasts, *J. Biol. Chem.* **248:**138–143.

Worthy, T. E., Grobner, W., and Kelley, W. N., 1974, Hereditary orotic aciduria: Evidence for a structural gene mutation, *Proc. Nat. Acad. Sci. U.S.A.* **71:**3031–3035.

Wyngaarden, J. B., and Kelley, W. N., 1972, Gout, *in: The Metabolic Basis of Inherited Disease,* Third Ed. (J. B. Stanbury, J. B. Wyngaarden, and D. S. Fredrickson, eds.), pp. 889–968, McGraw-Hill, New York.

Yanai, J., Kakimoto, Y., Tsujio, T., and Sano, I., 1969, Genetic study of beta-aminoisobutyric acid excretion by Japanese, *Amer. J. Hum. Genet.* **21:**115–132.

Yount, J., Nichols, P. Ochs, H. D., Hammer, S. P., Scott, C. R., Chen, S.-H., Giblett, E. R., and Wedgwood, R. J., 1974, Absence of erythrocyte adenosine deaminase associated with severe combined immunodeficiency, *J. Pediatr.* **84:**173–177.

Zöllner, N., and Gröbner, W., 1971, Influence of oral ribonucleic acid on orotaciduria due to allopurinol administration, *Z. Gesante Exp. Med.* **156:**317–319.

Zoref, E., de Vries, A., and Sperling, O., 1975, Mutant feedback-resistant phosphoribosylpyrophosphate synthetase associated with purine overproduction and gout. Phosphoribosylpyrophosphate and purine metabolism in cultured fibroblasts, *J. Clin. Invest.* **56:**1093–1099.

What's New—
Vitamins and Minerals

Louis V. Avioli

9.1. Introduction

A detailed, unbiased analysis of publications relating to "vitamin and mineral metabolism" could result only in an exhaustive, rambling potpourri of seemingly unrelated notes and comments. Advances in divalent ionic control of membrane transport, enzymatic activity, and hormonal synthesis and release are detailed elsewhere in this volume. Similarly, publications concerned with disorders of mineral metabolism and excretion and their relationship to human nutrition, growth, and the formation of renal calculi are reviewed in Chapter 11. In 1975, considerable efforts were expended to evaluate the effectiveness of vitamin C in preventing the common cold. Many significant advances were also made with respect to the metabolism, molecular response, and biological activity of vitamin D

LOUIS V. AVIOLI • Division of Bone and Mineral Metabolism, Washington University School of Medicine, St. Louis, Missouri 63110.

metabolites. For the sake of completion and uniformity, therefore, only these advances will be emphasized and reviewed in detail this year.

9.2. Vitamin C

Since vitamin C was isolated and crystallized in 1932 and proved to be antiscorbutic for guinea pigs (Waugh and King, 1932), it has been established as an essential antioxidant and cofactor in a variety of biological reactions (Birch and Parker, 1974). In man, vitamin C deficiency is prevented with intakes of 50–100 mg/day, although subjects with achlorhydria, chronic diarrhea, neoplastic disease, burns and surgical wounds, or hyperthyroidism may have increased needs. Similarly, ascorbic acid requirements may also be increased during pregnancy and lactation, and during the administration of oral contraceptives, salicylates, and antibiotics. It has still not been established, however, that these situations require or would benefit from adjunctive therapy with ascorbic acid. In 1975, it was reported that vitamin C in doses of 1 g/day led to a significant fall in plasma cholesterol and triglycerides (Ginter, 1976); identical doses in diabetic subjects also reportedly decreased cutaneous capillary fragility (Cox and Butterfield, 1975). These latter observations are of interest, since insulin does normally affect vitamin C metabolism in peripheral tissues, and the response is blunted in diabetic patients (Cox et al., 1974).

The reported effects of vitamin C on cholesterol and triglyceride metabolism are still contradictory, however. Crawford et al. (1975) reported an increase in cholesterol during vitamin C ingestion. These data confirm the results of Klevay (1976), who reported a hypercholesterolemic effect of ascorbic acid in rats in doses equivalent to 82–630 mg capsular ascorbic acid ingested by an average man. The mechanism or mechanisms underlying the vitamin C–induced hypercholesterolemia are still unknown. A malabsorption of copper attributed to vitamin C in the past (Evans, 1973) has been implicated in this regard, since an increase in the ratio of ingested zinc to copper produces hypercholesterolemia experimentally (Klevay, 1975), and the rise in serum cholesterol is greater when human scurvy is treated with oral rather than intramuscular vitamin C (Bronte-Stewart et al., 1963).

In 1970, it was claimed that the daily intake of 1 g vitamin C would lead to a 45% reduction in the incidence of colds and a 60% reduction of total days of illness (Pauling, 1970). It was later suggested that the adult intake be increased to 250–4000 mg/day (Pauling, 1974). In 1972, double-blind studies were performed in over 800 volunteers to test this hypothesis. The results revealed no significant decrease in the number of colds of persons taking 1.0 g vitamin C/day, although the "days confined to house," a measure of the severity of the cold, were significantly fewer (Anderson *et al.*, 1972). In 1975, these same investigators studied the effect of relatively lower doses of vitamin C in 622 volunteers. Confirming their early observations, the authors noted that low-dose supplementary vitamin C (500 mg/day), while ineffective in preventing the common cold, significantly reduced "the burden of winter illness" (Anderson *et al.*, 1975). A detailed evaluation of the efficacy and toxicity of ascorbic acid for the prevention of the common cold was reported by Dykes and Meier (1975) after they had reviewed all published clinical data on this subject. They concluded that "no clear, reproducible pattern of efficacy has emerged from the review of all the evidence," and that "the unrestricted use of ascorbic acid for these purposes cannot be advocated on the basis of the evidence currently available." Similar conclusions were reached by Chalmers (1975), although he noted that in most of the reported 14 clinical trials reviewed, "the severity of symptoms was significantly worse in the patients who received the placebo." The results of studies using D-isoascorbic acid, an isomer of L-ascorbic acid that has limited antiscorbutic activity, were also reported in 1975. On 1-g doses of either D-isoascorbic acid, L-ascorbic acid, or placebo, subjects taking D-isoascorbic acid reportedly suffered 34% fewer colds than the other two groups (Clegg and MacDonald, 1975). Although the controversy regarding beneficial effects of supplemental vitamin C therapy for the common cold still rages, and the results of innumerable surveys are controversial, to say the least, megavitamin C therapy continues to be advocated. This practice could prove hazardous and potentially deleterious, since megadose levels of vitamin C induce hemolysis in patients with G-6-DP deficiency (Campbell *et al.*, 1975), alter electroencephalographic driving responses to photic stimulation (Kerxhalli *et al.*, 1975), decrease the availability of dietary vitamin B_{12} (Herbert and Jacob, 1974), induce uricosuria in doses of 4–8 g/day (Stein *et al.*, 1976), and may, in certain persons with high ascorbic–oxalate conversion rates, lead to 8-fold increments in urinary oxalate excretion (Harris, 1976; Briggs, 1976; Briggs *et al.*, 1973) and renal calculi (Briggs, 1973). Finally, it should be emphasized that whereas the ingestion of 1 g ascorbic acid/day for 1 week significantly increases plasma and whole blood levels, larger doses do not further increase plasma and whole blood ascorbic acid levels (Angel *et al.*, 1975).

The role of vitamin C in collagen biosynthesis had been well established in the past, with ascorbate involved both in the conversion of an inactive to an active form of prolyl hydroxylase and as a cofactor in the hydroxylation of collagen proline residues by prolyl hydroxylase (Stassen *et al.*, 1973). Ascorbic acid is also an essential cofactor for the hydroxylation of lysine residues of the collagen molecule, an observation that may have clinical import, since cultured fibroblasts from skin biopsy samples of

some patients with Ehlers-Danlos syndrome are deficient in lysyl hydroxylase activity (Krane *et al.*, 1972). Although the nature of the defect
exhibited by these fibroblasts is yet undetermined, a recent study of the
effect of ascorbate on lysyl and prolyl hydroxylase activity of cultured
fibroblasts by Miller (1975) bears noting. He reported that unlike previous
reports of an active form of prolyl hydroxylase that is activated by
ascorbate, ascorbate does not activate lysyl hydroxylase in cultured L-929
fibroblasts. The data are consistent with the hypothesis that lysyl hydroxylase is not normally synthesized in an inactive precursor form. Thus, they
tentatively rule out one hypothesis offered to explain the decreased lysyl
hydroxylase activity observed in skin fibroblasts of patients with Ehlers-
Danlos syndrome, i.e., an inherited defect in the activation of an inactive
lysyl hydroxylase.

Although collagen is the major component of bone matrix, and
ascorbic acid is considered essential for the hydroxylation of proline and
lysine residues in the collagen molecule, there are few studies detailing the
specific effects of vitamin C on bone and cartilage collagen and minerali-
zation. The formation and stability of the collagen triple helix are condi-
tioned by the hydroxyproline residues (Jimenez *et al.*, 1973; Ramachandran *et al.*, 1973), and the cross-linkage of collagen is dependent on
hydroxylysine (Ayer and Glimcher, 1973). Using 18-day fetal rat radii
culture systems, Chen and Raisz (1975) reported that ascorbic acid deficiency decreased the hydroxylation of proline in bone and cartilage,
although calcification was unaffected. Using a collagenase assay for the
identification of both hydroxylated and underhydroxylated collagen,
these same investigators demonstrated an accumulation of poorly hydroxylated collagen in bone and the culture media, and an overall decrease in
synthesis of total collagen. The data are consistent with previous observations of Jeffrey and Martin (1966), who observed an overall decrease in
protein, RNA, and DNA synthesis in ascorbic acid–deficient cartilaginous
chick bone rudiments, and argue for a vitamin C–dependent translation
of the collagen in cartilage and bone. The studies of Chen and Raisz
(1975) conflict however, with previous reports indicating that underhydroxylated collagen is not normally released in cell culture systems (Margolis and Lukens, 1971).

9.3. Vitamin D

McCollum *et al.* (1922) reported that cod liver oil oxidized for 12-20
hr caused the deposition of calcium in the bones of rachitic rats. The role
of vitamin D as an antirachitic substance was subsequently established, and
the vitamins (D_2 and D_3) were crystallized. For years thereafter, the

vitamin was considered to act directly on the intestine and bone. As detailed in earlier (Avioli and Haddad, 1973) and more recent (DeLuca, 1975; Hill and Stanbury, 1975) reviews of vitamin D metabolism, considerable knowledge then accumulated (especially within the last decade) regarding the metabolism of vitamin D, sites of vitamin D activation, hormonal and ionic control of tissue-specific activating enzymes, and the biological effects of the metabolically active form of the vitamin. Specific assays for 25-hydroxycholecalciferol (25-OHD$_3$) and 1,25-dihydroxycholecalciferol [1,25-(OH)$_2$D$_3$] have been developed and applied in disorders of mineral and skeletal metabolism; structure–function relationships have been explored in target-specific tissues, and the nature of the biological response has been evaluated. The availability of synthetic preparations of 25-OHD$_3$, 1,25-(OH)$_2$D$_3$, and structurally related analogues also prompted detailed analyses of their biological effectiveness in patients with renal disease, vitamin D–resistant rickets, osteoporosis, hepatocellular damage, hypoparathyroidism, and pseudohypoparathyroidism. Surely, within the last decade, few fields of scientific endeavor have progressed from the isolated mitochondria–renal tubule–gut sac *in vitro* investigational stage to well-organized clinical therapeutic trials with such alacrity!

Following the identification of a biologically active renal metabolite of 25-OHD$_3$ by Kodicek *et al*, (1970) and Fraser and Kodicek (1970), which was later identified as 1,25-OHD$_3$, considerable interest centered about the ionic and hormonal control of the renal 24- and 1-hydroxylase enzymes (Tanaka *et al.*, 1975a). 25-OHD$_3$-24-Hydroxylase will convert 25-OHD$_3$ to 24,25-dihydroxycholecalciferol [24,25-(OH)$_2$D$_3$] (Holick *et al.*, 1972), and 1,25-(OH)$_2$D$_3$ to 1,24,25-trihydroxycholecalciferol [1,24,25-(OH)$_3$D$_3$] (Kleiner-Bossaller and DeLuca, 1974). As documented earlier for the 25-OHD$_3$-1-hydroxylase, the 24-hydroxylase was identified in the renal mitochondria. Unlike the 1-hydroxylase, the 24-hydroxylase is not inhibited by cytochrome P-450 inhibitors or carbon monoxide/oxygen mixtures (Knutson and DeLuca, 1974). Tanaka *et al.* (1975c), having previously established that parathyroid hormone (Garabedian *et al.*, 1972) and inorganic phosphate (Tanaka and DeLuca, 1973) regulated the renal synthesis of 1,25-(OH)$_2$D$_3$, advanced an intriguing hypothesis regarding the intrinsic renal enzymatic control of 25-OHD$_3$ metabolism. They argued that there is no regulation of the renal hydroxylase enzyme systems by alterations in calcium or phosphorus metabolism in the vitamin D–deficient state, and concluded that only after 1,25-(OH)$_2$D$_3$ is produced is enzymatic regulation possible. The authors presented data in defense of the hypothesis that 1,25-(OH)$_2$D$_3$ suppresses the 25-OHD-1-hydroxylase and stimulates the 25-OHD-24-hydroxylase (Tanaka *et al.*, 1975c). In the same report, it was demonstrated that parathyroid hormone also suppressed the $25\text{-OHD}_3\text{-}24$-hydroxylase, an effect that could not be ascribed to changes in serum calcium and inorganic phosphate. Since actinomycin D and cyclohexamide blocked these responses in $25\text{-OHD}_3\text{-}24$-hydroxylase activity, the authors inferred that the observed changes in the $25\text{-OHD}_3\text{-}1$- and $25\text{-OHD}_3\text{-}4$-hydroxylase were dependent on *de novo* protein synthesis, rather than on ionic activation or inhibition of existing hydroxylases. This hypothesis was confirmed by Evans *et al.* (1975) in experiments demonstrating inhibition of $25\text{-OHD}_3\text{-}1$-hydroxylase and stimulation of $25\text{-OHD}_3\text{-}24$-hydroxylase in kidney homogenates of rachitic chicks fed either vitamin D_3 or 1α-hydroxycholecalciferol.

Reports regarding the regulatory role of calcium and inorganic phosphate on the renal mitochondrial 25-OHD_3 hydroxylases also appeared in 1975. Hughes *et al.* (1975), utilizing a radioreceptor assay to quantify changes in serum concentrations in $1,25\text{-}(OH)_2D_3$ in rats fed either low-calcium or low-phosphate diets, reported that the rise in circulating $1,25\text{-}(OH)_2D_3$ concentration in calcium-deficient animals was dependent on parathyroid hormone. In contrast, the response to phosphate deficiency was independent of parathyroid hormone activity. Studies on the *in vitro* hydroxylation of $25\text{-}(OH)_2D_3$ by isolated kidney mitochondria or tubules of vitamin D–deficient chicks by Horiuchi *et al.* (1975) revealed that calcium, in 0.05–0.2-mM concentrations, produced a marked and dose-related stimulation of the $25\text{-OHD}_3\text{-}1$-hydroxylase. This ionic effect was not observed in renal tubules prepared from vitamin D–deficient parathyroidectomized chicks. The authors concluded that calcium activation of the chick renal mitochondrial $25\text{-OHD}_3\text{-}1$-hydroxylase—and $25\text{-OHD}_3\text{-}24$-hydroxylase, as reported in an earlier publication (Horiuchi *et al.*, 1974)—was independent of the delayed, actinomycin D–sensitive, adaptive responses of the hydroxylase enzymes to $1,25\text{-}(OH)_2D_3$, and attributed the observation to rapid alterations in existing enzymatic activities. The results of more detailed studies of the ionic control of $1,25\text{-}(OH)_2D_3$ synthesis in isolated chick renal mitochondria and tubules were also reported by Bikle and Rasmussen (1975). Renal tubules isolated from chicks raised on a vitamin D–deficient diet containing 0.43% calcium and 0.3% phosphate demonstrated maximal $1,25\text{-}(OH)_2D_3$ synthesis rates (Bikle *et al.*, 1975). Production of $1,25\text{-}(OH)_2D_3$ was decreased by diets containing more or less of either calcium or phosphate. In their studies, calcium concentrations of 0.5–1.0 mM were necessary for optimal 1-hydroxylase activity, with greater concentrations inhibiting $1,25\text{-}(OH)_2D_3$ synthesis. Enzymatic inhibition by the calcium ion was enhanced by increasing the media phosphate concentration. Of special interest was the observation that *increasing* media phosphate concentrations from 0 to 6 mM *in the absence of calcium* also stimulated $25\text{-OHD}_3\text{-}1$-hydroxylase activity, an effect that was blocked by 4 mM calcium. In both isolated tubules and mitochondria, the stimulation of $1,25\text{-}(OH)_2D_3$ produced by calcium was less at pH 6.7 than at 7.4 (Bikle *et al.*, 1975). Since neither $LaCl_3$ nor oligomycin altered the stimulating effects of the calcium ion on 1-hydroxylase activity, the accumulated data were considered consistent with the hypothesis that the $[Ca^{+2}]$ in the mitochondrial matrix conditions the activity of this enzyme.

Since it had been well documented that parathyroid hormone stimulates the renal production of $1,25\text{-}(OH)_2D_3$ in animals and humans (Mawer *et al.*, 1975), it seemed appropriate to evaluate the potential negative feedback control hypothesis; i.e., does $1,25\text{-}(OH)_2D_3$ in turn suppress parathyroid hormone secretion? Care *et al.* (1975) offered convincing data in this regard when they reported that direct perfusion of goat parathyroid glands with $1,25\text{-}(OH)_2D_3$ at a concentration of 125 pg/ml suppressed hormonal secretion. These findings were later confirmed in the rat by Chertow *et al.* (1975), who demonstrated *in vivo* suppression of parathyroid hormone secretion in the rat following the injection of a physiological dose (130 pmol or 2 IU) of $1,25\text{-}(OH)_2D_3$, as well as calcium-independent *in vitro* suppression of hormonal secretion from bovine parathyroid glands with media $1,25\text{-}(OH)_2D_3$ concentrations of 1.0 nM. The isolation of specific cytoplasmic and nuclear binding components for $1,25\text{-}(OH)_2D_3$ from chick parathyroid glands is also consistent with the hypothesis that the dihydroxyvitamin D_3 metabolite regulates parathyroid hormone synthesis and release (Brumbaugh *et al.*, 1975).

Although $1,25\text{-}(OH)_2D_3$ is presently considered an essential regulator of skeletal and mineral metabolism, the physiological or functional significance of the other $25\text{-}OHD_3$ hydroxylated derivative, $24,25\text{-}(OH)_2D_3$, is still uncertain. It had been previously established that 24-hydroxylated forms of the vitamin D_3 molecule are inactive until they are hydroxylated to $1,24,25\text{-}(OH)_3D_3$ (Boyle *et al.*, 1973). Whereas $24,25\text{-}(OH)_2D_3$ appears to function as a disposal pathway for $25\text{-}OHD_3$ in the chick (Holick *et al.*, 1976a), its function in the rat is still unclear, since in this species, the "24R" stereoisomer of $24,25\text{-}(OH)_2D_3$ possesses biological activity similar to its precursor, $25\text{-}OHD_3$ (Tanaka *et al.*, 1975a), and is cleared from plasma at a rate slower than that observed in the chick (Boyle *et al.*, 1973). Naturally occurring $24,25\text{-}(OH)_2D_3$ in the rat appears to be the "R" isomer (Tanaka *et al.*, 1975a). Stereo-selectivity for the biological action of $24,25\text{-}(OH)_2D_3$ was also reported in 1975 (Tanaka *et al.*, 1975a). Of the two isomeric forms, $24R,25\text{-}(OH)_2D_3$, the "R" configuration, is the most biologically potent. The primary site of discrimination is apparently not the end-organ response, but rather the 1-hydroxylation, since the "24S" and "24R" configurations of $1,24,25\text{-}(OH)_3D_3$ possess similar biological activity (DeLuca, 1976). The importance of the stereochemical position of the 24-hydroxyl group in the rat was described by Tanaka *et al.* (1975b) in a report comparing the biological activities of chemically synthesized 24(S)-OHD$_3$ and 24(R)-OHD$_3$. Both stereoisomers of 24-OHD$_3$ were equally effective in stimulating intestinal calcium transport; unlike 24R-OHD$_3$, the 24S isomer was ineffective in raising the serum phosphorus of rachitic rats, calcifying bone, or mobilizing calcium from bone. *In vitro* studies with the "R" and "S" isomers of 24-OHD$_3$ and 24,25-(OH)$_2$D$_3$ by Stern *et al.* (1975) were confirmatory in this regard. Analyzing the rate of calcium-45 release from fetal rat long bones, the investigators showed that 24R,25-(OH)$_2$D$_3$ and 24R-OHD$_3$ were more active than their respective "S" isomers. The bone-resorbing activities of 24R-OHD$_3$ and 25-OHD$_3$ were identical; 24R,25-(OH)$_2$D$_3$ was less potent than either one. Although the selectivity for the 24R isomer of 24-OHD$_3$ suggests that 24-hydroxylated forms of vitamin D$_3$ are biologically active in the rat, their relationship to the reported effects of biologically synthesized 24,25-(OH)$_2$D$_3$ is still virtually unknown. Lam *et al.* (1975) reported on the structural synthesis and biological activity of another dihydroxyvitamin D$_3$ metabolite, 25,26-(OH)$_2$D$_3$. In rats maintained on vitamin D–deficient, low-calcium diets, 0.25-μg doses of 25,26-(OH)$_2$D$_3$ stimulated intestinal calcium transport, but had no effect on bone calcium immobilization (Lam *et al.*, 1975). Further modification of the 25,26-(OH)$_2$D$_3$ appeared essential for biological activity, since the intestinal effect was abolished by nephrectomy. Continued interest in the metabolic fate of vitamin D$_2$ metabolites led to the isolation and identification of 1,25-(OH)$_2$D$_2$ in the chick (Tanaka *et al.*, 1975b) and the discovery of a new metabolic pathway in which carbons 26 and 27 of 1,25-(OH)$_2$D$_3$ are removed from the molecule and lost as carbon dioxide (DeLuca, 1976). The biological activity of this new vitamin D$_3$ metabolite is presently unknown.

Aforementioned studies with isomeric forms of 24-OHD$_3$ and 25,26-(OH)$_2$D$_3$ reveal that structural modifications in the vitamin D$_3$ molecule do lead to varied differences in biological activity. Utilizing relatively specific cytoplasmic and nuclear chromatin receptors obtained from chick intestinal tissue, Norman *et al.* (1975b) described the results of a series of elegant experiments comparing the relative biological activities of 1α,25-(OH)$_2$D$_3$ with those of the structurally related analogues 1α-OHD$_3$, 3D-1α-OH-D$_3$, 5,6-*trans*-D$_3$, and dihydrotachysterol (DHT$_3$). The structure–function relationships of the analogues of 1α,25-(OH)$_2$D$_3$ were presented, with emphasis on the A-ring, which consists of a pair of rapidly equilibrating chain conformers. A minimal planar blueprint necessary for biological activity of vitamin D$_3$ metabolites or structurally similar analogues was defined as a molecule that incorporates a 1α-OH (or pseudo 1α-OH) and a side chain, R, on a secosteroid backbone without a 3β-OH or C-19 carbon atom. A "secosteroid" is one in which one of the rings has undergone fission—the "B" ring in the case of vitamin D$_3$. A "pseudo 1α-OH" refers to compounds with carbon frameworks established by a 180° rotation about the 5,6 bond of vitamin D_3; as such, the 3β-OH group is in the same geometric position as the 1α-OH of the natural $1\alpha,25$-$(OH)_2D_3$ metabolite. Pseudo-1-hydroxyl-containing analogues include isotachysterol$_3$, 5,6-*trans*-D_4, DHT$_3$, and 25-OHDHT$_3$. According to the authors, either $1\alpha,25$-$(OH)_2D_3$ or any of its pseudo-1-hydroxyl structurally related synthetic analogues exist as a pair of dynamically interconverting chair-conformers, in that the pseudo-1-hydroxyl assumes either an equitorial or an axial orientation. The relative proportions of these conformers apparently depend on either or both the nature and stereochemistry of the C-10–C-19 bond. It is proposed in this excellent report that the 1-hydroxyl of 1α-25-$(OH)_2D_3$, or its geometric equivalent in analogues, must occupy the equitorial orientation for maximal biological activity in the intestine. Subsequent biological studies by Norman *et al.* (1975a), using chemically synthesized 3-dcoxy-1α-hydroxy-vitamin D_3, stress the importance of the conformations of the A-ring of vitamin D steroids with regard to biological activity (Okamura *et al.*, 1975). In these studies, the 3-deoxy-1α-hydroxyvitamin D analogues, with most of the 1α-hydroxyls in the equitorial conformer, were more effective in stimulating intestinal calcium transport than 1α-OHD$_3$ or 1α-25-$(OH)_2D_3$, compounds with a 1:1 equilibrium mixture of axial and equitorial orientations. Studies with the newly synthesized 1α-hydroxy-3-epivitamin D_3 should also shed light on these fascinating structure–function studies, since, in this compound, the A-ring exists predominantly in the conformation with the hydroxyl groups diaxial (Okamura and Pirio, 1975).

Molecular structural constraints that are essential for the maximal biological activity of vitamin D and synthetic analogues are apparently not limited to ring A of the molecule. Earlier studies revealed that reduction of the side chain of vitamin D_2 decreases its biological effectiveness by 25% (McDonald, 1936), and analogues with side chains of stigmasterol and sitosterol retained only 5–10% of the antirachitic activity of the intact vitamin D_3 molecule (Grab, 1936). Holick *et al.* (1975a) reported on experiments with synthetic forms of 25-OHD$_3$ that lacked either carbon 26, carbons 26 and 27, or the entire side chain. Both 27-nor-25-OHD$_3$ and 26,26-bisnor-25-OHD$_3$ analogues proved biologically active in stimulating calcium transport and bone calcium mobilization in intact but not anephric rats (Holick *et al.*, 1975a). Since these observations were consistent with the hypothesis that 1-hydroxylation was also an essential prerequisite for biological activity, the investigators synthesized the corresponding 5,6-*trans* isomers, the latter containing the 3β-hydroxyl in the pseudo-1α-hydroxy position (see above). Experimental confirmation of their initial hypothesis was obtained in that the 5,6-*trans* isomers of the 27-nor- and 26,27-bisnor-25-OHD$_3$ compounds exhibited biological activity in anephric animals. In contrast to these observations, the 22–27-hexanor-25-OHD$_3$ and its corresponding 5,6-*trans* isomer proved incapable of stimulating either bone calcium mobilization or intestinal calcium transport. The results of these studies, combined with others in which the biological effects of pregcalciferol and 5,6-*trans*-pregcalciferol were tested, led these authors to conclude that: (1) the 3β-hydroxyl is not required for biological activity of the vitamin D molecule, once there is a 1α-hydroxyl 'or a hydroxyl in a pseudo-1α position; (2) all 27 carbons in the vitamin D structure are not essential for the vitamin's activity; (3) 5,6-*cis*-triene and the C-19 methylene are not absolute requirements for biological activity; (4) part of the side chain is essential for biological activity, since replacement of the side chain with a hydroxyl eliminates the effects on intestine and bone; and (5) appropriate side-chain structure is more essential for the mobilization of bone calcium than for stimulation of intestinal calcium transport. These conclusions are still tentative, since, as the authors note, the relatively poor biological activity of the 27-nor- and 26,27-bisnor-25-OHD$_3$ compounds, compared with that of the parent 25-OHD$_3$, could also result either from reported incomplete binding of the side-chain analogues to circulating 25-OHD$_3$-binding proteins (Hadded and Stamp, 1974) or from more rapid *in vivo* degradation or from both.

Additional studies regarding the synthesis and biological activity of 1,24,25-(OH)$_3$D$_3$ were also reported in 1975. It had been previously demonstrated in 1973 that 24,25-(OH)$_2$D$_3$ could be further metabolized to a more polar metabolite in the rat (Boyle *et al.*, 1973; Holick *et al.*, 1973a). Subsequently, Kleiner-Bossaller and DeLuca (1974) reported that rats fed either normal (0.6%) or high (3%) calcium diets produced 1,24,25-(OH)$_3$D$_3$ *in vivo* in response to physiological doses of 25-OHD$_3$. Friendlander and Norman (1975), demonstrating that the chick kidney can also convert 24,25-(OH)$_2$D$_3$ to 1,24,25-(OH)$_3$D$_3$, were unable to isolate this compound *in vivo* from the intestine, liver, kidney, or blood of chickens raised on high (3%) or low (0.05%) calcium diets. In the past, species differences in the metabolism and biological activity of vitamin D metabolites have resulted in a confusing array of information regarding enzyme activation and intestinal response. This being the case, this new controversial information regarding dietary control of 1,24,25-(OH)$_2$D$_3$ production in the chick is no longer unique. The chick, unlike the rat, also responds poorly to vitamin D$_2$ and 25-OHD$_2$ (Drescher *et al.*, 1969), and metabolizes vitamin D$_2$ rapidly (Imrie *et al.*, 1967). In 1975, it was established by Jones *et al.* (1975) that vitamin D$_2$ can be converted to 1,25-(OH)$_2$D$_2$ by the chick. It was subsequently demonstrated that vitamin D$_2$ hydroxylation reactions in the chick are identical with those observed with the vitamin D$_3$ series (Jones *et al.*, 1976), thus disproving the hypothesis that the discriminations against vitamin D$_2$ seen in chicks result from an acquired defect in the enzymatic hydroxylation mechanisms for the vitamin D_2 molecule.

Following the demonstration of 25 hydroxylation of vitamin D by perfused rat livers and in rat liver homogenates (Horsting and DeLuca, 1969) and its inhibition by vitamin D_3 feeding (Bhattacharyya and DeLuca, 1973), relatively little information accumulated regarding the hepatic 25-hydroxylase system. The availability of a synthetic analogue of vitamin D_3, 1α-hydroxylated D_3 (1α-OHD$_3$) (Holick et al., 1973b), with in vivo biological effectiveness almost identical to the naturally occurring 1,25-$(OH)_2D_3$ (Holick et al., 1973b; Holick et al., 1975c) led to renewed interest in the role of the liver 25-hydroxylation mechanism. Studies by Holick et al. (1973b) confirmed earlier observations of Zerwerk et al. (1974), and demonstrated that 1α-OHD$_3$ must be hydroxylated to 1α-25-$(OH)_2D_3$ in vivo before biological activity is detectable (Holick et al., 1976b; Holick et al., 1975b). Isolated rat liver perfusion studies of Fukushima et al. (1975) were consistent with these results, linear increments of 1α-25-$(OH)_2D_3$ being noted during 120 min of hepatic perfusion with 1α-OHD$_3$. Arnaud et al. (1975) also reported additional information regarding the fate of 25-OHD$_3$. As previously demonstrated for vitamin D_3 by Avioli et al. (1967), a significant portion of circulating 25-OHD$_3$ is also secreted into the intestinal lumen, with over 85% of the endogenously secreted 25-OHD$_3$ reabsorbed (Arnaud et al., 1975). These investigators suggested that gastrointestinal disease may interfere with the normal enterohepatic recycling of 25-OHD$_3$, and thereby contribute to associated alterations in bone and mineral metabolism.

The antirachitic activity of plasma is due almost entirely to protein-bound forms of vitamin D_3 and 25-OHD$_3$. Although an α-globulin serves as the transport protein for vitamin D_3 and 25-OHD$_3$ in most mammals, β-globulins, albumin, and lipoproteins have also been shown to bind these sterols in a variety of vertebrates. Thus, the chick has two transport proteins that exhibit β-globulin mobility on gel electrophoresis (Edelstein et al., 1972), with weaker binding affinities for vitamin D_2 and 25-OHD$_2$ (Belsey et al., 1974). Two types of New World monkeys—Crebus albifrons and C. capucinus—use albumin as the circulating transport protein, whereas other New World monkeys—Aotus trivirgatus and Callithrix jaccus—as well as Old World primates—Erythocebus patas, Macaca mulatta, and Papio anubis—use an α-globulin fraction (Hay and Watson, 1975). Of note were the observations that the albumin transport protein of New World monkeys (Cebus albifrons) displayed a lower affinity for 25-OHD$_3$ than the α-globulin protein of Old World monkeys (Erythrocebus patas) (Hay, 1975), although the binding affinities of each primate species for 25-OHD$_3$ and 25-OHD$_2$ were similar (Hay and Watson, 1975). These latter findings are of significant interest, since New World primates, like chicks, utilize vitamin D_2 less efficiently than vitamin D_3 (Hunt *et al.*, 1967). Unlike the chick, however, the species resistance to vitamin D_2 observed in New World monkeys cannot be explained on weaker binding affinities of 25-OHD$_2$ to the transport protein (Belsey *et al.*, 1974).

The relationship between the protein-bound forms of vitamin D_3 and 25-OHD$_3$ and their tissue-specific receptors is still conjectural. In 1973, Haddad *et al.* (1973) isolated a soluble macromolecule from the intestine of rachitic rats with a molecular weight of 100,000 daltons. The binding affinity of the intestinal cytosol receptor for 25-OHD$_3$ (K_a) was 2.10 $\times$ 10^{-9} M. Subsequently, in 1975, these same authors reported the results of studies designed to evaluate 25-OHD$_3$ binding in extraintestinal tissues. They reported a mean K_a for serum of 1×10^{-9} M and binding affinities of 4×10^{-9} M for kidney and muscle cytosol (Haddad and Birge, 1975). Their findings that muscle and kidney contain binding sites of higher affinity than serum for 25-OHD$_3$ *in vitro* are consistent with prevailing hypotheses that muscle serves as a reservoir for 25-OHD$_3$ and is metabolically responsive to this metabolite (Birge and Haddad, 1975). They are also consistent with the fact that the kidney is an organ essential for the biological activation of 25-OHD$_3$ to 1,25-(OH)$_2$D$_3$, and for the hyperphosphatemic response to 25-OHD$_3$ (Puschett *et al.*, 1975; Popovtzer and Robinette, 1975).

Another provocative report regarding circulating vitamin D_3 and 25-OHD$_3$ binding properties that appeared in 1975 was that of Daiger *et al.* (1975). These authors reported that group-specific component (Gc) proteins are capable of binding large quantities of vitamin D_3 and 25-OHD$_3$ under physiologically normal conditions. Moreover, they also isolated plasma vitamin D-binding proteins immunologically similar to human Gc from the mouse, rat, cow, horse, rhesus monkey, and chimpanzee. Their proposal that the "vitamin D-binding α-globulin and Gc represent the same molecular protein species" is intriguing, since, although it was detected immunologically some 15 years ago (Hirschfeld, 1962), no physiological role had yet been assigned to the circulating Gc protein component.

Accumulated evidence in the past supported the view that 1,25-(OH)$_2$D$_3$ is primarily responsible for the stimulated intestinal absorption of calcium when physiological doses of vitamin D_3 are fed to rachitic animals. However, the exact sequence of subcellular molecular events that characterize the response to 1,25-(OH)$_2$D$_3$ and the mechanism whereby 1,25-(OH)$_2$D$_3$ initiates calcium absorption are still conjectural. The results of experiments with inhibitors of DNA-directed RNA synthesis are consistent with the interpretation that 1,25-(OH)$_2$D$_3$ stimulates the synthesis of RNA and an intestinal calcium-binding protein (CaBP) (Tsai and Norman, 1973). Since this mechanism of action of 1,25-(OH)$_2$D$_3$ resembles the action of other steroid hormones that control the expression of genetic information in target tissues, a number of investigators have attempted to isolate 1,25-(OH)$_2$D$_3$ cytosol and nuclear binding proteins from intestinal mucosal cells in rats and chicks. Haussler *et al.* (1968) concluded that in the chick, 1,25-(OH)$_2$D$_3$ was bound predominantly to the nuclear chromatin of intestinal cells, an observation that was strengthened by the reports of Tsai *et al.* (1973). These latter investigators subsequently isolated from chick intestine a cytoplasmic receptor highly specific for 1,25-(OH)$_2$D$_3$ with an association constant of 1×10^{-7} M, and noted that 1,25-(OH)$_2$D$_3$ binding to this cytoplasmic receptor was a prerequisite for its subsequent binding to the intestinal nuclei (Tsai and Norman, 1973). DeLuca, having previously championed the hypothesis that 1,25-(OH)$_2$D$_3$ was associated primarily with the outer nuclear membranes, reported that the chromatin preparation of Haussler *et al.* (1968) was, in fact, contaminated with nuclear membranes, and that pure homogeneous intestinal chromatin preparations from chicks and rats did not bind an appreciable amount of 1,25-(OH)$_2$D$_3$ (Chen *et al.*, 1970). In 1973, Chen and DeLuca (1973) reported that following a 62.5-pmole dose of ^{3}H-labeled 1,25-(OH)$_2$D$_3$ to rachitic rats, 30–45% of the ^{3}H-1,25-(OH)$_2$D$_3$ was bound to pure intestinal nuclear chromatin, while more than 50% was bound to a low-density lipoprotein extranuclear complex. Both the chromatin and the lipoprotein complex demonstrated highly specific binding activity for 1,25-(OH)$_2$D$_3$, in that the binding of 1,25-(OH)$_2$D$_3$ was some 30–40 times greater than that of 25-OHD$_3$. A series of rather elegant experiments were performed by Lawson and Wilson (1974) in an attempt to resolve the discrepancies regarding the intracellular localization of 1,25-(OH)$_2$D$_3$ in the chick. They also reported that intestinal chromatin prepared by the procedure of Haussler *et al.* (1968) was heavily contaminated with brush border membranes, and resorted to the more definite techniques of Dingman and Sporn (1964) and Marushige and Bonner (1966). At high doses of vitamin D$_3$ (up to 2.5 μg), both vitamin D$_3$ and 25-OHD$_3$ were isolated from intestinal nuclei, the major portion of the sterols associated with nuclear membranes. Although 1,25-(OH)$_2$D$_3$ was demonstrated with cell nuclei irrespective of the dose of vitamin D$_3$ administered to the rachitic chicks, significant amounts could not be found with chromatin isolated free of nuclear membranes. The studies on the nature of 1,25-(OH)$_2$D$_3$ nuclear binding revealed two nuclear proteins capable of binding 1,25-(OH)$_2$D$_3$, one of which was an acidic protein with saturable binding sites, an association constant of 2×10^{-9} M, and high specificity. The sedimentation coefficient of 3.5S observed for this protein was similar to that seen with the nuclear protein that binds 1,25-(OH)$_2$D$_3$ *in vivo* after vitamin D$_3$ feeding. These investigators also isolated a cytoplasmic receptor for 1,25-(OH)$_2$D$_3$ with an association constant of 1×10^{-9} M and a sedimentation coefficient of 3.0S. They concluded that in the chick, the intestinal nuclear $1,25\text{-}(OH)_2D_3$ receptor complex existed as an equilibrium mixture of $DNA\text{-}1,25\text{-}(OH)_2D_3\text{-}receptor$ and $1,25\text{-}(OH)_2D_3\text{-}receptor$. In 1975, Brumbaugh and Haussler (1975), using the chromatin preparation techniques previously published in 1968 and cited above, reported the isolation of specific cytosol and nuclear $1,25\text{-}(OH)_2D_3$ binders that had identical sedimentation coefficients of 3.7S and an association constant of 2.2×10^{-9} M. As noted previously in the rat by Haddad *et al.* (1973), Brumbaugh and Haussler (1975) also isolated a chick intestinal cytosol $25\text{-}OHD_3$ binder that differed from the cytosolic $1,25\text{-}(OH)_2D_3$ binder in that it sedimented at 5–6S and was observed in organs (kidney, liver) other than the intestine. As suggested in an earlier report (Brumbaugh and Haussler, 1974), these investigators concluded once again that in the chick, cytosol $1,25\text{-}(OH)_2D_3$ binding component(s) [not the cytosol $25\text{-}OHD_3$ binding component(s)] are essential for the nuclear migration of $1,25\text{-}(OH)_2D_3$. Later, Frolick and DeLuca (1975), detailing the procedures for solubilization and partial purification of the low-density lipoprotein $1,25\text{-}(OH)_2D_3$ binding complex isolated previously (Chen and DeLuca, 1973), reported that the binding complex had a molecular weight greater than 10,000 daltons.

Although considerable advances have been made during 1975 regarding enzymatic control of the metabolism of vitamin D_3 and the molecular response of target tissues to vitamin D_3 metabolites, contradictions and inconsistencies continue to cloud many important issues. Obviously, species differences and the use of varied *in vitro* preparations should be considered while interpreting the accumulated results. It seems more than obvious to this reviewer that the control mechanisms of a chick, which is normally hypercalcemic during the egg-laying cycle and has circulating inorganic phosphate levels of 3–4 mg/dl, may differ substantially from those governing the bioactivation of vitamin D_3 and the intestinal response to its metabolites in a nonegg-laying, nocturnal-feeding, hyperphosphatemic rodent. Is it in fact appropriate to extrapolate *in vitro* data obtained from isolated renal mitochondria or tubules and renal homogenates of chicks to rats, in which attempts to demonstrate $25\text{-}OHD_3\text{-}1\text{-}hydroxylase$ activity *in vitro* have been unsuccessful (Botham *et al.*, 1974)? Further, is there any reason to assume that data derived from *in vitro* experiments in rachitic chicks or rats apply to man? In humans, circulating $25\text{-}OHD_3$ levels approximate 20 ng/ml, and probably less than 5% of the circulating $25\text{-}OHD_3\text{-}binding$ protein is normally saturated (Haddad and Birge, 1975; Bayard *et al.*, 1972), whereas circulating $1,25\text{-}(OH)_2D_3$ levels in man average 4 ng/dl (Brumbaugh *et al.*, 1974). With a 500-fold increment in circulating $25\text{-}OHD_3$, is it not possible that the human $25\text{-}OHD_3$ intestinal cytosol receptor is as important as (or more important than!) the 1,25-$(OH)_2D_3$-binding complex in conditioning the intestinal absorption of calcium? We know now that 25-OHD_3 can directly stimulate calcium uptake and the synthesis of an intestinal calcium-binding protein; at certain concentrations, 25-OHD_3 is as effective as 1,25-$(OH)_2D_3$ in this regard (Corradino, 1973). Surely, additional studies need to be performed before a reasonably coherent and universally accepted concept of vitamin D_3 metabolism is established. We can only hope and await the reports of 1976 for review and consolation.

References

Angel, J., Alfred, B., Leichter, J., Lee, M., and Marchant, L., 1975, Effect of oral administration of large quantities of ascorbic acid on blood levels and urinary excretion of ascorbic acid in healthy men, *Int. J. Vitam. Nutr. Res.* **45**:237.

Anderson, T. W., Reid, D. B. W., and Beaton, G. H., 1972, Vitamin C and the common cold: A double-blind trial, *Can. Med. Assoc. J.* **107**:503.

Anderson, T. W., Beaton, G. H., Corey, P. N., and Spero, L., 1975, Winter illness and vitamin C: The effect of relatively low doses, *Can. Med. Assoc. J.* **112**:823.

Arnaud, S. B., Goldsmith, R. S., Lambert, P. W., and Go, V. L. W., 1975, 25-Hydroxyvitamin D_3: Evidence of an enterohepatic circulation in man, *Proc. Soc. Exp. Biol. Med.* **149**:570.

Avioli, L. V., and Haddad, J. G., 1973, Vitamin D: Current concepts, *Metabolism* **22**:507.

Avioli, L. V., Lee, S. W., McDonald, J. E., Lund, J., and DeLuca, H. F., 1967, Metabolism of vitamin D_3-^{3}H in human subjects: Distribution in blood, bile, feces and urine, *J. Clin. Invest.* **46**:983.

Bayard, F., Bec, P., and Louvet, J. P., 1972, Measurement of plasma 25 hydroxycholecalciferol in man, *Eur. J. Clin. Invest.* **2**:195.

Belsey, R. E., DeLuca, H. F., and Potts, J. T., Jr., 1974, Selective binding properties of vitamin D transport protein in chick plasma *in vitro*, *Nature* **247**:208.

Bhattacharyya, M. H., and DeLuca, H. F., 1973, The regulation of rat liver calciferol-25-hydroxylase, *J. Biol. Chem.* **248**:2969.

Bikle, D. D., and Rasmussen, H., 1975, The ionic control of 1,25-dihydroxyvitamin D_3 production in isolated chick renal tubules, *J. Clin. Invest.* **55**:292.

Bikle, D. D., Murphy, E. W., and Rasmussen, H., 1975, The ionic control of 1,25-dihydroxyvitamin D_3 synthesis in isolated chick renal mitochondria: The role of calcium as influenced by inorganic phosphate and hydrogen ion, *J. Clin. Invest.* **55**:299.

Birch, G. G., and Parker, K., 1974, *Vitamin C: Recent Aspects of Its Physiological and Technological Importance*, John Wiley & Sons, New York.

Birge, S. H., and Haddad, J. G., 1975, 25-Hydroxycholecalciferol stimulation of muscle metabolism, *J. Clin. Invest.* **56**:1100.

Botham, K. M., Tanaka, Y., and DeLuca, H. F., 1974, 25-Hydroxyvitamin D_3-1-hydroxylase. Inhibition *in vitro* by rat and pig tissues, *Biochemistry* **13**:4961.

Boyle, I. T., Omdahl, J. L., Gray, R. W., and DeLuca, H. F., 1973, The biological activity and metabolism of 24,25-dihydroxyvitamin D₃, *J. Biol. Chem.* **248:**4174.

Briggs, M. H., 1973, Side-effects of vitamin C, *Lancet* **2:**1439.

Briggs, M. H., 1976, Vitamin-C–induced hyperoxaluria, *Lancet* **1:**154.

Briggs, M. H., Garcia-Webb, P., and Davies, P., 1973, Urinary oxalate and vitamin-C supplements, *Lancet* **2:**201.

Bronte-Stewart, B., Roberts, B. and Wells, V. M., 1963, Serum cholesterol in vitamin C deficiency in man, *Br. J. Nutr.* **17:**61.

Brumbaugh, P. F., and Haussler, M. R., 1975, Nuclear and cytoplasmic binding components for vitamin D metabolites, *Life Sci.* **16:**353.

Brumbaugh, P. F., Haussler, D. H., Bursac, K. M., and Haussler, M. R., 1974, Filter assay for 1α,25-dihydroxyvitamin D₃. Utilization of the hormone's target tissue chromatin receptor, *Biochemistry* **13:**4091.

Brumbaugh, P. F., Hughes, M. R., and Haussler, M. R., 1975, Cytoplasmic and nuclear binding components for 1α,25-dihydroxyvitamin D₃ in chick parathyroid glands, *Proc. Nat. Acad. Sci. U.S.A.* **72:**4871.

Campbell, G. D., Jr., Steinberg, M. H., and Bower, J. D., 1975, Ascorbic acid–induced hemolysis in G-6-PD deficiency, *Ann. Intern. Med.* **82:**810.

Care, A. D., Bates, R. F. L., Swaminathan, R., Scanes, C. G., Peacock, M., Mawer, E. B., Taylor, C. M., DeLuca, H. F., Tomlinson, S., and O'Riordan, J. L. H., 1975, The control of parathyroid hormone and calcitonin secretion and their interaction with other endocrine systems, *in: Calcium-Regulating Hormones* (R. V. Talmage, M. Owen, and J. A. Parsons, eds.), pp. 100–110, Excerpta Medica, American Elsevier Publishing Co., New York.

Chalmers, T. C., 1975, Effects of ascorbic acid on the common cold, *Amer. J. Med.* **58:**532.

Chen, T. C., and DeLuca, H. F., 1973, Receptors of 1,25-dihydroxycholecalciferol in rat intestine, *J. Biol. Chem.* **248:**4890.

Chen, T. C., and Raisz, L. G., 1975, The effects of ascorbic acid deficiency on calcium and collagen metabolism in cultured fetal rat bones, *Calcif. Tissue Res.* **17:**113.

Chen, T. C., Weber, J. C., and DeLuca, H. F., 1970, On the subcellular location of vitamin D metabolites in intestine, *J. Biol. Chem.* **245:**3776.

Chertow, B. S., Baylink, D. J., Wergedal, J. E., Su, M. H. H., and Norman, A. W., 1975, Decrease in serum immunoreactive parathyroid hormone in rats and in parathyroid hormone secretion *in vitro* by 1,25-dihydroxycholecalciferol, *J. Clin. Invest.* **56:**668.

Clegg, K. M., and Macdonald, J. M., 1975, L-ascorbic acid and D-isoascorbic acid in a common cold survey, *Amer. J. Clin. Nutr.* **28:**973.

Corradino, R. A., 1973, Embryonic chick intestine in organ culture: Response to vitamin D₃ and its metabolites, *Science* **179:**402.

Cox, B. D., and Butterfield, W. J. H., 1975, Vitamin C supplements and diabetic cutaneous capillary fragility, *Br. Med. J.* **3:**205.

Cox, B. D., Whichelow, M. J., Butterfield, W. J. H., and Nicholas, P., 1974, Peripheral vitamin C metabolism in diabetics and non-diabetic: Effect of intra-arterial insulin, *Clin. Sci. Mol. Med.* **47:**63.

Crawford, G. P., Warlow, C. P., Bennett, B., Dawson, A. A., Douglas, A. S., Kernidge, D. F., Ogston, D., 1975, The effect of vitamin C supplements on serum cholesterol, coagulation, fibrinolysis and platelet adhesiveness, *Atherosclerosis* **21**:451.

Daiger, S. P., Schanfield, M. S., and Cavalli-Sforza, L. L., 1975, Group-specific component (Gc) proteins bind vitamin D and 25-hydroxyvitamin D, *Proc. Nat. Acad. Sci. U.S.A.* **72**:2076.

DeLuca, H. F., 1975, The kidney as an endocrine organ involved in the function of vitamin D, *Amer. J. Med.* **58**:39.

DeLuca, H. F., 1976, Recent advances in our understanding of the vitamin D endocrine system, *J. Lab. Clin. Med.* **87**:7.

Dingman, C. W., and Sporn, M. B., 1964, Studies on chromatin. I. Isolation and characterization of nuclear complexes of deoxyribonucleic acid, ribonucleic acid, and protein from embryonic and adult tissues of the chicken, *J. Biol. Chem.* **239**:3483.

Drescher, D., DeLuca, H. F., and Imrie, M. H., 1969, On the site of discrimination of chick against vitamin D_2, *Arch. Biochem. Biophys.* **130**:657.

Dykes, M. H. M., and Meier, P., 1975, Ascorbic acid and the common cold: Evaluation of its toxicity, *J. Amer. Med. Assoc.* **231**:1073.

Edelstein, S., Lawson, D. E. M., and Kodicek, E., 1972, Separation of binding proteins for cholecalciferol and 25-hydroxycholecalciferol from chick serum, *Biochim. Biophys. Acta* **270**:570.

Evans, G. W., 1973, Copper, homeostasis in the mammalian system, *Physiol. Rev.* **53**:535.

Evans, I. M. A., Colston, K. W., Galante, L., and MacIntyre, I., 1975, Feedback regulation of 25-hydroxycholecalciferol metabolism by vitamin D_3, *Clin. Sci. Mole. Med.* **48**:227.

Eyre, D. R., and Glimcher, M. J., 1973, Collagen cross-linking. Isolation of cross-linked peptides from collagen of chicken bone, *Biochem. J.* **135**:393.

Fraser, D. R., and Kodicek, E., 1970, Unique biosynthesis by kidney of a biologically active vitamin D metabolite, *Nature* **228**:764.

Friedlander, E. J., and Norman, A. W., 1975, Studies on the metabolism of calciferol XII, *Arch. Biochem. Biophys.* **170**:731.

Frolik, C. A., and DeLuca, H. F., 1975, Solubilization and partial purification of a rat intestinal 1,25-dihydroxyvitamin D_3 binding protein, *Steroids* **26**:683.

Fukushima, M., Suzuki, Y., Tohira, Y., Matsunaga, I., Ochi, K., Nagano, H., Nishii, Y., and Suda, T., 1975, Metabolism of 1α-hydroxyvitamin D_3 to 1α,25-dihydroxyvitamin D_3 in perfused rat liver, *Biochem. Biophys. Res. Commun.* **66**:632.

Garabedian, M., Holick, M. F., DeLuca, H. F., and Boyle, I. T., 1972, Control of 25-hydroxycholecalciferol metabolism by the parathyroid glands, *Proc. Nat. Acad. Sci. U.S.A.* **69**:1673.

Ginter, E., 1976, Vitamin C and plasma lipids, *N. Engl. J. Med.* **294**:559.

Grab, W., 1936, Die Auswertung der antirachitischen Wirksamkeit neuer Sterinderivate im Versuch an Ratten und Kuken, *Hoppe-Seyler's Z. Physiol. Chem.* **243**:63.

Haddad, J. G., and Birge, S. J., 1975, Widespread, specific binding of 25-hydroxy-cholecalciferol in rat tissues, *J. Biol. Chem.* **250:**299.

Haddad, J. G., and Stamp, T. C. B., 1974, Circulating 25-hydroxyvitamin D in man, *Amer. J. Med.* **57:**57.

Haddad, J. G., Hahn, T. J., and Birge, S. J., 1973, Vitamin D metabolites: Specific binding by rat intestinal cytosol, *Biochim. Biophys. Acta* **329:**93.

Harris, A. B., 1976, Vitamin C–induced hyperoxaluria, *Lancet* **1:**366.

Haussler, M. R., Myrtle, J. F., and Norman, A. W., 1968, The association of a metabolite of vitamin D_3 with intestinal mucosa chromatin *in vivo*, *J. Biol. Chem.* **243:**4055.

Hay, A. W. M., 1975, The transport of 25-hydroxycholecalciferol in a New World monkey, *Biochem. J.* **151:**193.

Hay, A. W. M., and Watson, G., 1975, Binding of 25-hydroxyvitamin D_2 to plasma protein in New World monkeys, *Nature* **256:**150.

Herbert, V., and Jacob, E., 1974, Destruction of vitamin B_{12} by ascorbic acid, *J. Amer. Med. Assoc.* **230:**241.

Hill, L. F., and Stanbury, S. W., 1975, Vitamin D and the kidney, *Nephron* **15:**369.

Hirschfeld, J., 1962, The Gc system. Immunoelectrophoretic studies of normal human sera with special reference to a new genetically determined system (Gc), *Prog. Allergy* **6:**1.

Holick, M. F., Schnoes, H. K., DeLuca, H. F., Gray, R. W., Boyle, I. T., and Suda, T., 1972, Isolation and identification of 24,25-dihydroxycholecalciferol: A metabolite of vitamin D_3 made in the kidney, *Biochemistry* **11:**4251.

Holick, M. F., Kleiner-Bossaller, A., Schnoes, H. K., Kasten, P. M., Boyle, I. T., and DeLuca, H. F., 1973a, 1,24,25-Trihydroxyvitamin D_3, a metabolite of vitamin D_3 effective on intestine, *J. Biol. Chem.* **248:**6691.

Holick, M. F., Semmler, E. J., Schnoes, H. K., and DeLuca, H. F., 1973b, 1α-hydroxy derivative of vitamin D_3: A highly potent analogue of 1α,25-dihydroxyvitamin D_3, *Science* **180:**190.

Holick, M. F., Garabedian, M., Schnoes, H. K., and DeLuca, H. F., 1975a, Relationship of 25-hydroxyvitamin D_3 side chain structure to biological activity, *J. Biol. Chem.* **250:**226.

Holick, M. F., Holick, S. A., Tavela, T., Gallagher, B., Schnoes, H. K., and DeLuca, H. F., 1975b, Synthesis of $(6-{}^3H)$-1α-hydroxyvitamin D_3 and its metabolism *in vivo* to $({}^3H)$-1α,25-dihydroxyvitamin D_3, *Science* **190:**576.

Holick, M. F., Kasten-Schraufrogel, P., Tavela, T., and DeLuca, H. F., 1975c, Biological activity of 1α-hydroxyvitamin D_3 in the rat, *Arch. Biochem. Biophys.* **166:**63.

Holick, M. F., Baxter, L. A., Schraufrogel, P. K., Tavela, T. E., and DeLuca, H. F., 1976a, Metabolism and biological activity of 24,25-dihydroxyvitamin D_3 in the chick, *J. Biol. Chem.* **251:**397.

Holick, M. F., Tavela, T. E., Holick, S. A., Schnoes, H. K., and DeLuca, H. E., 1976b, Synthesis of 1α-hydroxy$(6-{}^3H)$-vitamin D_3 and its metabolism to 1α,25-dihydroxy-$(6-{}^3H)$-vitamin D_3 in the rat, *J. Biol. Chem.* **251:**1020.

Horiuchi, N., Suda, T., Sasaki, S., Ezawa, I., Sano, Y., and Ogata, E., 1974, Direct involvement of vitamin D in the regulation of 25-hydroxycholecalciferol metabolism, *FEBS Lett.* **43:**353.

Horiuchi, N., Suda, T., Sasaki, S., Ogata, E., Ezawa, I., Sano, Y., and Shimazawa, E., 1975, The regulatory role of calcium in 25-hydroxycholecalciferol metabolism in chick kidney *in vitro*, *Arch. Biochem. Biophys.* **171:**540.

Horsting, M., and DeLuca, H. F., 1969, *In vitro* production of 25-hydroxycholecalciferol, *Biochem. Biophys. Res. Commum.* **36:**251.

Hughes, M. R., Brumbaugh, P. F., Haussler, M. R., Wergedal, J. E., and Baylink, D. J., 1975, Regulation of serum $1\alpha,25$-dihydroxyvitamin D_3 by calcium and phosphate in the rat, *Science* **190:**578.

Hunt, R. D., Garcia, F. G., Hegsted, D. M., and Kaplinsky, N., 1967, Vitamins D_2 and D_3 in New World primates: Influence on calcium absorption, *Science* **157:**943.

Imrie, M. H., Neville, P., Snellgrove, A. W., and DeLuca, H. F., 1967, Metabolism of vitamin D_2 and vitamin D_3 in the rachitic chick, *Arch. Biochem. Biophys.* **120:**525.

Jeffrey, J. J., and Martin, G. R., 1966, The role of ascorbic acid in the biosynthesis of collagen. I. Ascorbic acid requirement by embryonic chick tibia in tissue culture, *Biochim. Biophys. Acta* **121:**269.

Jimenez, S., Harsch, M., and Rosenbloom, J., 1973, Hydroxyproline stabilizes the triple helix of chick tendon collagen, *Biochem. Biophys. Res. Commun.* **52:**106.

Jones, G., Schnoes, H. K., and DeLuca, H. F., 1975, Isolation and identification of 1,25-dihydroxyvitamin D_2, *Biochemistry* **14:**1250.

Jones, G., Schnoes, H. K., and DeLuca, H. F., 1976, An *in vitro* study of vitamin D_2 hydroxylases in the chick, *J. Biol. Chem.* **251:**24.

Kerxhalli, J. S., Vogel, W., Broverman, D. M., and Klaiber, E. L., Effect of ascorbic acid on the human electroencephalogram, *J. Nutr.* **105:**1356.

Kleiner-Bossaller, A., and DeLuca, H. F., 1974, Formation of 1,24,25-trihydroxyvitamin D_3 from 1,25-dihydroxyvitamin D_3, *Biochim. Biophys. Acta* **338:**489.

Klevay, L. M., 1975, The ratio of zinc to copper of diets in the United States, *Nutr. Rep. Int.* **11:**237.

Klevay, L. M., 1976, Hypercholesterolemia due to ascorbic acid, *Proc. Soc. Exp. Biol. Med.* **151:**579.

Knutson, J. C., and DeLuca, H. F., 1974, 25-Hydroxyvitamin D_3-24-hydroxylase: Subcellular location and properties, *Biochemistry* **13:**1543.

Kodicek, E., Lawson, D. E. M., and Wilson, P. W., 1970, Biological activity of a polar metabolite of vitamin D_3, *Nature* **228:**763.

Krane, S. M., Pinnell, S. R., and Erbe, R. W., 1972, Lysyl-protocollagen hydroxylase deficiency in fibroblasts from siblings with hydroxylysine-deficient collagen, *Proc. Nat. Acad. Sci. U.S.A.* **69:**2899.

Lam, H. Y., Schnoes, H. K., and DeLuca, H. F., 1975, Synthesis and biological activity of $25\zeta,26$-dihydroxycholecalciferol, *Steroids* **25:**247.

Lawson, D. E. M., and Wilson, P. W., 1974, Intranuclear localization and receptor proteins for 1,25-dihydroxycholecalciferol in chick intestine, *Biochem. J.* **144:**573.

Margolis, R. L., and Lukens, L. N., 1971, The role of hydroxylation in the secretion of collagen by mouse fibroblasts in culture, *Arch. Biochem. Biophys.* **147:**612.

Marushige, K., and Bonner, J., 1966, Template properties of liver chromatin, *J. Mol. Biol.* **15**:160.

Mawer, E. B., Backhouse, J., Hill, L. F., Lumb, G. A., De Silva, P., Taylor, C. M., and Stanbury, S. W., 1975, Vitamin D metabolism and parathyroid function in man, *Clin. Sci. Mole. Med.* **48**:349.

McCollum, E. V., Simmonds, N., and Becker, J. E., 1922, Studies on experimental rickets. XXI. An experimental demonstration of the existence of a vitamin which promotes calcium deposition, *J. Biol. Chem.* **53**:293.

McDonald, F. G., 1936, The multiple nature of vitamin D. III. Irradiation of 22-dihydroergosterol, *J. Biol. Chem.* **114**:lxv.

Miller, R. L., 1975, The effect of ascorbic acid on lysyl and prolyl hydroxylase activity of cultured fibroblasts, *Arch. Biochem. Biophys.* **170**:341.

Norman, A. W., Mitra, M. N., Okamura, W. H., and Wing, R. M., 1975a, Vitamin D: 3-Deoxy-1α-hydroxyvitamin D_3, biologically active analog of 1α,25-dihydroxyvitamin D_3, *Science* **188**:1013.

Norman, A. W., Procsal, D. A., Okamura, W. H., and Wing, R. M., 1975b, Structure–function studies of the interaction of the hormonally active form of vitamin D_3, 1α-25-dihydroxyvitamin D_3, with the intestine, *J. Steroid Biochem.* **6**:461.

Okamura, W. H., and Pirio, M. R., 1975, Studies on vitamin D (calciferol) and its analogs. IX. 1α-hydroxy-3-epivitamin D_3: Its synthesis and conformational analysis, *Tetrahedron Lett.* **49**:4317.

Okamura, W. H., Mitra, M. N., Procsal, D. A., and Norman, A. W., 1975, Studies on vitamin D and its analogs. VIII. 3-deoxy-1α,25-dihydroxyvitamin D_3, a potent new analog of 1α,25-$(OH)_2$-D_3, *Biochem. Biophys. Res. Commun.* **65**:24.

Pauling, L. 1970, *Vitamin C and the Common Cold*, W. H. Freeman and Co., San Francisco.

Pauling, L., Are recommended allowances for vitamin C adequate?, *Proc. Nat. Acad. Sci. U.S.A.* **71**:4442.

Popovtzer, M. M., and Robinette, M. J., 1975, Effect of 25-(OH)-vitamin D_3 on urinary excretion of cyclic adenosine monophosphate, *Amer. J. Physiol.* **229**:907.

Puschett, J. B., Beck, W. S., Jr., and Jelonek, A., 1975, Parathyroid hormone and 25-hydroxy vitamin D_3: Synergistic and antagonistic effects on renal phosphate transport, *Science* **190**:473.

Ramachandran, G. N., Bansal, M., and Bhatnagar, R. S., 1973, A hypothesis on the role of hydroxyproline in stabilizing collagen structure, *Biochim. Biophys. Acta* **322**:166.

Stassen, F. L. H., Cardinale, G. J., and Udenfriend, S., 1973, Activation of prolyl hydroxylase in L-929 fibroblasts by ascorbic acid, *Proc. Nat. Acad. Sci. U.S.A.* **70**:1090.

Stein, H. B., Hasan, A., and Fox, I. H., 1976, Ascorbic acid–induced uricosuria, *Ann. Intern. Med.* **84**:385.

Stern, P. H., DeLuca, H. F., and Ikekawa, N., 1975, Bone resorbing activities of 24-hydroxy stereoisomers of 24-hydroxyvitamin D_3 and 24,25-dihydroxyvitamin D_3, *Biochem. Biophys. Res. Commun.* **67**:965.

Tanaka, Y., and DeLuca, H. F., 1973, The control of 25-hydroxyvitamin D metabolism by inorganic phosphorus, *Arch. Biochem. Biophys.* **154**:566.

Tanaka, Y., DeLuca, H. F., Ikekawa, N., Morisaki, M., and Koizumi, N., 1975a, Determination of stereochemical configuration of the 24-hydroxyl group of 24, 25-dihydroxyvitamin D_3 and its biological importance, *Arch. Biochem. Biophys.* **170**:620.

Tanaka, Y., Frank, H., DeLuca, H. F., Koizumi, N., and Ikekawa, N., 1975b, Importance of the stereochemical position of the 24-hydroxyl to biological activity of 24-hydroxyvitamin D_3, *Biochemistry* **14**:3293.

Tanaka, Y., Lorenc, R. S., and DeLuca, H. F., 1975c, The role of 1,25-dihydroxyvitamin D_3 and parathyroid hormone in the regulation of chick renal 25-hydroxyvitamin D_3-24-hydroxylase, *Arch. Biochem. Biophys.* **171**:521.

Tsai, H. C., and Norman, A. W., 1973, Studies on calciferol metabolism. VIII. Evidence for a cytoplasmic receptor for 1,25-dihydroxy vitamin D_3 in the intestinal mucosa, *J. Biol. Chem.* **248**:5967.

Waugh, W. A., and King, C. G., 1932, Isolation and identification of vitamin C, *J. Biol. Chem.* **97**:325.

Zerwekh, J. E., Brumbaugh, P. F., Haussler, D. H., Cork, D. J., and Haussler, M. R., 1974, 1α-Hydroxyvitamin D_3. An analogue of vitamin D which apparently acts by metabolism to 1α,25-dihydroxyvitamin D_3, *Biochemistry* **13**:4097.

10

Nutrition, Growth, and Development

Myron Winick

10.1. Introduction

This chapter will attempt to review briefly those areas in nutrition, growth, and development in which major advances have been made during the last few years. Of necessity, the areas covered are highly selective and the selection both arbitrary and subjective. No attempt is being made to cover the entire literature in any of the areas. Rather, a number of studies related to an area will be discussed and, it is hoped, placed in context of the major advances that have occurred in that area and the direction that future studies are likely to take. Where there are still major gaps, this will be noted and approaches designed to fill these gaps commented on.

The chapter is divided into two main parts, one covering normal

MYRON WINICK • Institute of Human Nutrition, College of Physicians and Surgeons of Columbia University, New York, New York 10032.

nutrition, the other abnormal nutrition. The nature of the material is such that overlap will occur. When such material is presented, it will be covered wherever it seems to fit best.

10.2. Normal Nutrition

10.2.1. Nutrition and Cellular Growth

During the past few years, a number of concepts have become firmly established. Normal growth in any nonregenerating organ goes through three phases: (1) an early phase pf pure hyperplasia (characterized by a rapid increase in total organ DNA content, with the protein DNA ratio remaining constant); (2) a phase of combined hyperplasia and hypertrophy (characterized by a slowing in the rate of DNA synthesis and a concomitant rise in the protein DNA ratio); and (3) a phase of pure hypertrophy or cell enlargement (characterized by a cessation of DNA synthesis and continued accretion of protein, resulting in marked increases in the protein DNA ratio). These phases merge into each other, but their time of occurrence varies from organ to organ and from species to species. In the rat, for example, DNA synthesis ceases in brain by 21 days after birth, whereas in the heart it continues to 65 days. In the human, while the rate of DNA synthesis slows shortly after birth, the most recent data available suggest that cells continue to divide until 18 months to 2 years of age. In addition, it has been shown that two peaks occur in the rate of cell division in human brain, one at about 26 weeks of gestation, and a second at around birth. These peaks have been interpreted as neuronal and glial proliferation, respectively. In both rat and human brain, cells divide most rapidly in cerebellum during early postnatal growth. In the rat, cerebellar cell division ceases by 17 days; in the human, it continues to 18 months.

Restriction of total caloric intake during the period of hyperplastic growth will result in a curtailment in the rate of cell division, and if the restriction is for a sufficient period of time, the final number of cells attained is reduced. The most marked effects occur in those regions that are proliferating at the greatest rate; hence, cerebellum is particularly vulnerable. Any cell type undergoing division will be affected. Thus, caloric restrictions appears to have a general effect on the rate of division in all dividing cells. The mechanisms by which this effect occurs have recently come under study. The enzymatic synthesis of DNA during normal growth of mammalian tissues has been partially examined. The activity of both DNA polymerase and thymidine kinase has been shown to parallel the rate of cell division in liver and in brain (Brasel et al., 1970). Moreover, this parallel relationship holds in the case of DNA polymerase for each of the brain regions studied. Restriction of calories during hyperplastic growth reduces the activity of thymidine kinase in brain and of DNA polymerase in both liver and brain (Jasper and Brasel, 1974). In addition, when such animals are rehabilitated during the proliferative phase, the activity of DNA polymerase increases to supranormal levels before any evidence of cell division (as measured by increased tissue incorporation of radioactive thymidine or by increase in total tissue DNA) can be detected (Jasper and Brasel, 1974).

There is evidence that RNA metabolism and protein synthesis are markedly altered by early undernutrition. There is a shift in the polysome profile in the direction of free ribosomes, and a concomitant decrease in the ability to synthesize protein both *in vitro* and *in vivo* (Wunner *et al.*, 1966). The rate of RNA turnover is increased by what appears to be an increased rate of both synthesis and degradation. Studies of synthesis are only beginning, but should provide important results within the next year. Studies of degradation have demonstrated an increased decay rate in previously labeled RNA in tissues from malnourished animals, and a marked elevation in the activity of alkaline RNAse in the tissues of these animals (Rosso and Winick, 1975). A recent report has indicated that the concentration of polyamines and the activity of those enzymes involved in polyamine synthesis are profoundly altered by malnutrition (Rozovski *et al.*, 1976). Since polyamines are important in RNA metabolism, future studies in this area should be of great interest.

Thus, it can be said at present that the retardation of cell division in undernourished animals involves a lowering of the activity of enzymes involved in DNA synthesis, as well as an alteration in RNA metabolism and a decrease in protein synthesis. The exact sequence of events has yet to be worked out.

Central nervous system myelination is retarded by early malnutrition imposed during the period of active myelination. The mechanisms by which this occurs have not yet been carefully studied. So far, the activity of certain enzymes involved in myelination have been found to be reduced. Many more data are necessary, however, before we can begin to understand how myelination is affected by undernutrition. Recent studies have used the concentration of gangliocides as an indication of dendritic arborizations, the reason being that these glycolipids are localized to the ends of the dendrites. Early malnutrition reduces the gangliocide concentration in both rat and human brain (Dickerson, personal communication). The quality of myelin can also be changed by early changes in the quality of the diet. Feeding a diet devoid of essential fatty acids results in the deposition of myelin with an abnormal fatty acid composition. These changes, however, appear reversible when the diet is returned to normal (Galli *et al.*, 1971).

10.2.1.1. Specific Nutrient Deficiencies

The changes in cellular growth so far described have been induced mainly by limiting the total amount of food available to the growing animal. Certain specific nutrient deficiencies have also been shown to retard cellular growth. Both vitamin B_6 and zinc deficiency have been shown to result in a reduction in brain cell number (Bhagavan and Coursin, 1971).

Studies in adipose tissue have demonstrated that a similar pattern of hyperplasia only, combined hyperplasia and hypertrophy, and hypertrophy (fat filling of existing cells) only occurs during development. The timing of these phases is still unclear because of the technical problem of being able to identify fat cells positively only after fat droplets have been deposited within them. This problem is being approached by looking for "markers" of fat cell proliferation that do not depend on lipid filling. Recent studies have shown that thymidine kinase and perhaps DNA polymerase may be useful as such markers (Cleary *et al.*, 1975). The importance of fat cell number and size in the overall problem of obesity is discussed fully in Chapter 5.

10.2.2. Nutrition and Neurohormones

The neurohormones, seretonin, norepinephrine, and acetylcholine, appear in localized areas of the brain during the early postnatal life of the rat. Undernutrition will delay the appearance of both serotonin and norepinephrine. Certain enzymes involved in the synthesis of these hormones are reduced in activity. Acetylcholine esterase activity is initially depressed by early undernutrition, but subsequently increases to supranormal levels, where it remains for a long time (Im *et al.*, 1972).

Recent experiments have shown that the levels of serotonin are dependent on the brain levels of its precursor amino acid, tryptophan. Tryptophan, in turn, is dependent on serum levels, which respond directly to the amount of this amino acid available from the diet. This is the first demonstration of the production of a neural hormone, or of any hormone, being under the direct control of a precursor supplied directly by the diet. Thus, under normal conditions, the concentration of serotonin will fluctuate with dietary intake of proteins, specifically, of tryptophan, which is often the limiting amino acid in proteins consumed. In malnourished animals, especially those on a marginal protein intake, brain serotonin levels remain chronically low. This low level of brain serotonin may have particular significance in human populations in which chronic malnutrition is prevalent. There is some evidence at present that acetylcholine levels are similarly controlled by the quantity of choline in the diet through the amount of choline present in the brain (Wurtman and Fernstrom, 1975). This system has been studied only in the CNS, and whether or not similar control mechanisms are present in the autonomic nervous system is unknown. The synthesis of norepinephrine does not appear to be controlled by a similar mechanism, and hence the reason for its reduced concentration during malnutrition is still unclear.

10.2.3. Nutrition and Pregnancy

Data in rats, pigs, dogs, and monkeys have shown that undernutrition in the mother will result in a curtailment in the rate of cell division in all fetal organs, including the brain. By contrast, vascular insufficiency, produced in rats by ligating the uterine artery and in monkeys by excising a portion of the placenta, results in a form of fetal growth failure in which the brain is spared. In rats, this result has been shown to be due to a reflex vasodilation in the fetal carotid artery, which preferentially allows more blood to reach the brain. The liver has only 50% of the expected number of cells, and is totally devoid of glycogen. By contrast, the brain has a normal number of cells, and shows only transient changes in RNA metabolism.

In the human, severe chronic maternal undernutrition produces retarded cell division in placenta, a shift in polysomes to free ribosomes, and a marked elevation of placental RNAse activity (Laga *et al.*, 1972). Thus, changes are induced in placenta and fetus by maternal undernutrition similar to those produced in the young animal by postnatal undernutrition. Recent evidence in the rat has demonstrated that placental transport of α-aminobutyric acid (a nonmetabolized amino acid) and of glucose are reduced by undernutrition (Rosso, 1975). Data in the guinea pig would suggest that during undernutrition, transport of α-aminobutyric acid to each fetus is maintained by resorbing a number of fetuses, thereby cutting down the total amount of material to be transported (Young and Widdowson, 1975). Thus, it would appear that at least part of the mechanism leading to fetal growth failure in malnourished mothers involves a "shutting down" of placental transport of essential nutrients. These data help to explain previous studies demonstrating that maternal undernutrition during pregnancy actually affects the fetus more than the mother.

In a recently published volume reviewing the outcome of the Dutch famine of 1945 (Stein *et al.*, 1975), it was shown that mothers in the last trimester of pregnancy gave birth to infants of lower birth weight (about 250 g less than expected), and that infant mortality was higher at that time. By the time these infants reached adulthood, they had attained normal heights, suggesting that catch-up growth had occurred. In addition, their psychological development was normal when tested at age 21. The implications of this finding will be discussed in Section 10.3.2. In chronically malnourished populations, the reduction in birth weight is greater (around 400 g). In addition, these infants remain stunted throughout their lives. Supplementation during pregnancy will increase birth weight to normal. In the study from Guatemala (Lechtig *et al.*, 1975) in which this was demonstrated, the type of supplement had very little influence, as long as 20,000 extra calories were consumed during the course of the pregnancy. In view of the animal studies on placental transport, one wonders whether these increased calories were able to restore placental transport of nutrients to normal, and thereby allow the maternal stores of nutrients to become available for the fetus.

The problem of "fetal malnutrition" is being approached from another direction by several groups who are trying to develop "prenatal markers" of fetal growth and to examine the effect of maternal malnutrition on these "markers." At present, the evidence suggests that the activity of pyruvate kinase and the ATP:ADP ratio in maternal leukocytes may be useful in this regard (Metcoff *et al.*, 1973). In addition, studies in maternal serum and urine and in amniotic fluid are being conducted, although no definitive answers have as yet been forthcoming. This area, while in its early stages, should give important results in the next few years.

Another area that is beginning to yield important findings is a reevaluation of the nutrient requirements during pregnancy. Studies in pregnant teenagers suggest that their nitrogen (protein) requirements may be much greater than we previously believed. Even at the highest nitrogen intakes given, subjects continue to increase the rate of nitrogen deposition into tissues. Thus, the amount of protein necessary for maximum nitrogen deposition has not yet been established (Calloway, 1974).

As more studies of the effects of various nutritional manipulations on pregnancy are carried out, it is becoming more and more evident that certain changes in the maternal physiology and biochemistry take place, and that many of these changes can be influenced by the maternal nutritional state. For example, in rats, urea synthesis is depressed both *in vitro* and *in vivo* during normal gestation (Naismith and Fears, 1972). In addition, nitrogen retention in muscle and other tissues increases during the first 14 days of pregnancy, perhaps as a result of the nitrogen conserved by the decreased urea production (Naismith, 1966). Since previous studies have not taken into account nitrogen retention in organs other than carcass, the scope of nitrogen retention during pregnancy has been underestimated. This conceivably could explain the higher nitrogen retention findings in the human metabolic studies referred to above. Some studies have been completed examining enzymatic mechanisms that might control the changes in nitrogen metabolism referred to. Argininosuccinate and alanine amino acid transferase activities are reduced (Naismith and Fears, 1972). Malnutrition does not seem to affect these mechanisms, however, since less nitrogen is available, less is deposited, and the deposition that is made is qualitatively changed, in that muscle is most affected (Naismith, 1966).

In addition, changes occur during pregnancy within the mother that presumably are in preparation for lactation. For example, fat is deposited, primarily in deep tissue depots, during the last trimester of pregnancy and used up. presumably as a source of energy, during the lactation period. Severe malnutrition during pregnancy markedly retards the deposition of such fat (Widdowson, 1975). However, whether the deposition of this fat is preferentially spared in milder forms of malnutrition is as yet unknown.

10.2.4. Early Infant Nutrition

There has been evidence that breast milk contains not only immunoglobulins but also maternal macrophages and lymphocytes throughout the first few months of lactation. These cells have *in vitro* activity against human enteric pathogens, which may protect the infant against gastrointestinal infection (Goldman and Smith, 1973; Ahlstedt *et al.,* 1975). In addition, serial measurements of breast-fed vs. bottle-fed infants indicate that the latter are heavier at the end of the first year of life (Fomon, 1974); this is true even if the formula is isocaloric to breast milk. These data suggest that the quantity of formula fed by the average mother exceeds the amount normally consumed by the infant who is breast-feeding. Data from several developing countries consistently support the fact that children who are breast-fed only will grow adequately for the first 4 months of life.

There are data from the U.S. that also suggest that the early introduction of solid foods may lead to excessive weight gain during the first year of life. This appears to result from the use of solid foods in addition to the usual amount of formula or breast milk. Thus, the total caloric consumption is increased (*Ten-State Nutrition Survey,* 1972).

Iron deficiency anemia is still the most prevalent single nutrient deficiency in infants. However, recent data would suggest that its prevalence is declining. This may be due to the widespread use of iron-fortified formulas, the incorporation of iron into infant cereals in a more absorbable form, or a combination of the two. In older children, iron deficiency anemia is also prevalent, especially among poorer populations. The data from recent surveys suggest, contrary to previous ideas, that this prevalence is equal among boys and girls (*Ten-State Nutrition Survey,* 1972). Other nutrient deficiencies, while not common, have been described in infant populations. Zinc can now be determined extremely accurately in hair, and such determinations are useful in assessing body Zn stores. In poorer populations, such determinations have suggested at least marginal Zn deficiencies in infants. One deficiency syndrome that is clinically important is a hemolytic anemia induced by vitamin E deficiency in premature infants. Finally, several cases of essential fatty acid deficiency have been reported in parenterally nourished infants and adults, and in a few infants on an extremely low fat intake (Forget *et al.*, 1975; Richardson and Sgoutas, 1975; Wene *et al.*, 1975).

What may be a new syndrome in infants whose mothers are ingesting large quantities of vitamin C has been reported. Two infants who were given adequate amounts of vitamin C after birth developed scurvy, suggesting that a "dependency" might have been induced (Cochrane, 1965). During the past year, studies in guinea pigs have confirmed these findings, and demonstrated that the breakdown of ascorbate to CO_2 occurs at an increased rate in such pups. This leads to a more rapid development of scurvy, and ultimately to more rapid death (Norkus and Rosso, 1975).

10.2.5. Nutrition and Muscle Metabolism

The major advance in this area has been the use of 3-methyl histidine as a marker for muscle catabolism (Munro, personal communication). Since histidine is methylated during its incorporation into muscle protein, there is no body pool of 3-methyl histidine outside of muscle. When muscle tissue breaks down, the 3-methyl histidine is released into serum and excreted in urine, since it cannot be reutilized for the synthesis of muscle protein. Normal serum and urine values have been measured, and the effects of certain environmental conditions that result in muscle breakdown are also being examined. This method theoretically will markedly improve quantitation of muscle breakdown in various conditions. Another area that is quite new, but that should result in the acquisition of considerable quantitative data, is the measurement of intracellular amino acid concentration on minute muscle biopsy specimens. These measurements are making it possible to study amino acid transport into muscle under normal and abnormal conditions.

10.2.6. Interaction of Nutrition and the Endocrine System

During the past two years, more and more data have accumulated demonstrating an interaction of nutrition with the function of various endocrine glands. During this year, the effects of protein–calorie malnutrition (PCM) in adults on cortisol metabolism and the pituitary–adrenal axis have been examined (Smith *et al.*, 1975a). The rate of cortisol production was found to be reduced, and, in addition, the chloroform-extractable 17-hydroxycorticosteroid metabolites is disproportionately small. The pituitary–adrenal axis is intact, and ACTH secretion is maintained, producing elevated plasma cortisol levels. The stimulus for maintaining ACTH secretion is not hypoglycemia and is not blocked by dexamethasone. The nature of the stimulus remains unknown. Another study on adult males with PCM has examined the pituitary–gonadal axis (Smith *et al.*, 1975b). The authors conclude that the hypogonadism of PCM is primarily on the basis of diminished Leydig cell function. Elevation of FSH in malnutrition may be secondary to the reduced Leydig's cell function. In children with edemetous PCM, calorie expenditure was found to be low on admission, and correlated linearly with increased calorie intake throughout the study. On admission, these children failed to respond to arginine or glucose by altering insulin secretion. In addition, growth hormone levels were elevated, but not increased by arginine or suppressed by intravenous glucose. Serum thyroxine values were low, but free thyroxine index and serum TSH levels were normal. The 24-hr dopamine and norepinephrine excretion was low when compared to epinephrine excretion. All these abnormalities were corrected during recovery. The authors suggest that in kwashiorkor, insulin acts as the primary regulator of peripheral fuel release, and that the high, nonsuppressible growth hormone levels may form part of an important homeostatic mechanism to provide substrates for brain metabolism via lipolysis (Parra *et al.*, 1975).

A number of studies have dealt with thyroid hormone and undernutrition. Starvation reduces the concentration of circulating T_3 and T_4 (Merimee and Fineberg, 1976; Moshang *et al.*, 1975). Protein–calorie malnutrition results in the same findings (Pain and Phillips, 1976). Very little change in TSH, however, is demonstrable in PCM (Chopra and Smith, 1975), and although basal prolactin levels are low, they respond normally to TSH (Becker *et al.*, 1975). Some of the mechanisms by which these changes occur have been explored in rats. Starvation decreases fecal and urinary excretion of T_4. The increased T_4 levels in these experiments resulted from an impairment of peripheral deiodinization (Ingbar and Galton, 1975).

Studies with growth hormone and malnutrition indicate that (hGH) drops rapidly after somatostatin in infants with PCM (Pimstone *et al.*, 1975).

10.3. Abnormal Nutrition

10.3.1. Parenteral Nutrition in Small Infants

The use of parenteral nutrition in small infants has become much more prevalent. Until this year, intralipid preparations have not been available in the United States except for research purposes. Studies conducted on young infants and on newborn puppies hyperalimented with glucose, amino acids, and vitamins and minerals have demonstrated that essential fatty acid deficiency will develop if therapy is prolonged. This deficiency is manifested by abnormal serum lipids in which the triene:tetratene ratio is elevated. In addition, brain myelination is affected in the puppies, with the deposition of myelin containing a distorted fatty acid pattern, again showing the elevated triene:tetracene ratio. It is interesting that these manifestations of fatty acid deficiency develop much more rapidly in the hyperalimented animals than in animals starved for an equal period of time. The data would suggest that if rapid growth is maintained and essential fatty acids not supplied, deficiency will ensue rapidly. By contrast, if little or no growth is occurring, the essential fatty acid requirements are much less.

10.3.2. Nutrition and Physical and Mental Development

During the past few years, a number of articles have focused attention on the changes in physical growth and mental development induced by early malnutrition. These data are reviewed extensively in a recent book (Winick, 1976). In general, they have shown that malnutrition contributes to retarded growth and development as part of a complex of poverty and low socioeconomic status. In children, severely malnourished but of high socioeconomic status, i.e., children with cystic fibrosis, retarded mental development is not seen (Lloyd-Still et al., 1972). This is also true in acute malnutrition affecting well-nourished populations during pregnancy (Stein et al., 1975). By contrast, chronic malnutrition either during pregnancy or during early infancy will result in retarded physical and mental development (Winick, 1976). Because of these and previous findings, a theory has been put forth (Levitsky and Barnes, 1972) suggesting that malnutrition may exert its major effect on brain function by functionally isolating the person from his environment and thereby producing a lack of stimulation at a critical point in development. This hypothesis implies that it might be possible to reverse some of the effects of early malnutrition by enriching the environment either during or after the malnutrition. Results in animals (Levitsky and Barnes, 1975; Frankova, 1975) suggest that this is true. Animals stimulated either by increased handling or by introducing a surrogate mother into the cage, together with the real mother, develop normally even if previously malnourished. During the past year, a study examining the effects of environmental enrichment on the development of previously malnourished children has been completed (Winick et al., 1975). In this study, Korean children who were malnourished during the first 18 months of life and then adopted before age 2 were compared to Korean children adopted at the same age, but not previously malnourished. The results showed that although slight differences remained by ages 6–12 in both height and performance, the malnourished children showed remarkable recovery in an enriched environment when compared to what would be expected had they been returned to the environment from which they came.

10.3.3. Childhood Obesity

Criteria for predicting childhood obesity are still being actively pursued. Recently, rapid weight gain in the first 6 months has been considered as an obesity index (Crawford *et al.*, 1974; Huenemann, 1974a). However, no follow-up of the infants was undertaken in the first study, and a follow-up study of the second group at 3 years of age indicated that of 14 "fat" 6-month-olds, 9 were normal for height and 5 were overweight (110–120% above standard weight for height) (Huenemann, 1974b). Another study reports a high incidence (44.4%) of overweight and obesity during the first year of life (Shukla *et al.*, 1972). When the data are examined carefully, the highest incidence of obesity is at 6 months (54.6%), and the lowest incidence of obesity is at 1 year (27.3%) (Shukla *et al.*, 1972).

Two studies have evaluated obesity and overweight status in children from 5 to 8 years of age whose pattern of weight gain in infancy was known (Eid, 1970; Mellbin and Viulle, 1973). Eid claims a significantly higher incidence of obesity in a group of infants who were rapid weight-gainers in the first 6 months of life when compared with a combined sample of children who gained weight around the 50th percentile or whose weight fell below the 10th percentile. However, examining the data in detail leaves certain doubts about these conclusions. The second study by Mellbin and Viulle concludes that weight gain in the first year of life is not a suitable index of predicting weight problems in later childhood.

Although it is frustrating that there is still no tool for predicting childhood onset obesity, since both Knittle (1974) and Brook *et al.* (1972) report that by 2 years of age, it is possible for an obese child to have fat cell number in the normal adult range, we must await further results in this area.

10.3.4. Nutrition and Cancer

This area is one in which work is just beginning. The most significant reports are contained in a special issue of the journal *Cancer Research* (1976) and in a report in the *Annals of the New York Academy of Sciences* (1974). The reader is referred to these two issues for comprehensive coverage of the subject. Some of the most important findings are studies relating carcinoma of the colon to high-fat, low-fiber diets, and implicating some as yet undefined dietary practice in the high incidence of gastric cancer in Japanese.

Studies have also begun to define the physiological changes that occur in cancer cachexia. In addition, there are several reports indicating that parenteral nutrition may have an important role both in maintaining patients with cancer and in allowing more comprehensive chemotherapy.

References

Ahlstedt, S., Carlsson, B., Hanson, L. A., and Goldblun, R. M., 1975, Antibody production by human colosterol cells, I. Immunoglobin class, specificity, and quantity, *Scand. J. Immunol.* **4**:535.

Annals of the New York Academy of Sciences, 1974, Symposium: Paraneoplastic syndromes, **230**:1.

Becker, D. J., Vinik, A. I., Pimstone, B. L., and Paul, M., 1975, Prolactin responses to thyrotropin-releasing hormone in protein–calorie malnutrition, *J. Clin. Endocrinol. Metab.* **41**:782.

Bhagavan, H. N., And Coursin, D. B., 1971, Effect of pyridoxine deficiency on nucleic acid and protein contents of brain and liver in rats, *Int. J. Vitamin Res.* **43**:419.

Brasel, J. A., Ehrenkranz, R. A., and Winick, M., 1970, DNA polymerase activity in rat brain during ontogeny, *Dev. Biol.* **23**:424.

Brook, C. D. G., Lloyd, J. K., and Wolf, O. H., 1972, Relation between age of onset of obesity and size and number of adipose cells, *Br. Med. J.,* **2**:25.

Calloway, D. H., 1974, Nitrogen balance during pregnancy, *in: Current Concepts in Nutrition,* Vol. 2, *Nutrition and Fetal Development* (M. Winick, ed.), pp. 79–94, John Wiley & Sons, New York.

Cancer Research, 1976, Symposium: Immunological control of virus-associated tumors in man: Prospects and problems, **36**:2, Part II, p. 559.

Chopra, I. J., and Smith, S. R., 1975, Circulating thyroid hormones and thyrotropin in adult patients with protein-calorie malnutrition, *J. Clin. Endocrinol. Metab.* **40**:21.

Cleary, M. P., Greenwood, M. R. C., and Brasel, J. A., 1975, Thymidine kinase as a measure of adipocyte proliferation in normal and obese rats, *Fed. Proc. Fed. Amer. Soc. Exp. Biol.* **34**:908 (abstract).

Cochrane, W. A., 1965, Overnutrition in prenatal and neonatal life: A problem?, *Can. Med. Assoc. J.* **93**:893.

Crawford, P. B., Keller, C. A., Hampton, M. C., Pacheco, F. P., and Huenemann, R. L., 1974, An obesity index for six-month-old children, *Amer. J. Clin. Nutr.* **27**:706.

Eid, E. E., 1970, Follow up study of physical growth of children who had excessive weight gain in the first six months of life. *Br. Med. J.* **2**:74.

Fomon, S. J., 1974, *Protein in Infant Nutrition,* Second Ed., W. B. Saunders, Philadelphia.

Forget, P. P., Fernandes, J., and Haverkamp Begemann, P., 1975, Utilization of fat emulsion during total parenteral nutrition in children, *Acta Paediatr. Scand.* **64:**377.

Frankova, S., 1975, Behavioral consequences of early malnutrition and environmental stimuli, presented at the Cornell Conference on Malnutrition and Behavior, November 6–8, 1975, Ithaca, New York.

Galli, C., White, H. B., Jr., and Paoletti, R., 1971, Lipid alterations and their reversion in the central nervous system of growing rats deficient in essential fatty acids, *Lipids* **6:**378.

Goldman, A. S., and Smith, C. W., 1973, Host resistance factors in human milk, *J. Pediatr.* **82:**1082.

Huenemann, R. L., 1974a, Environmental factors associated with preschool obesity. I, *J. Amer. Diet. Assoc.* **64:**480.

Huenemann, R. L., 1974b, Environmental factors associated with preschool obesity. II, *J. Amer. Diet. Assoc.* **64:**488.

Im, H. S., Barnes, R. H., Levitsky, D., Krook, L., and Pond, W. C., 1972, Postnatal malnutrition and regional cholinesterase activities in brain of pigs, *Fed. Proc. Fed. Amer. Soc. Exp. Biol.* **31:**697 (abstract).

Ingbar, D. H., and Galton, V. A., 1975, The effect of food deprivation on the peripheral metabolism of thyroxine in rats, *Endocrinology* **96:**1525.

Jasper, H. G., and Brasel, J. A., 1974, Rat liver DNA synthesis during the "catch-up" growth of nutritional rehabilitation, *J. Nutr.* **104:**405.

Knittle, J. L., 1974, Obesity and the cellularity of the adipose depot, *Triangle* **13:**57.

Laga, E. M., Driscoll, S. G., and Munro, H. N., 1972, Comparison of placentas from two socioeconomic groups. II. Biochemical characteristics, *Pediatrics* **50:**33.

Lechtig, A., Habicht, J. P., Delgado, H., Klein, R. E., Yarbrough, C. and Martorell, R., 1975, Effect of food supplementation during pregnancy on birthweight, *Pediatrics* **56:**508.

Levitsky, D. A., and Barnes, R. H., 1972, Nutritional and environmental interactions in the behavioral development of the rat: Long-term effects, *Science* **176:**68.

Levitsky, D. A., and Barnes, R. H., 1975, Malnutrition and the hunger to learn, presented at the Cornell Conference on Malnutrition and Behavior, November 6–8, 1975, Ithaca, New York.

Lloyd-Still, J. D., Wolff, P. H., Hurwitz, I., and Schwachman, H., 1972, Studies on intellectual development after severe malnutrition in infancy in cystic fibrosis and other intestinal lesions, presented at the Ninth International Congress of Nutrition, September 3–9, 1972, Mexico City.

Mellbin, T., and Vuille, J. C., 1973, Physical development at 7 years of age in relation to velocity of weight gain in infancy with special reference to incidence of overweight, *Br. J. Prev. Med.* **27:**225.

Merimee, T. J., and Fineberg, E. S., 1976, Starvation-induced alterations of circulating thyroid hormone concentrations in man, *Metabolism* **25:**79.

Metcoff, J., Wikman-Coffelt, J., Yoshida, T., Bernal, A., Rosado, A., Yoshida, P., Urrusti, J., Frenk, S., Madrazo, R., Velasco, L., and Morales, M., 1973, Energy metabolism and protein synthesis in human leukocytes during pregnancy and in placenta related to fetal growth, *Pediatrics* **51:**866.

Moshang, T., Jr., Parks, J. S., Baker, L., Vaidya, V., Utiger, R. D., Bongiovanni, A. M., and Snyder, P. J., 1975, Low serum triiodothyronine in patients with anorexia nervosa, *J. Clin. Endocrinol. Metab.* **40**:470.

Naismith, D. J., 1966, The requirement for protein and the utilization of protein and calcium during pregnancy, *Metabolism* **15**:582.

Naismith, D. J., and Fears, R. B., 1972, Adaptations in the metabolism of protein during pregnancy in the rat, *Proc. Nutr. Soc.* **31**:8A.

Norkus, E. P., and Rosso, P., 1975, Changes in ascorbic acid metabolism of the offspring following high maternal intake of this vitamin in the pregnant guinea pig, *Ann. N.Y. Acad. Sci.* **258**:401.

Pain, R. W., and Phillips, P. J., 1976, Thyroid-hormone levels in protein–calorie malnutrition, *Lancet* **1**:202.

Parra, A., Klish, W., Cuellar, A., Serrano, P. A., Garcia, G., Argote, R. M., Canseco, L., and Nichols, B. L., 1975. Energy metabolism and hormonal profile in children with edematous protein–calorie malrutrition, *J. Pediatr.* **87**:307.

Pimstone, B. L., Becker, D., and Kronheim, S., 1975, Disappearance of plasma growth hormone in acromegaly and protein-calorie malnutrition after somatostatin, *J. Clin. Endocrinol. Metab.* **40**:168.

Richardson, T. J., and Sgoutas, D., 1975, Essential fatty acid deficiency in four adult patients during total parenteral nutrition, *Amer. J. Clin. Nutr.* **28**:258.

Rozovski, S. J., Winick, M., and Rosso, P., 1976, Adaptive changes in polyamine metabolism during malnutrition and refeeding, *Fed. Proc. Fed. Amer. Soc. Exp. Biol.* **35**:341.

Rosso, P., 1975, Maternal malnutrition and placental transfer of alpha-amino isobutyric acid in the rat, *Science* **187**:648.

Rosso, P., and Winick, M., 1975, Effects of early undernutrition and subsequent refeeding on alkaline ribonuclease activity of rat cerebrum and liver, *J. Nutr.* **105**:1104.

Shukla, A., Forsyth, H. A., Anderson, C. M., and Marwah, S. M., 1972, Infantile overnutrition in the first year of life: A field study in Dudley, Worcestershire, *Br. Med. J.* **4**:507.

Smith, S. R. Bledsoe, T., and Chhetri, M. K., 1975a, Cortisol metabolism and the pituitary–adrenal axis in adults with protein–calorie malnutrition, *J. Clin. Endocrinol. Metab.* **40**:43.

Smith, S. R., Chhetri, M. K., Johanson, A. J., Radfar, N., and Migeon, C. J., 1975b, The pituitary–gonadal axis in men with protein–calorie malnutrition, *J. Clin. Endocrinol. Metab.* **41**:60.

Stein, Z., Susser, M., Saenger, G., and Marolla, F., 1975, *Famine and Human Development: The Dutch Hunger Winter of 1944–45*, Oxford University Press, New York.

Ten-State Nutrition Survey, 1968–70, 1972, U.S. DHEW, Center for Disease Control, Publication No. (HSM) 72-8130, July 1972.

Wene, J. D., Connor, W. E., and DenBesten, L., 1975, The development of essential fatty acid deficiency in healthy men fed fat-free diets intravenously and orally, *J. Clin. Invest.* **56**:127.

Widdowson, E. M., 1975, Nutrition and lactation, presented at the Symposium on

Nutritional Disorders of American Women, presented by the Institute of Human Nutrition, Columbia University, November 1975, New York.

Winick, M., 1976, *Malnutrition and Brain Development*, Oxford University Press, New York.

Winick, M., Meyer, K. K., and Harris, R. C., 1975, Malnutrition and environmental enrichment by early adoption, *Science* **190**:1173.

Wunner, W. H., Bell, J., and Munro, H. N., 1966, The effect of feeding with a tryptophane-free amino acid mixture on rat-liver polysomes and ribosomal ribonucleic acid, *Biochem. J.* **101**:417.

Wurtman, R. J., and Fernstrom, J. D., 1975, Control of brain monoamine synthesis by diet and plasma amino acids, *Amer. J. Clin. Nutr.* **28**:638.

Young, M., and Widdowson, E. M., 1975, The influence of diet deficient in energy, or in protein, on conceptive weight and the placental transfer of a non-metabolistic amino acid in the guinea pig, *Biol. Neonate* **27**:184.

Additional Selected Reading List

Ashwell, M., 1975, The relationship of the age on onset of obesity to the success of its treatment in the adult, *Br. J. Nutr.* **34**:201.

Barkai, A., Mahadik, S., and Rapport, M., 1974, Flow *in vivo* of glucose carbon to brain protein in rats: Effect of starvation, *J. Neurochem.* **22**:511.

Bøhmer, T., and Havel, R. J., 1975, Genesis of fatty liver and hyperlipemia in the fetal guinea pig, *J. Lipid Res.* **16**:454.

Burger, R. L., Waxman, S., Gilbert, H. S., Mehlman, C. S., and Allen, R. H., 1975, Isolation and characterization of a novel vitamin B_{12}-binding protein associated with hepatocellular carcinoma, *J. Clin. Invest.* **56**:1262.

Connell, A. M., 1976, Dietary fiber and diverticular disease, *Hospital Practice* (March 1976), p. 119.

Davidson, M. B., 1975, Insulin sensitivity of the large human adipocyte *in vitro*, *Diabetes* **24**:1086.

Deb, S., and Martin, R. J., 1975, Effects of exercise and of food restriction on the development of spontaneous obesity in rats, *J. Nutr.* **105**:543.

DeGuglielmone, A., Soto, A., and Duvilanski, B., 1974, Neonatal undernutrition and RNA synthesis in developing rat brain, *J. Neurochem.* **22**:529.

Demeyer, D. I., Tan, W. C., and Privett, O. S., 1974, Effect of essential fatty acid deficiency on lipid metabolism in isolated fat cells of epididymal fat pads of rats, *Lipids* **9**:1.

Felix, E. L., Loyd, B., and Cohen, M. H., 1975, Inhibition of the growth and development of a transplantable murine melanoma by vitamin A, *Science* **189**:886.

Gitlin, J. D., and Gitlin, D., 1974, Protein binding by specific receptors on human placenta, murine placenta, and suckling murine intestine in relation to protein transport across these tissues, *J. Clin. Invest.* **54**:1155.

Greenman, J., and Jacobs, A., 1975, The effect of iron stores on iron absorption in the rat: The possible role of circulating ferritin, *Gut* **16**:613.

Grummt, I., 1975, Synthesis of RNA molecules larger than 45 S by isolated rat-liver nucleoli, *Eur. J. Biochem.* **57:**159.

Hansen, F. M., Nielson, J. H., and Gliemann, J., 1974, The influence of body weight and cell size on lipogenesis and lipolysis of isolated rat fat cells, *Eur. J. Clin. Invest.* **4:**411.

Harrell, J., Decastro, J. M., and Balagura, S., 1975, A critical evaluation of body weight loss following lateral hypothalamic lesions, *Physiol. Behav.* **15:**133.

Holm, G., Jacobsson, B., Bjorntorp, P., and Smith, U., 1975, Effects of age and cell size on rat adipose tissue metabolism, *J. Lipid Res.* **16:**461.

Holzbach, R. T., Wieland, R. G., Lieber, C. S., DeCarli, L. M., Koepke, K. R., and Green, S. G., 1974, Hepatic lipid in morbid obesity: Assessment at and subsequent to jejunoileal bypass, *N. Engl. J. Med.* **290:**296.

Ingelbleek, Y., and Beckers, C., 1975, Triiodothyronine and thyroid stimulating hormone in protein–calorie malnutrition in infants, *Lancet* **2:**845.

Jason, C. J., Polokoff, M. A., and Bell, R. M., 1976, Triacylglycerol synthesis in isolated fat cells. An effect of insulin on microsomal fatty acid coenzyme A ligase activity, *J. Biol. Chem.* **251:**1488.

Jeejeebhoy, K. N., Anderson, G. H., Nakhooda, A. F., Greenberg, G. R., Sanderson, I., and Marliss, E. B., 1976, Metabolic studies in total parenteral nutrition with lipid in man. Comparison with glucose, *J. Clin. Invest.* **57:**125.

Kovanen, P. T., Nikkilä, E. A., and Miettinen, T. A., 1975, Regulation of cholesterol synthesis and storage in fat cells, *J. Lipid Res.* **16:**211.

Law, D. K., Dudrick, S. J., and Abdou, N. T., 1974, The effect of dietary protein depletion on immunocompetence, *Ann. Surg.* **179:**168.

Martin, R. J., 1974, Characterization of enzyme and metabolic patterns in mice selected for rapid postweaning growth rate, *Growth* **38:**53.

Nestel, P. J., Homma, Y., Scott, T. W., Cook, L. J., and Havenstein, N., 1976, Effect of dietary polyunsaturated pork on plasma lipids and sterol excretion in man, *Lipids* **11:**42.

Ogundipe, O. O., and Bray, A., 1974, The influence of diet and fat cell size on glucose metabolism, lipogenesis and lipolysis in the rat, *Horm. Metab. Res.* **6:**351.

Ong, D. E., Page, D. L., and Chytil, F., 1975, Retinoic acid binding protein: Occurrence in human tumors, *Science* **190:**60.

Opsahl, C. A., and Powley, T. L., 1974, Failure of vagotomy to reverse obesity in the genetically obese Zucker rat, *Amer. J. Physiol.* **226:**34.

Pittman, R. C., Khoo, J. C., and Steinberg, D., 1975, Cholesterol esterase in rat adipose tissue and its activation by cyclic adenosine 3',5'-monophosphate-dependent protein kinase, *J. Biol. Chem.* **250:**4505.

Raghuramulu, N., and Rao, K. S. J., 1974, Growth hormone secretion in protein–calorie malnutrition, *J. Clin. Endocrinol. Metab.* **38:**176.

Rowland, N. E., and Antelmon, S. M., 1976, Stress-induced hyperphagia in obesity in rats: A possible model for understanding human obesity, *Science* **191:**310.

Spaulding, S. W., Chopra, I. J., Sherwin, R. S., and Lyall, S. S., 1976, Effect of caloric restriction and dietary composition on serum T_3 and reverse T_3 in man, *J. Clin. Endocrinol. Metab.* **42:**197.

Sullivan, A. C., Triscari, J., Hamilton, J. G., and Miller, O. N., 1974, Effect of (-)-

Hydroxycitrate upon the accumulation of lipid in the rat: II. Appetite, *Lipids* **9:**129.

Sullivan, A. C., Triscari, J., Hamilton, J. G., Miller, O. N., and Wheatly, V. R, 1974, Effect of (-)-Hydroxycitrate upon the accumulation of lipid in the rat: I. Lipogenesis, *Lipids* **9:**121.

Van Campen, D., 1974, Regulation of iron absorption, *Fed. Proc. Fed. Amer. Soc. Exp. Biol.* **33:**100.

Waterlow, J. C., 1975, Protein turnover in the whole body, *Nature* **253:**157.

Wilmore, D. W., Moylan, J. A. Helmkamp, G. M., and Pruitt, B. A., Jr., 1973, Clinical evaluation of a 10% intravenous fat emulsion for parenteral nutrition in thermally injured patients, *Ann. Surg.* **178:**503.

Wolfe, B. M., Havel, J. R., Marliss, E. B., Kane, J. P., Seymour, J., and Ahuja, S. P., 1976, Effects of a 3-day fast and of ethanol on splanchnic metabolism of FFA, amino acids and carbohydrates in healthy young men, *J. Clin. Invest.* **57:**329.

Young, V. R., Steffee, W. P., Pencharz, P. B., Winterer, J. G., and Scrimshaw, N. S., 1975, Total human body protein synthesis in relation to protein requirements at various ages, *Nature* **253:**192.

11

Metabolic Aspects of Renal Stone Disease

Hibbard E. Williams

11.1. Introduction

Renal stone disease continues to represent one of the most common medical disorders encountered in medical practice. Estimates of the frequency of this disorder suggest that one person in every thousand will be hospitalized each year for an episode of renal colic. This clearly underestimates the true incidence of nephrolithiasis when it is realized that many stones are quiescent and asymptomatic for many years, and in addition, many patients with renal colic are treated in outpatient departments and physicians' offices and are not hospitalized. Despite the recognition of renal stone disease since antiquity, adequate preventive treatment often remains as elusive today as it did for the Egyptian Pharaohs and ancient Greek scribes.

HIBBARD E. WILLIAMS • Medical Service, San Francisco General Hospital; Department of Medicine, University of California, San Francisco, California.

Most renal stone episodes in this country are isolated events that fortunately never recur. The pathogenesis of these episodes is not known and is difficult to study. Most of our knowledge concerning the formation, growth, and treatment of renal stones comes from studies of patients with recurrent stone disease. These studies and patients will be reviewed and discussed in this chapter.

11.2. Types of Renal Stones

Although no recent studies of the composition of renal stones have been carried out, there is little reason to suspect any change in composition. Calcium oxalate remains the single most common type of renal stone passed by patients in this country. Approximately two-thirds of all renal stones are composed of calcium oxalate, usually as the monohydrate. In approximately half the stones, significant amounts of calcium phosphate in the form of hydroxyapatite are mixed with the calcium oxalate. It is unusual to see pure calcium phosphate stones excreted from the urinary tract.

Stones composed of magnesium ammonium phosphate, usually mixed with hydroxyapatite, represent about 15% of the total number of stones, and are found mainly in patients with recurrent urinary tract infections. Uric acid stones and cystine stones account for no more than 10% of the total, and the remaining stones are composed of a variety of less common components, such as xanthine, silicates, matrix, and urinary pigments.

11.3. Pathogenesis of Renal Stones

11.3.1. Basic Mechanisms of Stone Formation

There appear to be at least three events in the development of a renal stone: nucleation, crystal growth, and crystal aggregation. Factors controlling these three processes continue to be studied, debated, and reviewed. Supersaturation of urine with certain urinary crystalloids clearly accounts for crystal formation in most patients with uric acid, cystine, and mixed magnesium ammonium phosphate–hydroxyapatite stones. The low solubility of these compounds in urine and the dependence of their solubility on urine pH accounts for the initial nucleation of these crystals and eventual stone formation.

The situation with the more common calcium oxalate stone is more confusing. It has been difficult to demonstrate consistently that urine is supersaturated with respect to calcium oxalate in all patients with stone disease of this variety. Supersaturation undoubtedly leads to nucleation in patients with hyperoxaluria and profound hypercalciuria, but what happens in the large number of patients who do not have elevated levels of either of these constituents? Recent studies of recurrent calcium oxalate stone–formers showed that the urine is frequently supersaturated with calcium oxalate, although overlap with values found in the urine of normal nonstone-formers does exist (Robertson *et al.*, 1976). For this reason, searches have been carried out for other pathogenetic mechanisms of stone formation. One such mechanism is the inhibitor-absence mechanism, which relates stone disease to the absence of one or more specific inhibitors of calcium oxalate crystal formation. Although a large number of compounds have been identified as inhibitors of calcium oxalate crystallization (pyrophosphate, mucopolysaccharides, trace metals, diphosphonates, organic acids), it has not been possible to incriminate the absence of any *one* of these substances consistently in patients with recurrent calcium oxalate stone disease. Recently, it was demonstrated that patients with idiopathic calcium oxalate stone disease have a tendency of reduced inhibitory activity in the urine, but a great deal of overlap with normal values existed in this study (Robertson *et al.*, 1976). This finding again emphasizes the difficulty in assigning a primary role to the absence of an inhibitor of crystallization in the etiology of renal stone disease. This does not deny the potential importance of urinary inhibitors in the control of crystal growth and aggregation once nucleation has occurred, a theory supported by the finding of larger urinary crystals in stone-formers with low inhibitory activity (Robertson *et al.*, 1972a).

In summary, the single most common mechanism controlling stone formation in patients with recurrent stone disease appears to be supersaturation of urine with various urinary crystalloids. Reduction of crystal inhibitory activity may play a role in stone episodes, but rarely is this the only or primary mechanism.

11.3.2. Specific Causes of Renal Stone Disease

11.3.2.1. Hypercalciuria

Because of the common finding of calcium in over 90% of renal stones, it is obvious that this crystalloid is of major importance in stone disease. Calcium-containing renal stones are common in most conditions associated with persistent hypercalciuria, i.e., more than 300 mg/24 hr in men and more than 250 mg/24 hr in women on a normal calcium intake. Therefore, a wide variety of hypercalciuric states have been associated with recurrent renal stone disease, usually of the calcium oxalate variety. Primary hyperparathyroidism remains one of the more frequent hypercalciuric conditions associated with stone disease, and estimates of the frequency of stones in hyperparathyroid patients vary between 50 and 80%. The finding of recurrent calcium oxalate stones in an adult with hypercalciuria requires a serious effort by the physician to rule out hyperparathydroidism.

The most common hypercalciuric syndrome associated with recurrent calcium oxalate stones is idiopathic hypercalciuria. This syndrome undoubtedly represents a group of disorders, all characterized by recurrent stones occurring after the age of 20 years, and mostly in men who often have a family history of stone disease and have persistent hypercalciuria. The most commonly accepted mechanism for the hypercalciuria in these patients is increased gastrointestinal absorption of dietary calcium (Coe et al., 1973). In normal subjects, increasing dietary calcium affects urinary calcium excretion very little; in these patients, increases in dietary calcium lead to direct and proportional increases in urinary calcium, presumably secondary to increased absorption. The specific mechanism for increased absorption of calcium remains unknown. Because of the finding of increased parathyroid hormone levels in some patients with this syndrome, increased intestinal absorption has been thought to be a secondary phenomenon (Pak et al., 1974b). Two conditions that might lead to increased parathyroid hormone levels have been found in small numbers of patients with the diagnosis of idiopathic hypercalciuria: normocalcemic primary hyperparathyroidism, and a renal tubular leak of calcium. The former has been documented by surgical demonstration of a parathyroid adenoma in a small number of these patients. In this group of patients, parathyroid hormone levels are not affected by maneuvers that lower urinary calcium levels, and serum ionized calcium levels are persistently elevated despite a normal total calcium concentration.

In patients with a renal tubular leak of calcium, hypercalciuria may be reduced by administration of thiazide diuretics that in turn reduce the high circulating levels of parathyroid hormone and return them to the normal range (Coe et al., 1973). The specific molecular mechanism involved in the renal tubular leak has not been identified. Recently, a preliminary report suggests a defect in vitamin D metabolism in patients with idiopathic hypercalciuria, but proof of this theory must await more definitive confirmation (Shen et al., 1976).

It has been difficult to determine the relative frequencies of these various abnormalities in patients with idiopathic hypercalciuria because of differences in the various reported series. In the author's opinion, hyperparathyroidism and the renal leak mechanism represent relatively uncommon mechanisms in patients with idiopathic hypercalciuria, and increased intestinal absorption of calcium remains the most frequent and consistent

Table I.   Causes of Hyperoxaluria

Increased endogenous production
   Pyridoxine deficiency
   Primary hyperoxaluria, types I and II
   Ingestion of oxalate precursor
      Ethylene glycol
      Methoxyflurane
      Ascorbic acid

Increased exogenous oxalate
   Massive oxalate ingestion
   Enteric hyperoxaluria

finding, albeit one not well delineated on a pathophysiological or molecular basis.

11.3.2.2. Hyperoxaluria

Increased excretion of oxalic acid in the urine represents a rather uncommon cause of recurrent renal stone disease, perhaps accounting for no more than 5% of patients with recurrent calcium oxalate stones. However, changes in urinary oxalate excretion within the so-called normal range of 10–50 mg/24 hr may be more important in the initiation of calcium oxalate stones than has previously been thought (see Section 11.3.3).

The causes of increased urinary oxalate excretion (more than 50 mg/24 hr) are outlined in Table I. In this classification, the types of hyperoxaluria are separated into two major categories: those due to increased endogenous production of oxalate, occurring predominantly in the liver; and those secondary to increased exogenous dietary oxalate or increased gastrointestinal absorption.

In the first category, a number of interesting disorders have been identified. The primary hyperoxalurias, types I and II, are two genetically distinct metabolic errors leading to the same phenotypic picture—early onset of recurrent renal stone disease leading eventually to renal damage, either through oxalate deposits in renal parenchyma or secondary to associated chronic pyelonephritis (Williams and Smith, 1976). Severe renal damage leading to chronic renal failure early in life has been seen only in the type I syndrome. Both syndromes are transmitted by an autosomal recessive mode of inheritance. In both syndromes, oxalate excretion usually exceeds 100 mg/24 hr, and may be as high as 400 mg/24 hr. The two syndromes may be differentiated by the pattern of organic

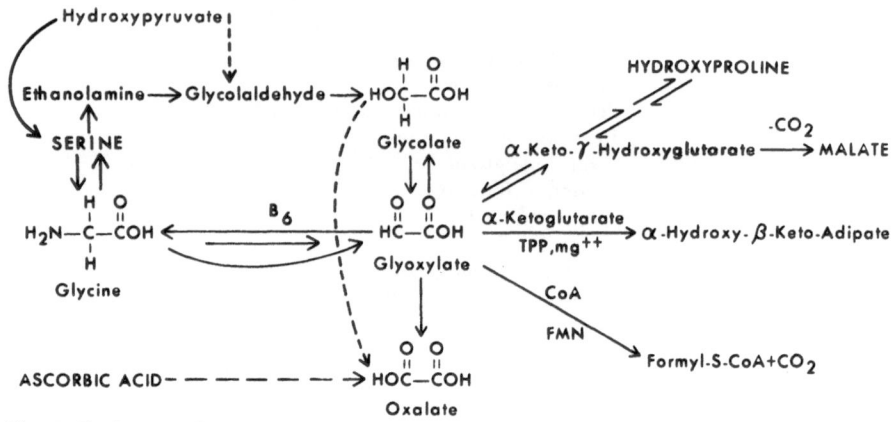

Fig. 1. Pathways of oxalate metabolism in man. (From Williams and Smith, 1976. Reproduced with permission of the publisher.)

acid excretion. In type I, glycolic acid is excreted in excess; in type II, glycolate excretion is within normal limits, but the urine contains large amounts of L-glyceric acid. The metabolic defect in type I primary hyperoxaluria occurs in the metabolism of the immediate precursor of oxalate, glyoxylate, to α-hydroxy-β-ketoadipate, a reaction catalyzed by the enzyme α-ketoglutarate:glyoxylate carboligase. This defect leads to accumulation of glyoxylate behind the enzymatic block, with subsequent increased synthesis and excretion of oxalate (Fig. 1) (Williams and Smith, 1976).

In the type II syndrome, a block in the metabolism of hydroxypyruvate to D-glyceric acid in the gluconeogenic pathway of serine metabolism leads to excessive synthesis of L-glyceric acid brought about by the action of lactic dehydrogenase on the accumulated hydroxypyruvate. The mechanism of the hyperoxaluria in this syndrome continues to be debated. There is evidence to suggest a linked reaction between hydroxypyruvate conversion to L-glycerate and increased conversion of glyoxylate to oxalate, the latter reaction also controlled primarily by lactic dehydrogenase (Williams and Smith, 1971). In rats, hydroxypyruvate is converted to urinary oxalate, but this reaction has not yet been demonstrated in man (Richardson and Liao, 1973).

Other causes of hyperoxaluria secondary to increased oxalate synthesis include pyridoxine deficiency and ingestion of precursors of oxalate: ethylene glycol, ascorbic acid, and methoxyflurane. Pyridoxine deficiency has been demonstrated to produce significant hyperoxaluria in both man and experimental animals (Gershoff, 1964). The mechanism for this effect relates to the role pyridoxine plays as a cofactor in the transamination of glyoxylate to glycine. A block in this step leads to increased diversion of glyoxylate into oxalate synthesis. Clinical examples of hyperoxaluria secondary to pyridoxine deficiency are very rare.

Ethylene glycol and ascorbic acid can both be metabolized to oxalate by the human liver. Hyperoxaluria and intrarenal obstructive uropathy secondary to massive oxalate crystalluria have been observed following ingestion of ethylene glycol (Parry and Wallach, 1974). Conversion of this substance to oxalate occurs through its metabolism to glycoaldehyde, glycolate, and hence oxalate. Ascorbic acid in very large doses (more than 5 g/24 hr) may lead to some modest increase in urinary oxalate (Briggs *et al.*, 1973), but there is no proof to date of an increased incidence of renal stone disease in patients who are heavy users of this vitamin.

Administration of the anesthetic agent methoxyflurane has resulted in hyperoxaluria and deposits of oxalate in the kidneys (McIntyre *et al.*, 1973). This two-carbon fluorinated compound is presumably converted *in vivo* to oxalate, and then is not only excreted in excess in the urine, but also deposited in the renal parenchyma, leading to transient renal failure. Small doses of methoxyflurane administered periodically to a patient with extensive burns during wound debridement (Jensen and Williams, unpublished observations) resulted in gradual development of renal failure and urinary excretion of oxalate crystals and hyperoxaluria in excess of 250 mg/24 hr. The drug was discontinued, and urinary oxalate eventually returned to normal levels over a 2-week period.

Of particular interest is the recognition of a new hyperoxaluric syndrome in patients with a variety of malabsorptive states (Admirand, 1972; Smith *et al.*, 1972b) in which gastrointestinal absorption of oxalate is increased. The syndrome was originally observed in patients with ileal resection of more than 50 cm. Recurrent calcium oxalate nephrolithiasis first developed in these patients soon after surgery, and was related to marked hyperoxaluria in the absence of glycolic or glyceric aciduria. This syndrome was subsequently recognized in patients with significant fat malabsorption secondary to a variety of chronic gastrointestinal disorders—i.e., chronic inflammatory bowel disease, chronic pancreatic and biliary tract diseases, bacterial overgrowth syndrome—and after jejunoileal bypass procedures. Hyperoxaluria in these patients usually ranges between 100 and 300 mg/24 hr.

Patients with this syndrome hyperabsorb dietary oxalate (Chadwick *et al.*, 1972; Earnest *et al.*, 1974): more than 40% of an orally administered dose of isotopic oxalate was absorbed by most patients, compared with a mean of 12% of normal subjects (Fig. 2).

The degree of hyperabsorption and the amount of oxalate excreted

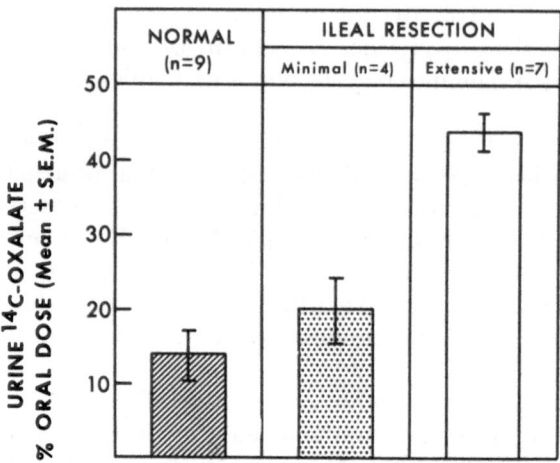

Fig. 2. Forty-eight-hour urinary excretion of orally administered [^{14}C]oxalate in normal subjects, in patients with minimal ileal resection (<50 cm), and in patients with extensive ileal resection (≤100 cm). (From Earnest *et al.*, 1974. Reproduced with permission of the publisher.)

in the urine appear to be proportional to the degree of fat malabsorption (Earnest *et al.*, 1974). Control of the fat malabsorption by dietary administration of medium-chain triglycerides, reduction of dietary oxalate, and administration of oral calcium supplements reduces oxalate excretion to normal levels in these patients (Earnest and Williams, unpublished observations). Thus, the oxalate hyperabsorption and hyperoxaluria in these patients may result from oxalate and fatty acids in the lumen of the small intestine competing for intraluminal calcium ion. In the presence of normal fat absorption and adequate intraluminal calcium, most oxalate in the intestine exists as the insoluble and relatively nonabsorbable calcium salt, which accounts for the very small amount of oral oxalate absorbed in normal subjects. In the presence of significant fat malabsorption, the intraluminal fatty acid concentration increases dramatically, binding calcium to form calcium–fatty acid soaps and lowering the concentration of intraluminal free calcium ion. Therefore, more oxalate is in solution as the sodium salt, and as such can diffuse freely across the gastrointestinal wall (Binder, 1974), enabling hyperabsorption of oxalate. This hypothesis is supported by *in vitro* studies of oxalate solubility in the presence of fatty acids (Earnest, unpublished observations), as well as by the aforementioned *in vivo* studies in which luminal concentrations of fatty acids, oxalate, and calcium were altered in patients with the syndrome (Earnest and Williams, unpublished observations).

11.3.2.3. Recurrent Urinary Tract Infections

Patients with recurrent infections of the urinary tract with urea-splitting microorganisms have an increased incidence of stone formation. In this situation, the stones are composed of mixtures of magnesium ammonium phosphate and hydroxyapatite. The mechanism of stone formation in this situation appears to be supersaturation of the urine due to increased production of ammonia by the urea splitters and, in addition, chronic alkalinization of the urine, which favors precipitation of these crystals from solution. Rates of stone formation in this situation may be quite high, and bilateral staghorn calculi are not an unusual finding in these patients, particularly when stasis secondary to obstructive uropathy is also present.

11.3.2.4. Hyperuricosuria

Recurrent uric acid stones occur in two settings: chronic hyperurico-suria, and chronic acidification of the urine favoring the crystallization of free uric acid owing to its very poor solubility below pH 5.5. (For further information concerning the factors controlling urate production and excretion, see Chapter 8.) In short, any condition associated with chronic hyperuricosuria (more than 600 mg/24 hr) will be associated with an increased incidence of uric acid stones. Uric acid stones occur in about 25% of patients with a history of gout, and in approximately 40% of patients with hyperuricemia secondary to myeloproliferative disorders (Gutman and Yü, 1968).

Recurrent uric acid stones also occur in the setting of chronic acidification of the urine, either because of a chronic metabolic acidosis or because of medications that acidify the urine. In addition, there are a small number of patients with a "renal tubular alkalosis" syndrome in whom normal alkalinization of the urine in the postprandial periods cannot be carried out because of a presumed disorder of renal tubular function; this leads to chronic urinary acidification and recurrent uric acid stones at normal concentrations of urinary uric acid.

A role for uric acid in the formation of calcium oxalate stones has been proposed recently (Coe and Kavalach, 1974). It is based on the observations of a high incidence of hyperuricemia and hyperuricosuria in recurrent calcium oxalate stone-formers, and of the apparent reduction in stone episodes when these patients are treated with allopurinol to reduce urinary uric acid. The uric acid is thought to act as the nucleus for the calcium oxalate stone formation in this setting. However, it has been extremely difficult to demonstrate uric acid nuclei in calcium oxalate stones, making this theory tenuous. Additional studies will be needed to confirm this interesting speculation concerning the role of uric acid in the genesis of calcium oxalate stones.

11.3.2.5. Cystinuria

This rare genetic disease accounts for approximately 2% of all renal calculi. The cystine stone formation in the urinary tract of these patients is a direct result of supersaturation of the urine with cystine. The excessive excretion of cystine is due to a genetically determined defect in the renal tubular transport of cystine, and, in most cases, transport of the dibasic amino acids lysine, ornithine, and arginine. The intestinal mucosa shares this same transport defect in patients with cystinuria. The disease is inherited as an autosomal recessive trait, although different subtypes of the disease have been characterized as completely or incompletely recessive, based on differences in the pattern of urinary amino acid excretion in parents of patients with the disease (Thier and Segal, 1972).

11.3.2.6. Xanthinuria

Xanthine, the immediate metabolic precursor of uric acid, shares with uric acid the same insolubility in an acid medium. Therefore, conditions associated with xanthinuria have been associated with xanthine stone disease. These include two conditions: hereditary xanthinuria, a hereditary metabolic defect in xanthine oxidase leading to xanthine accumulation and increased excretion of xanthine in urine, and certain hyperuricemic states in which allopurinol therapy has been used to reduce serum uric acid levels. In the latter condition, allopurinol, through its inhibitory effect on xanthine oxidase, allows massive accumulation and excretion of xanthine. This has been observed clinically in two settings: patients with malignant myeloproliferative disorders being treated with chemotherapy, leading to marked increases in nucleoprotein turnover; and patients with the Lesch-Nyhan disease, in whom marked hyperuricemia results from a defect in the salvage pathway of uric acid synthesis (see Chapter 8). Despite the physicochemical similarity of xanthine to uric acid, xanthine calculi have not been observed in patients with persistently acid urine.

11.3.3. Idiopathic Stone Disease

Approximately 25% of patients with recurrent calcium oxalate stone disease will have one of the well-described hypercalciuric or hyperoxaluric conditions described earlier. However, the majority of patients with calcium oxalate stones remain an enigma relative to the etiology of the stone

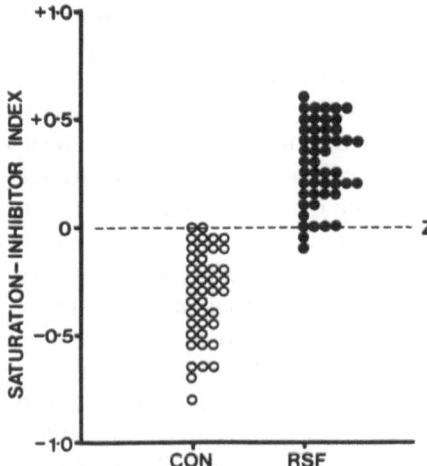

Fig. 3. Saturation–inhibition indexes of the patients with recurrent stone formation (RSF) and the controls (CON) in relation to the discriminant line (----). (From Robertson *et al.*, 1976. Reproduced with permission of the authors and publisher.)

formation. Urinary calcium and oxalate values are generally within the published normal ranges in most of these patients, and a search for the lack of certain specific inhibitors of stone formation has been for the most part unsuccessful. This is not to deny the possibility of the lack of an inhibitor, only to emphasize that no definite proof now exists to incriminate any one of the known inhibitors in patients with recurrent stone disease. The recent study by Robertson *et al.* (1976) suggests that most stone-formers do have some abnormalities in the inhibition of crystal growth in *in vitro* studies of urine from such patients. This was particularly emphasized by comparing the urinary saturation–inhibition index of stone-formers and normal subjects. This index was defined by a discriminant line relating inhibitory activity and urine saturation with respect to calcium oxalate (Fig. 3). The specific mechanism for this diminished inhibitory activity in stone-formers' urine remains to be determined, as does its role relative to the importance of the saturation of calcium oxalate in urine.

The importance of supersaturation of calcium oxalate in urine has been emphasized by a number of studies during the past few years. The activity products for calcium oxalate in urine are clearly increased in stone-formers, as is the degree of supersaturation of the urine with respect to calcium oxalate (Robertson *et al.*, 1976; Marshall and Barry, 1973). More important, the degree of supersaturation has been correlated directly with the volume of calcium oxalate crystals in the stone-former's urine (Robertson *et al.*, 1972a).

If the degree of supersaturation of calcium oxalate in urine is the most important factor in controlling stone formation, then what factors affect the degree of supersaturation? In recent studies from the Leeds group (Robertson *et al.*, 1972b), it was shown that changes in urinary oxalate concentration have a much greater effect on supersaturation than changes in calcium. These effects occurred with changes of oxalate within the normal range of oxalate excretion. This represents a very important observation in the etiology of calcium oxalate stone disease; i.e., the relatively small change in urinary oxalate *within the normal range* may have a profound effect on the urinary supersaturation of calcium oxalate, and therefore on the volume of calcium oxalate crystals, and perhaps on the frequency of stone episodes. This theory is supported by the finding from several laboratories of a higher excretion of oxalate (within the normal range) in stone-formers than in normal subjects (Hodgkinson, 1974; Marshall *et al.*, 1972). The importance of this finding in the treatment of idiopathic renal stone disease by attempts to lower urinary oxalate is obvious (see Section 11.4.2.2).

One other theory of renal stone disease relates to the role of certain nucleators of stone formation, namely, calcium phosphate and uric acid. Calcium phosphate in the form of apatite is found in approximately half of all calcium oxalate stones. The effect of increasing urinary pH on decreasing solubility of calcium phosphate has raised the question of the importance of transient urinary alkalinization in precipitation of calcium phosphate, leading to subsequent growth of calcium oxalate on this crystalline nidus. The absence of calcium phosphate in many calcium oxalate stones and the general failure of urinary acidification to affect the frequency of stone episodes in calcium oxalate stone-formers has made it difficult to accept this theory as a major one in idiopathic renal stone disease. Persistent alkalinization of the urine may be important in the stone disease of distal renal tubular acidosis, in which the stones are mostly pure calcium phosphate (apatite), although hypercalciuria and diminished citrate excretion may also play a role. The role of uric acid in calcium oxalate stone disease was discussed earlier (see Section 11.3.2.4).

11.4. Treatment and Prevention of Renal Stones

11.4.1. General Measures

11.4.1.1. Fluids

Because supersaturation of various crystalloids represents a major mechanism for stone formation, the single most important approach to the treatment of stone disease must remain dilution of the urine with increased fluid intake. The greater the urine volume, the lower the concentration of urinary crystalloids and the less the likelihood that a stone will form, although experimental support for the last statement is difficult to muster. Because inhibitors of crystal formation will presumably be diluted by an increase in urine volume, urinary dilution could have a negative effect, although this has never been shown. Nevertheless, an increased fluid intake throughout the day and night should be advocated for the treatment of all stone-formers in an attempt to maintain evenly diluted urine throughout the entire 24-hr period.

11.4.1.2. Diet

Dietary approaches to the treatment of renal stone disease are important in several circumstances. In the syndrome of idiopathic hypercalciuria, reduction of dietary calcium will diminish calcium excretion, although not always into the normal range. Note, however, that in nonhypercalciuric stone-formers, dietary calcium restriction does not affect significant urinary calcium excretion, and this dietary limitation is therefore of little benefit in the nonhypercalciuric patient. In the syndrome of hyperoxaluria secondary to malabsorptive states, decreasing dietary oxalate can reduce urinary oxalate, and dietary purine restriction can modestly reduce urinary uric acid in some patients with hyperuricemia and hyperuricosuria.

One important observation needs emphasis at this point, namely, that reducing dietary calcium *raises* urinary oxalate excretion in patients with normal urinary oxalate (Marshall *et al.*, 1972). If, as just noted, modest changes in urinary oxalate even within the normal range are important in controlling crystal formation, then this effect of a low-calcium diet assumes importance. Potentially, a low-calcium diet could raise urinary oxalate sufficiently to increase new crystal formation, and thereby precipitate a stone episode. For this reason, dietary calcium restriction should not be used randomly in the treatment of renal stone disease, and new prospective studies must be carried out to evaluate the proper dietary calcium intake for patients with idiopathic calcium oxalate stone disease.

11.4.1.3. Urine pH

Manipulation of urine pH is of value in a relatively small number of patients with stone disease. Acidification is beneficial in patients with recurrent infections of the urinary tract and magnesium ammonium phosphate stones. Alkalinization of the urine should decrease stone episodes in patients with uric acid, xanthine, or cystine stones. Alterations of urine pH are of little benefit in patients with recurrent calcium oxalate stones, in view of the lack of any significant effect of changes in pH between 4.5 and 8.0 on oxalate solubility.

11.4.2. Specific Measures

11.4.2.1. Agents That Affect Calcium Excretion

Two approaches have been employed to affect urinary calcium excretion: (1) reducing the filtered load of calcium by the binding of calcium in the intestine, thereby reducing its absorption; and (2) decreasing the clearance of calcium by the kidney. In the first approach, the use of cellulose phosphate has been popularized by Pak *et al.* (1974a). Use of this compound has reduced urine calcium excretion significantly and decreased stone episodes in hypercalciuric patients. Minimal side effects such as mild diarrhea have been observed in some patients taking this drug. No long-term studies have been reported, although in short-term studies, no effect of this drug on serum alkaline phosphatase or parathyroid hormone levels was observed. However, recent work has shown an increase in urinary oxalate after cellulose phosphate administration (Hayashi *et al.*, 1975).

In the second approach, the major group of drugs known to affect urine calcium handling are the thiazide diuretics. Administration of these agents to hypercalciuric patients consistently reduces urinary calcium excretion into the normal range. Long-term studies to date have shown a persistent effect of these agents (Yendt, 1970), with some side effects. However, hypercalcemia has been observed in some patients taking diuretics, and clinically inapparent metabolic bone disease or hyperparathyroidism has been found in many of these patients. At this point, it is difficult to state how frequently hypercalcemia may occur in the absence of either bone disease or hyperparathyroidism.

The mechanism of action of diuretics in lowering urinary calcium is not completely understood. The effect seems to be coupled to the effect of these agents on salt and water depletion and on contraction of extracellular fluid volume. A direct effect of diuretics on renal calcium reabsorptive mechanisms has not been shown. Regardless of the mechanism of action of these drugs, they appear to be a safe and effective means of lowering urinary calcium excretion and reducing the incidence of stone disease in patients with hypercalciuria.

11.4.2.2. Agents That Affect Oxalate Excretion

The effect of dietary calcium on urinary oxalate was discussed in Section 11.4.1.2. This indirect relationship of dietary calcium and urinary oxalate has been of most importance in the syndrome of enteric hyperoxaluria. Dietary calcium supplements have proved beneficial in reducing urinary oxalate excretion in patients with this syndrome (Earnest and Williams, unpublished observations). If changes in urinary oxalate within the normal range are critical in stone formation in patients with idiopathic stone disease, then dietary calcium supplements may be of great importance in controlling urinary oxalate in those patients. At the present time, however, this possibility must remain theoretical, and careful studies of varying calcium intake in patients with stone disease must be performed before calcium supplements can be recommended in this situation. Despite the nearly heretical nature of this suggestion, it should be emphasized that random use of low-calcium diets in patients with idiopathic stone disease should be discouraged until long-term studies are performed.

Pyridoxine has a variable effect on reduction of oxalate excretion in certain patients with primary hyperoxaluria (Gibbs and Watts, 1970), but no consistent effect has been observed in nonhyperoxaluric subjects. For this reason, pyridoxine cannot be recommended routinely in the treatment of patients with idiopathic stone disease. Several *in vitro* inhibitors of oxalate synthesis from glyoxylate have been studied (Smith *et al.*, 1972a) and shown to be effective, but their potential toxicity has precluded their use in patients with stone disease. Nevertheless, the importance of oxalate in determining the state of saturation of urine with respect to calcium oxalate requires a serious search for safe and effective *in vivo* inhibitors of oxalate synthesis. Development of such a drug could potentially eliminate stone formation in patients with recurrent calcium oxalate stones, regardless of cause.

11.4.2.3. Agents That Affect Urate Excretion

Allopurinol is the only drug known to reduce urinary uric acid without producing a concomitant increase in serum uric acid. This potent xanthine oxidase inhibitor has been useful in reducing stone episodes in hyperuricosuric uric acid stone-formers, and is the drug of choice in this setting. Toxicity results in skin rashes, cholestatic jaundice, and precipitation of a vasculitis-like syndrome. The proposed role of urate as a nucleus for the epitaxial growth of calcium oxalate in urine has led to the use of allopurinol in patients with idiopathic stone disease. The variable results achieved by such therapy (Coe and Kavalach, 1974) have raised questions about the validity of this theory of stone formation, and have emphasized the need for additional studies. (For additional discussion of uric acid metabolism, see Chapter 8)

11.4.2.4. Agents That Affect Cystine Excretion

No recent studies of agents that affect cystine excretion have appeared in the last few years. D-Penicillamine and its analogue, N-acetyl-D-penicillamine, by forming mixed urinary disulfides, have reduced stone formation and enabled cystine stones to be dissolved in cystinuric subjects.

Unfortunately, the very high incidence of hypersensitivity reactions with these drugs has limited their long-term use, although the N-acetyl analogue may be somewhat less toxic than the parent drug.

11.4.2.5. Inhibitors of Stone Formation

As noted in section 11.3.1, a large number of inhibitors of stone formation are known to exist, and they have received extensive study over the past decade. Three such inhibitors have been used effectively in the clinical setting: (1) phosphate (through its effect on increasing urinary pyrophosphate); (2) magnesium, in the form of magnesium oxide; and (3) the diphosphonates. A high phosphate intake (utilizing either potassium acid phosphate or mixed sodium and potassium phosphate salts to supply 1–2 g phosphorus) and magnesium oxide have both been shown to be effective inhibitors of new stone formation. Clinical experience with both forms of therapy has demonstrated successful inhibition of new stone formation in recurrent calcium oxalate stone-formers (Smith et al., 1973; Silver and Breudler, 1971).

The diphosphonates represent a group of entirely new inhibitors of calcium oxalate crystal formation. *In vitro*, they are extremely potent inhibitors (Fleisch and Monod, 1973; Pak *et al.*, 1975). Their effects are currently under study in patients with stone disease, but no long-term studies have been reported to date. Unfortunately, these compounds mobilize bone calcium, and long-term effects must be carefully evaluated before their routine use in patients with stone disease can be recommended.

11.5. Summary

The riddle of renal stone disease is gradually bening unraveled through the application of careful analytical and physicochemical techniques to the urine of patients with recurrent stone disease. As knowledge of pathophysiological mechanisms in stone formation expands, new rational therapeutic approaches can be developed. The development of new inhibitors of stone formation and the introduction of drugs that can lower the content of various urinary crystalloids should eventually relegate renal stone disease to its rightful place in antiquity.

Acknowledgment

This work was supported in part by U.S. Public Health Service Grant GM-19527 from the National Institutes of Health, Bethesda, Maryland.

References

Admirand, W. H., 1972, Hyperoxaluria and bowel disease, *N. Engl. J. Med.* **286**:1412.

Binder, H. J., 1974, Intestinal oxalate absorption, *Gastroenterology* **67**:441.

Briggs, M. H., Garcia-Webb, P., and Davies, P., 1973, Urinary oxalate and vitamin-C supplements, *Lancet* **2**:201.

Chadwick, V. S., Modha, K., and Dowling, R. H., 1972, Pathogenesis of secondary hyperoxaluria in ileal resection, *Gut* **13**:840.

Coe, F. L., and Kavalach, A. G., 1974, Hypercalciuria and hyperuricosuria in patients with calcium nephrolithiasis, *N. Engl. J. Med.* **291**:1344.

Coe, F. L., Canterbury, J. M., Firpo, J. J., and Reiss, E., 1973, Evidence for secondary hyperparathyroidism in idiopathic hypercalciuria, *J. Clin. Invest.* **52**:134.

Earnest, D. L., Johnson, G., Williams, H. E., and Admirand, W. H., 1974, Hyperoxaluria in patients with ileal resection: An abnormality in dietary oxalate absorption, *Gastroenterology* **66**:1114.

Fleisch, H., and Monod, A., 1973, A new technique for measuring aggregation of calcium oxalate crystals *in vitro:* Effect of urine, magnesium, pyrophosphate and diphosphonates, *in: Urinary Calculi. Recent Advances in Aetiology, Stone Structure and Treatment* (L. Cifuentes Delatte, A. Rapado, and A. Hodgkinson, eds.), pp. 53–56, S. Karger, Basel.

Gershoff, S. N., 1964, Vitamin B_6 and oxalate metabolism, *Vitam. Horm. N. Y.* **22**:581.

Gibbs, D., and Watts, R. W. E., 1970, The action of pyridoxine in primary hyperoxaluria, *Clin. Sci.* **38**:277.

Gutman, A. B., and Yü, T. F., 1968, Uric acid nephrolithiasis, *Amer. J. Med.* **45**:756.

Hayashi, Y., Kaplan, R. A., and Pak, C. Y., 1975, Effect of sodium cellulose phosphate therapy on crystallization of calcium oxalate in urine, *Metabolism* **24**:1273.

Hodgkinson, A., 1974, Relations between oxalic acid, calcium, magnesium, and creatinine excretion in normal men and male patients with calcium oxalate kidney stones, *Clin. Sci. Mol. Med.* **46**:357.

Marshall, R. W., and Barry, H., 1973, Urine saturation and the formation of calcium-containing renal calculi: The effects of various forms of therapy, *in: Urinary Calculi, Recent Advances in Aetiology, Stone Structure and Treatment* (L. Cifuentes Delatte, A. Rapado, and A. Hodgkinson, eds.), p. 164, S. Karger, Basel.

Marshall, R. W., Cochran, M., and Hodgkinson, A., 1972, Relationships between calcium and oxalic acid intake in the diet and their excretion in the urine of normal and renal-stone-forming subjects, *Clin. Sci.* **43**:91.

McIntyre, J. W. R., Russell, J. C., and Chambers, M., 1973, Oxalemia following methoxyflurane anesthesia in man, *Anesth. Analg. Cleveland* **52**:946.

Pak, C. Y. C., Delea, C., and Bartter, F. C., 1974a, Successful treatment of recurrent nephrolithiasis (calcium stones) with cellulose phosphate, *N. Engl. J. Med.* **290**:175.

Pak, C. Y. C., Ohata, M., Lawrence, E. C., and Snyder, W., 1974b, The hypercalciurias: Causes, parathyroid functions, and diagnostic criteria, *J. Clin. Invest.* **54**:387.

Pak, C. Y. C., Ohata, M., and Holt, K., 1975, Effect of diphosphonate on crystallization of calcium oxalate *in vitro*, *Kidney Int.* **7**:154.

Parry, M. F., and Wallach, R., 1974, Ethylene glycol poisoning, *Amer. J. Med.* **57**:143.

Richardson, K. E., and Liao, L. L., 1973, Formation of oxalate from hydroxypyruvate by isolated perfused rat liver, *Fed. Proc. Fed. Amer. Soc. Exp. Biol.* **32**:565.

Robertson, W. G., Peacock, M., and Knowles, C. F., 1972a, Calcium oxalate crystallisation in recurrent renal stone formers, *in: Urinary Calculi. Recent Advances in Aetiology, Stone Structure and Treatment* (L. Cifuentes Delatte, A. Rapado, and A. Hodgkinson, eds.), pp. 302–306, S. Karger, Basel.

Robertson, W. G., Peacock, M., and Nordin, B. E. C., 1972b, Measurement of activity products in urine from stone-formers and normal subjects, *in: Urolithiasis—Physical Aspects* (B. Finlayson, L. L. Hench, and L. H. Smith, eds.), pp. 79–96, National Academy of Sciences, Washington, D.C.

Robertson, W. G., Peacock, M., Marshall, R. W., Marshall, D. H., and Nordin, B. E. C., 1976, Saturation–inhibition index as a measure of the risk of calcium oxalate stone formation in the urinary tract, *N. Engl. J. Med.* **294**:249.

Shen, F., Baylink, D., Nielsen, R., Sherrara, D., and Haussler, M., 1976, A study of the pathogenesis of idiopathic hypercalciuria (IH), *Clin. Res.* **24**:157A.

Silver, L., and Brendler, H., 1971, Use of magnesium oxide in management of familial hyperoxaluria, *J. Urol.* **106**:274.

Smith, L. H., Jr., Bauer, R. L., Craig, J. C., and Williams, H. E., 1972a, Inhibition of oxalate synthesis: *In vitro* studies using analogues of oxalate and glycolate, *Biochem. Med.* **6**:317.

Smith, L. H., Fromm, H., and Hofmann, A. F., 1972b, Acquired hyperoxaluria, nephrolithiasis, and intestinal disease. Description of a syndrome, *N. Engl. J. Med.* **286**:1371.

Smith, L. H., Thomas, W. C., Jr., and Arnaud, C. D., 1973, Orthophosphate therapy in calcium renal lithiasis, *in: Urinary Calculi. Recent Advances in Aetiology, Stone Structure and Treatment* (L. Cifuentes Delatte, A. Rapado, and A. Hodgkinson, eds.), pp. 188–197, S. Karger, Basel.

Thier, S. O., and Segal, S., 1972, Cystinuria, *in: The Metabolic Basis of Inherited Disease* (J. B. Stanbury, J. B. Wyngaarden, and D. S. Fredrickson, eds.), Third Ed., pp. 1504–1519, McGraw-Hill Book Co., New York.

Williams, H. E., and Smith, L. H., Jr., 1971, Hyperoxaluria in L-glyceric aciduria: Possible pathogenic mechanism, *Science* **171**:390.

Williams, H. E., and Smith, L. H., Jr., 1976, Primary hyperoxaluria, *in: The Metabolic Basis of Inherited Disease* (J. B. Stanbury, J. B. Wyngaarden, and D. S. Fredrickson, eds.), Fourth Ed., McGraw-Hill Book Co., New York (in press).

Yendt, E. R., 1970, Renal calculi, *Can. Med. Assoc. J.* **102**:479.

Metabolism and Metabolic Actions of Ethanol

Charles S. Lieber

12.1. Metabolism of Ethanol

It has been known for a long time that metabolism of ethanol is faster in the fed than in the fasted state. The mechanism of this effect has recently been clarified by the definition of some rate-limiting factors in the oxidation of ethanol in a study by Meijer *et al.* (1975). Ethanol oxidation in liver via its main alcohol dehydrogenase (ADH) pathway (Fig. 1) is limited by the rate of reoxidation of cytosolic NADH, not by the activity of ADH. Reoxidation of cytosolic NADH requires transport of reducing equivalents into the mitochondria via substrate shuttles and reoxidation of the reducing equivalents by the mitochondrial respiratory chain. There have been few attempts to determine whether the rate-limiting factor in

CHARLES S. LIEBER • Section of Liver Disease and Nutrition, Veterans Administration Hospital, Bronx, New York 10468; Department of Medicine, Mt. Sinai School of Medicine of the City University of New York, New York, New York 10029.

ethanol oxidation is the activity of the shuttles in transporting reducing equivalents, or the actual oxidation of these reducing equivalents by the respiratory chain. Data from Meijer *et al.* (1975) now suggest that each of these factors may be a rate-limiting step in ethanol oxidation, depending on whether rats were fed or starved prior to the experiment. Ethanol oxidation was studied in isolated rat liver cells. In cells from starved animals, the addition of the components of the malate–aspartate shuttle, e. g., glutamate or malate, resulted in a marked stimulation of ethanol oxidation; this effect was sensitive to inhibition by the transaminase inhibitor cycloserine. These results indicate that the malate–aspartate cycle does not operate at full capacity. Addition of dihydroxyacetone stimulated ethanol uptake by 45% and caused a 3-fold increase in glycerol-3-phosphate content. Since ethanol uptake under these conditions is insensitive to cycloserine, it may be assumed that hydrogen transport into mitochondria occurs by the glycerol-3-phosphate cycle. The increase of ethanol oxidation by the addition of components of the malate–aspartate cycle (and its inhibition by transaminase inhibitors) or of the glycerol-3-phosphate cycle suggests that in the fasting state, the oxidation of ethanol by isolated liver cells is limited by the rate of transfer of reducing equivalents from the cytosol (where they are generated by ADH) to the mitochondria, and that this transport is itself regulated by the intracellular concentrations of the intermediates of the shuttles. Inhibition of the electron transport chain by the addition of amytal resulted in a significant reduction of ethanol oxidation, suggesting that the flux through the respiratory chain also regulates the rates of ethanol metabolism. However, the actual reoxidation of reducing equivalents by the respiratory chain is not limiting under these conditions, since uncoupling agents, which stimulate oxygen consumption, did not stimulate ethanol oxidation.

In liver cells isolated from fed rats, the rate of ethanol oxidation was about twice that in the fasting state. Since the concentrations of malate, aspartate, and glycerol-3-phosphate in liver cells from fed rats were higher than in cells from starved rats, it seems likely that the higher rate of ethanol oxidation in liver cells from fed rats was caused by increased activities of the hydrogen-transport cycles. In contrast to the finding in starved rats, malate addition was rather ineffective in stimulating ethanol oxidation in liver cells of fed rats, indicating that the hydrogen-transport cycles were not rate-limiting. Under these conditions, it might be expected that reoxidation of reducing equivalents would be rate-limiting in ethanol oxidation. Indeed, addition of uncoupling agents now resulted in stimulation of ethanol oxidation. Contrasting with its lack of effect in cells of starved animals, addition of carbonyl cyanide *t*-trifluromethoxyphenyl hydrazone (a potent uncoupler of oxidative phosphorylation) caused a large stimulation of ethanol oxidation, suggesting that in livers of fed rats, the mitochondrial reoxidation of NADH, whether transported from the cytosol or generated directly in the mitochondria by acetaldehyde dehydrogenase, is a rate-limiting step in ethanol oxidation.

In addition to the main ADH pathway, ethanol is also oxidized in the liver by the microsomal ethanol-oxidizing system (MEOS) (Fig. 1). The nature of this process has recently been clarified, particularly its differentiation from ethanol oxidation via catalase and H_2O_2 generated by microsomal NADPH oxidase. One method for differentiation of MEOS from catalase was by the exploitation of differences in substrate specificity. Higher aliphatic alcohols (such as butanol) are not substrates for catalase–H_2O_2 (Chance, 1947; Chance and Oshino, 1971). By contrast, Teschke *et al.* (1975a) found such long-chain alcohols to be excellent substrates for MEOS—both in total microsomes and in microsomal fractions obtained by DEAE cellulose column chromatography—and devoid of catalase. MEOS was also differentiated from catalase by its insensitivity to catalase inhibitors such as azide. Similar results were obtained in liver microsomes of "acatalatic" mice, which contained a heat-labile catalase (Teschke *et al.*, 1975b). Differentiation of MEOS from NADPH oxidase activity was achieved *in vivo* by CCl_4 administration, which decreased the activity of the former, but not that of the latter. Conversely, phenobarbital treatment enhanced the specific activity of NADPH oxidase, and not that of MEOS (Hasumura *et al.*, 1975b). Both after chronic and after acute ethanol treatment, the activity of MEOS paralleled that of cytochrome P-450, particularly its cyanide-binding subform 1; it therefore appears that the MEOS activity may involve a mechanism akin to that of the cytochrome P-450–dependent drug detoxification in microsomes, possibly utilizing, at least in part, a different type of cytochrome P-450. The significance of this MEOS pathway results from the fact that chronic ethanol consumption produces an increase in its activity, which may contribute to the hypermetabolic state associated with alcoholism (see below); it may also explain, at least in part, the acceleration in ethanol metabolism after chronic ethanol feeding.

That chronic ethanol consumption may be associated with accelerated rates of ethanol clearance of the blood has been known for a long time. The mechanism of this effect, however, is still the subject of some debate. To elucidate possible biochemical changes involved, Khanna *et al.* (1975) fed ethanol as part of a totally liquid diet according to a modification of the procedure originally devised by Lieber *et al.* (1963, 1965). The lactate/pyruvate (L/P) and β-hydroxybutyrate/acetoacetate (β-HB/AcAc) ratios in the livers were determined under different experimental conditions. As expected, these ratios were significantly higher in the alcohol-fed animals than in the controls, when the animals were allowed to eat their respective diets up to the time of sacrifice. However, the most interesting

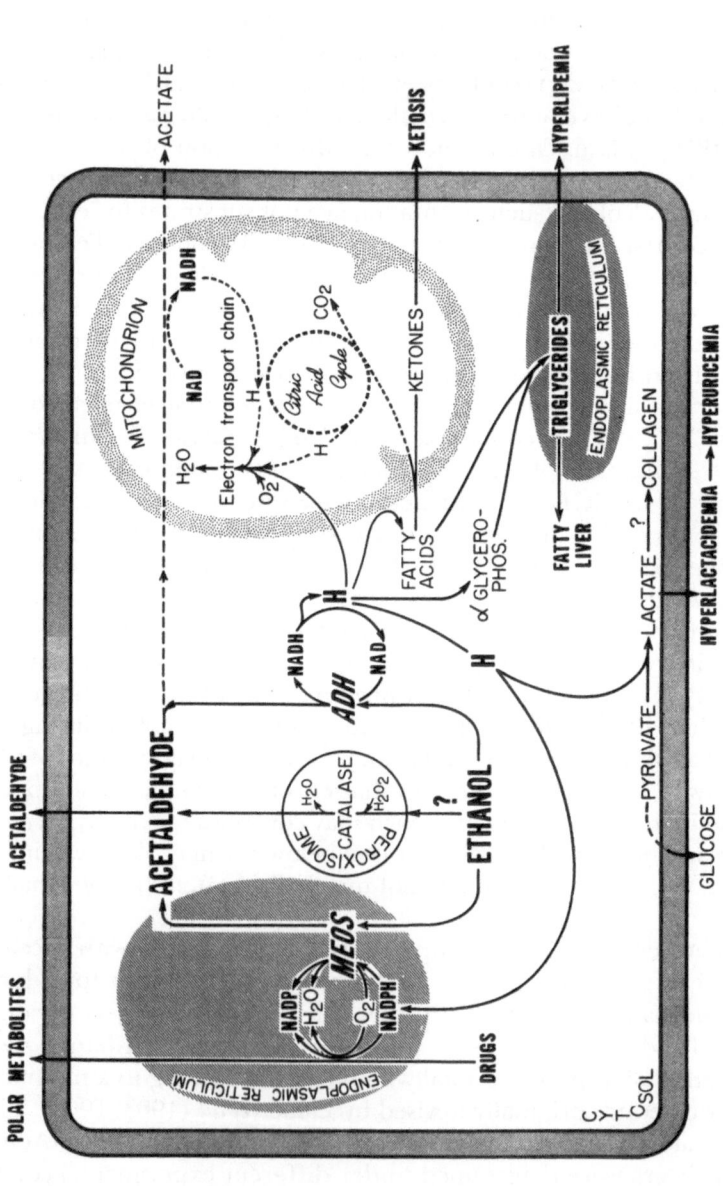

Fig. 1. Oxidation of ethanol in the hepatocyte and schematic representation of its link to: (ADH) alcohol dehydrogenase; (MEOS) microsomal ethanol-oxidizing system; (NAD) nicotinamide adenine dinucleotide; (NADH) nicotinamide adenine dinucleotide, reduced form; (NADP) nicotinamide adenine dinucleotide phosphate; (NADPH) nicotinamide adenine dinucleotide phosphate, reduced form. (From Lieber and DeCarli, 1976.)

results were obtained when the rats were studied after 24–48-hr discontinuation of the alcohol-containing diet and when an acute dose of ethanol was given intraperitoneally 1–3 hr prior to the sacrifice period under these conditions, the β-HB/AcAc ratio was significantly higher in the controls. The authors conclude that their results are compatible with "an adaptive increase in mitochondrial reoxidation of NADH in the chronic alcohol group," a change that could explain both the accelerated rates of ethanol metabolism and the difference in the redox state, although the authors admit that the possibility of a change due to alcohol withdrawal cannot be excluded. The attenuation of the redox change produced by acute alcohol administration in animals fed ethanol chronically essentially confirms the results of Domschke *et al.* (1974), which showed that an acute dose of ethanol orally administered causes much less extensive redox change in rats chronically fed ethanol than in their controls. Although the results were comparable, interpretation of the findings differed. Instead of increased NADH reoxidation by the mitochondria, hypothesized by Khanna *et al.* (1975), Domschke *et al.* (1974) postulated that the increased MEOS activity may be responsible, since MEOS is associated with NADPH utilization and in view of the fact that NADP/NADPH and NAD/NADH ratios are linked (Veech *et al.*, 1969). Indeed, if increased NADH reoxidation by the mitochondria were the only biochemical change involved, it would be difficult to understand how this could explain both the accelerated rates of metabolism and the altered redox change. The assumed increased metabolism via the ADH pathway would result in increased production of NADH, which, however, would be offset by the comparable increased NADH reoxidation postulated to have caused the accelerated ethanol oxidation in the first place. With the postulated ADH mechanism, the increase in NADH reoxidation should indeed be equivalent to the increase in NADH production via the ADH pathway and not exceed it, since NADH reoxidation is rate-limiting in the ADH pathway. Thus, one would expect as an overall result merely accelerated ethanol metabolism in ethanol-fed rats, but a redox potential comparable in ethanol-fed and control rats when both are given the same ethanol load. If, however, a non-ADH pathway (such as MEOS) is involved after chronic ethanol feeding, this might explain both the accelerated ethanol metabolism and the lesser redox change, since the accelerated ethanol metabolism would be secondary to increased activity of a non-ADH pathway, which, instead of generating NADH, actually consumes reducing equivalents. This interpretation is consistent with the findings that an acceleration in ethanol metabolism after chronic ethanol feeding persists even after the administration of an ADH inhibitor such as pyrazole (Lieber and DeCarli, 1972). However, this interpretation was recently questioned by Kalant *et al.* (1975). These authors observed that within the first few hours after ethanol and pyrazole administration, blood ethanol levels remained unchanged. From this lack of fall of blood ethanol levels, the authors concluded that pyrazole had inhibited ethanol metabolism completely, and therefore that the ADH pathway does account fully for the metabolism of alcohol. It must be pointed out, however, that during the study period, ethanol absorption had not been completed, and therefore that continuous absorption of ethanol could have offset any metabolism of alcohol due to the non-ADH pathway. The authors also assume the disappearance of blood ethanol at high levels to be linear, whereas inspection of their figures clearly shows a nonlinear disappearance similar to the one observed by others (Lieber and DeCarli, 1972). Moreover, analysis (from their figures) of the ethanol disappearance rate in the "MEOS" range (between 300 and 100 mg/100 ml) reveals a K_m value for ethanol similar to that obtained for MEOS *in vitro* (about 10 mM), rather than the low K_m value of 0.78 that the authors find when they include in their analysis data obtained at low ethanol concentrations, at which only the ADH pathway is fully saturated (since ADH has a low K_m for ethanol of about 1 mM). Although interpretation of the data may vary, the actual results are thus comparable to those previously published by other authors. The consensus also includes ADH: Kalant *et al.* (1975) now find that ADH activity does not increase after chronic ethanol feeding. This finally settles a long-standing debate kindled by several past studies (Hawkins *et al.*, 1966; Hawkins and Kalant, 1972) that reported liver ADH activity to be increased after chronic ethanol consumption, a finding that could not be verified by other investigators (Lieber and DeCarli, 1970; Singlevich and Barboriak, 1971; Raskin and Sokoloff, 1972).

Additional, albeit indirect, evidence in favor of the operation, *in vivo*, of a non-ADH pathway for ethanol metabolism can be derived from a study of Guynn and Pieklik (1975), who demonstrated dependence on dose of the acute effects of ethanol on liver metabolism *in vivo*. Ethanol was given to rats intraperitoneally in doses of 0.69, 1.7, and 3.0 g/kg. The liver was freeze-clamped 120 min after injection. Each group showed a significantly different pattern of metabolites, redox states, and phosphorylation potentials, although the rate of ethanol disappearance, at least between the two highest-dose groups, was not significantly different. The mitochondrial free $[NAD^+]/[NADH]$ ratios and the cytoplasmic free $[NADP^+]/[NADPH]$ ratio were paradoxically most reduced with the lowest dose of ethanol, and became progressively more oxidized with increasing dose. In a somewhat different pattern, the phosphorylation potential $([ATP]/[ADP]P_i)$ remained at the control level in the low-dose group, but was significantly elevated in the two higher-dose groups. Although these complex results may not be explained completely by any one hypothesis, the authors conclude that "the increasing oxidation of the cytoplasmic free [NADP$^+$]/[NADPH] ratio and the mitochondrial free [NAD$^+$]/ [NADH] ratios from the lowest to highest doses in the current study is compatible with a significant *in vivo* contribution by the microsomal ethanol-oxidizing system," and that "even though the important factors operative *in vivo* are yet to be resolved, it can at least be concluded from the differential effects of dose of the current study that the rate of NADH production alone cannot explain the findings." Thus, the evidence that has accumulated over the last few years clearly indicates that the ADH pathway alone cannot explain all effects of ethanol, especially at high concentrations and particularly after chronic ethanol consumption.

12.2. The Hypermetabolic State Produced by Ethanol

Several studies showed that both in rats (Mitchell, 1935; Lieber *et al.*, 1965) and in man (Pirola and Lieber, 1972), gain in body weight is significantly lower with ethanol than with isocaloric amounts of carbohydrate. One interpretation of this lack of weight gain with ethanol compared to other sources of dietary calories is the possibility that chronic alcohol intake increases the energy requirements of the body. If this were the case, it should be reflected in a higher rate of oxygen consumption. It was indeed found in rats fed alcohol as part of their total liquid diet that oxygen consumption was slightly but significantly higher than that of animals pair-fed the isocaloric diet containing carbohydrates instead of ethanol (Pirola and Lieber, 1976).

Among the many mechanisms that could be postulated to account for an inefficient use of ethanol calories, two have gained experimental support recently: one involves the energy wastage secondary to an induction of liver microsomal pathways; the other one supports the concept that chronic ethanol consumption may result in increased utilization of ATP by the Na$^+$–K$^+$-activated ATPase activity.

Efficient utilization of the calories of ethanol would be anticipated from a consideration of its major metabolic pathway, which involves the hepatic cytosolic enzyme alcohol dehydrogenase (ADH):

$$\left.\begin{array}{l} CH_3CH_2OH \\ \\ ADH \\ \\ CH_3CHO \end{array}\right) \left(\begin{array}{l} NAD^+ \\ \\ NADH \\ + \\ H^+ \end{array}\right. \xrightarrow[\text{electron transport chain}]{\overset{3\ ATP}{\uparrow}} \left(\begin{array}{l} H_2O \\ \\ \tfrac{1}{2}O_2 \end{array}\right.$$

From an energy point of view, this process appears to be an economical one, because the associated production of NADH supplies the electron transport chain with hydrogen equivalents, yielding high-energy phosphate bonds. As noted before, however, recent studies indicate the presence of a distinct hepatic microsomal ethanol-oxidizing system (MEOS) (Lieber and DèCarli, 1970). The exact quantitative significance of the enzyme system *in vivo* remains uncertain, but studies indicate that it could normally involve 20–25% of the oxidation of ethanol (Lieber and DeCarli, 1972). The potential importance of this in the body's caloric balance lies in the fact that in contrast to the ADH pathway, MEOS results in the loss of chemical energy from both the substrate and the cofactor (NADPH), without any known effective coupling to ATP synthesis:

$$CH_3CH_2OH + NADPH + H^+ + O_2 \longrightarrow CH_3CHO + NADP^+ + 2H_2O$$

Presumably, the loss of chemical energy is dissipated as heat and (insofar as it exceeds the body's thermoregulatory needs) represents an inefficient use of ingested calories. It is of interest that similar considerations apply to the oxidation of other drugs and endogenous substrates (such as steroids) by hepatic microsomal drug-metabolizing enzymes. These oxidations have the general formula:

$$RH + NADPH + H^+ + O_2 \rightarrow ROH + NADP^+ + H_2O$$

The proposed hypothesis (Pirola and Lieber, 1976) is that the inefficiency of microsomal drug-metabolizing enzymes could be of quantitative significance in the energy balance of the body during the repeated intake of drugs, especially ethanol. This view is supported by the following considerations:

1. The liver normally accounts for approximately one-fifth of the body's total oxygen consumption.
2. Hepatic microsomal enzymes are induced by the repeated intake of ethanol and other drugs.
3. Hepatic microsomal enzymes are responsible for the oxidation of numerous endogenous substrates as well as xenobiotic agents.
4. During alcohol ingestion, ethanol becomes the major fuel of hepatic metabolism, without any known mechanism of storage or of feedback control.
5. Ethanol can account for 50% or more of the caloric intake of some persons.

The hypothesis is in keeping with other animal studies in which metabolic rates were increased by the administration of ethanol and barbiturates in doses known to induce hepatic microsomal enzymes. Thus, pretreatment with barbiturates enhanced oxygen consumption in rats tested under various conditions: in the absence of drugs, during hexobarbital anesthesia, and after the administration of aminopyrine (Pirola and Lieber, 1975).

There are, of course, many metabolic pathways in the body that are not effectively linked to ATP synthesis. These pathways contribute to the net wastage of calories to give a less than optimal overall efficiency of the body. In this respect, the microsomal drug-metabolizing enzyme system is unique in its extraordinary versatility and in its ability to be induced by a wide variety of agents.

Another major theory for the explanation of the hypermetabolic state produced by ethanol is an increased utilization of ATP by the Na^+-K^+-activated ATPase after chronic ethanol feeding. Israel et al. (1975b) reported that in liver slices, ouabain, an inhibitor of the Na^+-K^+-activated ATPase, can completely block the extra ethanol metabolism elicited by chronic ethanol treatment. Dinitrophenol increased the rate of ethanol metabolism in the livers of the treated animals only in the presence of ouabain. Administration of thyroxine led to an increase in the rate of ethanol metabolism when measured both in vitro and in vivo. This effect was biphasic; activation occurred only with low doses of thyroxine, but disappeared after administration of larger doses. Alcohol dehydrogenase activity in the livers of the animals treated with large doses of thyroxine was found to be significantly reduced. With the doses used (50–1000 $\mu g/$ kg), thyroxine also increased the rate of oxygen consumption as measured in liver slices. However, a biphasic effect did not occur; near-maximum activation on the rate of oxygen consumption occurred with low doses of thyroxine (100 $\mu g/kg$). Oxygen consumption was also found to be increased in the liver of animals chronically treated with ethanol. A maximal effect was produced after 18–21 days of treatment. For both ethanol- and thyroxine-treated animals, an increased rate of oxygen consumption occurred with a concomitant loss of dinitrophenol effect. Mitochondrial α-glycerophosphate oxidase was found to be increased in the livers of animals treated with ethanol or with thyroxine. It was concluded that chronic treatment with ethanol produces many changes in the liver that are similar to those produced by thyroid hormones. Indeed, the hypermetabolic effect produced in the liver by chronic administration of ethanol was markedly reduced, but not completely suppressed, by thyroidectomy (Bernstein et al., 1975). Thus, the hypermetabolic condition that occurs in the livers of animals chronically treated with ethanol may be similar in some aspects to that found in the livers of animals treated with thyroid hormones, in which the hypermetabolic state also appears to be associated with an increased hydrolysis of ATP by the Na^+–K^+-ATPase system (Ismail-Beigi and Edelman, 1970, 1971).

It is also known that ethanol administration leads to an increase in the release of epinephrine from the adrenal glands, both in animals and in man (Klingman and Goodall, 1957; Perman, 1958, 1960, 1961; Anton, 1965; Ogata et al., 1971). Epinephrine is known to produce a calorigenic effect, which appears to be similar to the one produced by thyroid hormones (Harrison, 1964; Himms-Hagen, 1967; Gale, 1973). Moreover, it is known that administration of thyroid hormones produces a marked supersensitivity to many of the actions produced by norepinephrine and epinephrine (Harrison, 1964). The calorigenic effects produced by ethanol in the liver, as measured in liver slices, could be reproduced by a single large dose of epinephrine (Bernstein et al., 1975). Oxygen consumption by liver slices of animals given a 2-mg/kg dose of epinephrine bitartrate increased by 40–50%. In these livers, all the extra oxygen consumption, but not the basal respiration, could be abolished by ouabain, an inhibitor of the sodium pump. Dinitrophenol did not affect the respiratory rate in the livers of ephinephrine-treated animals, but markedly increased that in controls. In the livers of treated animals, the activating effect of dinitrophenol could be recovered in the presence of ouabain. The calorigenic effect of epinephrine in the liver was found to be completely abolished by phentolamine (an α-adrenergic blocker), but was not modified by D,L-propranolol (a β-adrenergic blocker).

The data cited above raise the question whether the hypermetabolic state found in the livers of ethanol-treated animals could also be mediated by catecholamines. That this could be the case is further suggested by the fact that adrenalectomy completely abolished, and pretreatment of the animals with phentolamine markedly decreased, the production of the ethanol-induced hypermetabolic state of the liver.

The theory that increased utilization of ATP by the Na^+–K^+-activated ATPase (and the resulting lowering of the phosphorylation potential) is responsible for the metabolic adaptation that occurs in rats after chronic ethanol treatment, and that a situation develops that is very similar to that found after administration of thyroid hormones or epinephrine, is intriguing. Certainly, the influence of ethanol consumption on hormonal actions deserves further investigation. To date, there have been few studies performed to confirm these observations, and to clear up some inconsistencies concerning the theory in connection with thyroxine effects, α-glycerophosphate changes, and conflicting data on ATPase activity.

In some studies in which the animals were pretreated with thyroxine for several days (Ylikahri and Mäenpää, 1968; Ylikahri, 1970), or even a single dose 24 hr before the experiment (Choisy and Potron, 1972), the rate of ethanol metabolism was found to be increased. Increases of up to 100% in humans with hyperthyroidism have also been reported recently (Ugarte *et al.*, 1975). However, other workers have found no effect or only slight inhibition after thyroxine pretreatment (Stokes and Lasley, 1967; Rawat and Lundquist, 1968; Hillbom and Pikkarainen, 1970; Hillbom, 1971). Goldberg *et al.* (1960) found that the rate of ethanol metabolism was more than doubled by triiodothyronine in conditions in which the hormone was administered almost simultaneously with the test dose of ethanol. These experiments are difficult to interpret, due to the well-known fact that the calorigenic effect of thyroid hormones is produced after a lag period of several hours or days (Tata, 1964; Hoch, 1974). In fact, no effect of triiodothyronine on the rate of ethanol metabolism was reported to occur by other authors using this procedure (Newman and Smith, 1959; Kalant *et al.*, 1962; Kinard *et al.*, 1962; Smith *et al.*, 1963).

Some of these discrepancies were attributed to the fact that higher levels of thyroxine inhibit ADH activity. In particular, Israel *et al.* (1975b) attribute the lack of increased ethanol metabolism after large doses of thyroxine under their experimental conditions to this ADH inhibition. It must be pointed out, however, that in another study carried out by the same group (Videla *et al.*, 1975), the ethanol disappearance rate *in vivo* was increased by cold acclimation, even though liver ADH activity was reduced to the same extent as after thyroxine (Israel *et al.*, 1975b). These results are consistent with the generally held view that normally, the rates of NADH reoxidation, rather than the ADH activity, are rate-limiting for ethanol oxidation via the ADH pathway. Thus, a moderate depression of ADH activity should not prevent the increase in ethanol metabolism, and this concept was verified in the case of cold acclimation (Videla *et al.*, 1975). The increased oxygen consumption but lack of acceleration in ethanol metabolism found by Israel *et al.* (1975b) is thus unexplained. Despite this discrepancy, the authors postulate that the same mechanism, namely, increased hydrolysis of ATP by the sodium pump system, is responsible for the increased oxygen consumption and ethanol metabolism in the livers of cold-acclimated animals, after chronic ethanol treatment and in hyperthyroidism.

Other discrepancies concern the changes of mitochondrial α-glycerophosphate oxidase: it was found increased by Israel *et al.* (1975b) after chronic ethanol feeding, whereas others found no change (Pilstrom and Kiessling, 1972), or even found decreases (Rubin *et al.*, 1972). It must be pointed out, however, that the experimental conditions were not identical; whereas Israel *et al.* (1975b) used a low-fat diet in association with ethanol administration, other studies were conducted with ethanol and a diet containing an amount of fat comparable to that of human consumption. As a consequence, under the conditions used by Israel *et al.* (1975b), ethanol consumption did not result in liver changes comparable to those seen in human alcoholic liver injury; for instance, no fatty liver was observed. Under conditions that mimic the clinical situation in development of fatty liver, chronic ethanol consumption was not found to be associated with increased ATPase activity (Gordon, in press), and the increase in the rates of ethanol metabolism after chronic ethanol consumption could not be abolished by ouabain (Cederbaum *et al.*, 1976), which indicates that the theory of enhanced ATPase activity may not be applicable to the situation that normally prevails after chronic alcohol consumption. One must also bear in mind that thyroid hormones may interact with the effects of ethanol in ways other than those postulated by Israel *et al.* (1975b). For instance, a single oral dose of ethanol (3g/kg) caused death within 12 hr after administration to rats pretreated with triiodothyronine (0.15 mg/kg per day on 6 successive days) (Hillbom and Pösö, 1975). However, pretreatment with the ADH inhibitor 4-methylpyrazole did not affect the mortality rate or the time course of mortality after ethanol administration in the triiodothyronine-intoxicated rats. It was concluded that tissue sensitivity in the CNS to high ethanol concentrations *per se* is increased in the hyperthyroid state, and that metabolism of ethanol was not involved in the observed effect.

12.3. Effects of Alcohol on the Liver and Development of Alcoholic Liver Injury

The long-standing debate whether the liver injury so commonly observed in the alcoholic is due to malnutrition rather than to alcohol *per se* was rekindled by a report of Patek *et al.* (1975). In this epidemiological study of 304 alcoholic patients, alcohol intake and dietary habits were evaluated. There were 195 patients with hepatic cirrhosis, 40 precirrhotics, and 69 noncirrhotics. By history, alcohol contributed 50–58% of total calories. Two-thirds of the patients had been drinking for more than 20 years. The duration and degree of alcoholic abuse were comparable in all three groups. The dietary intake, however, differed; over the 2-year period preceding the presenting illness, the noncirrhotics had higher food caloric intake and higher protein intake than the cirrhotics. The authors conclude that this study incriminates dietary factors in the pathogenesis of cirrhosis. This type of retrospective study, however, is complicated by the difficulty in differentiating cause and effect. It is well known that complications of severe liver disease, particularly cirrhosis, can by themselves be reasons for poor dietary intake. It is therefore not clear whether the differences in dietary intake between cirrhotics and noncirrhotics is the cause of, rather than a consequence of, that disease.

The etiological role of alcohol *per se* (in the absence of dietary deficiency) in the pathogensis of alcoholic liver injury was assessed in an experimental study carried out in the baboon. The study, by Lieber *et al.* (1975), reproduced in experimental animals the sequential development of all the liver lesions seen in the human alcoholic: in 15 baboons fed ethanol, all developed fatty liver, 5 progressed to mild hepatitis, and 5 had cirrhosis. Maintenance of a nutritionally adequate regimen despite the intake of inebriating amounts of ethanol (50% of total calories) was achieved by incorporation of the ethanol in a totally liquid diet. On ethanol withdrawal, signs of physical dependence, such as seizures and tremors, developed. Ultrastructural changes of the mitochondria and the endoplasmic reticulum were already present at the fatty liver stage, and persisted throughout the hepatitis and cirrhosis. The lesions were similar to those observed in alcoholics (including the inflammation and the central sclerosis), and differed from the alterations produced by choline and protein deficiencies. At the fatty liver stage, some "adaptive" increases in the activity of microsomal enzymes (aniline hydroxylase and MEOS) were observed, but these tended to disappear with the development of hepatitis and cirrhosis. Fat accumulation was also much more pronounced in the animals with the hepatitis, as compared with those with simple fatty liver (an 18-fold, compared with a 3–4-fold, increase in liver triglycerides). The demonstration that these lesions can develop despite an adequate diet indicates that in addition to correction of the nutritional status, control of alcohol intake is mandatory for the management of patients with alcoholic liver injury, and that ethanol *per se* must be considered a direct etiological agent in the pathogenesis of alcoholic liver injury, independent of dietary factors. This does not preclude, however, that dietary factors may contribute to and potentiate the alcohol effect, which had previously been shown to be the case in rats (Lieber *et al.*, 1969). No similar studies are available for man.

Because a hypermetabolic state, resembling that produced by thyroid hormones, exists in the livers of animals treated chronically with ethanol (see above), it was proposed that this alteration produces in the centrilobular zone of the liver a relative hypoxia that, if severe enough, leads to cellular death and to the production of hepatitis (Israel *et al.*, 1975a). Rats consuming ethanol for 30 days, in a nutritionally adequate diet, and exposed to reduced oxygen tensions for only 6 hr, did indeed develop histological and biochemical evidence of hepatocellular necrosis and inflammatory lesions confined to the centrilobular zone. The severity was proportional to the degree of hypoxia. Pair-fed (nonalcohol) controls showed no such lesions. Treatment of the animals with propylthiouracil for 3–10 days abolished the hypermetabolic state of the liver in ethanol-consuming animals, and drastically reduced the histological and biochemical effects of hypoxia in them. It was proposed that these findings may have implications for the pathogenesis and treatment of alcoholic hepatitis in man. However, no evidence is given that hypoxia of a degree comparable to that produced experimentally actually occurs in alcoholic liver injury. Moreover, it is possible that in the experiments of Israel *et al.* (1975a), hypoxia and ethanol have merely additive injurious effects on the liver and that the beneficial action of propylthiouracil may simply result from a nonspecific decrease in oxygen requirement, thereby diminishing the adverse effects of hypoxia. To what extent the involved hypoxic mechanism plays a role in the pathogenesis of alcoholic liver injury in man remains to be established. In baboons fed ethanol and which developed alcoholic liver injury, no evidence was found for hypoxemia in the hepatic vein, both after acute and chronic ethanol administration (Shaw *et al.*, 1976).

12.4. Interaction of Ethanol and Lipid Metabolism in Liver and Intestine

Since it was originally proposed (Lieber and Davidson, 1962), the concept that a number of the hepatic as well as metabolic effects of ethanol can be attributed to the change in the NADH/NAD ratio associated with the oxidation of ethanol has been shown to have widespread applicability, including enhanced lipid synthesis and decreased lipid oxidation. The latter can be viewed as the replacement of lipid, the normal fuel of the liver, by ethanol. Recent studies have indicated that in addition to decreased lipid oxidation resulting from inhibition of citric acid cycle activity secondary to the enhanced NADH/NAD ratio directly associated with the oxidation of ethanol, chronic ethanol ingestion also results in alterations of lipid metabolism that persist beyond the presence of ethanol. Rats were fed ethanol as part of a totally liquid diet (DeCarli and Lieber, 1967), and their mitochondria were isolated. It was found by Cederbaum *et al.* (1975a) that chronic ethanol consumption resulted in decreased fatty acid oxidation by the mitochondria, as evidenced by a reduction in oxygen uptake and CO_2 production associated with the oxidation of fatty acids. The State 3 (ADP-stimulated) rate of oxygen uptake was depressed to a greater extent than the State 4, or the uncoupler-stimulated, rate; the respiratory control ratio was also decreased. Therefore, one site of action of chronic ethanol feeding is on oxidative phosphorylation.

The reduction in fatty acid oxidation, in general, was not due to an effect on the activation or translocation of fatty acids into the mitochondria. There was no effect by ethanol feeding on the activity of palmitoyl

CoA synthetase, whereas carnitine palmitoyltransferase activity was increased. Total oxidation of fatty acids to Co_2 was depressed by chronic ethanol intoxication because of effects on oxidative phosphorylation or the citric acid cycle (or both). Neither nutritional deficiency, cofactor depletion, nor the presence of ethanol *in vitro* explains these effects. The impairment of mitochondrial oxidation of the fatty acids to CO_2 produced by chronic ethanol consumption may in turn contribute to the development of the fatty liver, in addition to the alteration in lipid metabolism resulting from the altered NAD/NADH ratio directly associated with the oxidation of ethanol in the liver. Although chronic ethanol consumption led to persistent reduction in the mitochondrial oxidation of fatty acids to CO_2, the oxidation of fatty acids to acetyl-CoA was not decreased by chronic ethanol consumption. This conclusion was reached with the use of an artificial system (formazan production) to study β-oxidation in the absence of the electron transport chain. In the presence of fluorocitrate, which inhibits citric acid cycle activity, ketogenesis and formazan production were increased by chronic ethanol consumption. A relative increase in ketogenesis may actually have been present, which in turn may play a role in explaining, at least in part, the previous observation that ethanol consumption is associated with an increase in circulating levels of ketone bodies (Lefevre *et al.*, 1972).

Not only does chronic ethanol consumption affect lipid metabolism, but the lipid content of the diet also influences the degree of the changes observed after chronic ethanol administration. In a study by Joly and Hetu (1975), female Sprague-Dawley rats were fed nutritionally adequate liquid diets without or with ethanol, at two ethanol concentrations, 5 and 6% (vol/wt). In other animals, various degrees of caloric deficiency were obtained by replacing ethanol by water in one animal of a pair. Ethanol given as a 5% (wt/vol) solution with high amounts of dietary fat increased cytochrome P-450, the activities of NADPH-cytochrome P-450 reductase, benzphetamine demethylase, aniline hydroxylase, and the MEOS. When ethanol was given with a low-fat diet as a 5% (wt/vol) solution, the increase in cytochrome P-450 and P-450 reductase was much less than with a high-fat diet; other microsomal enzyme activities, however, were enhanced to a level comparable to that achieved with the high-fat diet. When ethanol was administered as a 6% (wt/vol) solution in the presence of a low-fat diet, caloric deficiency was observed, and no significant induction of any parameter except aniline hydroxylation could be found. When it was given with a high-fat diet, in spite of caloric deficiency and lower ethanol ingestion, cytochrome P-450 and P-450 reductase activities were enhanced, while that of the MEOS was not. It is concluded that ethanol is associated with a greater induction of drug-metabolizing enzyme activities in the high-fat model than in the low-fat model. Similar results were reported in part in a preliminary study by DeCarli *et al.* (1972).

There are conflicting reports concerning the effects of ethanol on intestinal lipid metabolism. It has now been clarified that the action depends on both the duration and dose of ethanol administration. To assess the effects of ethanol on intestinal lipid metabolism, fatty acid oxidation and triacylglycerol synthesis were measured in intestinal slices incubated with ethanol (Baraona *et al.*, 1975). Ethanol, when used in concentrations likely to be achieved in the upper jejunum after moderate drinking, inhibited both palmitate and acetate oxidation and CO_2 production and triacylglycerol synthesis, whereas it enhanced the esterification of fatty acid with ethanol. The concentrations required for the inhibitory effect were much higher than those needed to saturate enzyme systems known to participate in ethanol oxidation.

In vivo administration of ethanol-containing diets produced persistent changes of the intestinal slices with respect to fatty acid oxidation and triacylglycerol synthesis. Acute intragastric administration of ethanol (3 g/kg) 1 hr prior to sacrifice inhibited both processes in slices obtained from the jejunum, but not in those derived from the ileum. By contrast, chronic ethanol feeding increased the ability for fatty acid oxidation and triacylglycerol synthesis both in the jejunum and in the ileum. This stimulatory effect was associated with significant enhancement of palmitoyl-CoA synthetase activity, suggesting increased fatty acid activation.

The inhibition of high ethanol concentrations of intestinal fatty acid oxidation and of triacylglycerol synthesis probably reflects epithelial cell damage; by contrast, prolonged administration of ethanol results in a persistent enhancement of lipid metabolism, which may reflect the presence of a different cell population in the intestine. The effects of ethanol on intestinal lymph formation and fat absorption were opposite to the changes observed in intestinal lipid metabolism. Indeed, Baraona and Lieber (1975) found that the acute administration of ethanol, either in lipid emulsions administered intraduodenally or in liquid diets given by gastric tube, increased the flow of intestinal lymph and the output of proteins and dietary lipids into the lymph, mainly in the first hour after administration. During this time, the intraduodenal administration of ethanol (0.75 g/kg body weight), without exogenous lipids, increased the flow of lymph without changing the lymph lipid output. Stimulation of the lymph flow with neostigmine or by increasing the fluid load also enhanced the output of lymph proteins and the transport of exogenous lipids from the intestinal lumen into the lymph. Contrasting with these acute effects of ethanol, chronic administration of ethanol for 3–4 weeks as part of a total liquid diet resulted in a reduced capacity to respond to the acute ethanol challenge. Indeed, the administration of an acute ethanol dose to rats chronically fed alcohol moderately increased the lymph flow, but did not change the output of dietary lipids. Furthermore, rats chronically fed alcohol responded to a dietary challenge devoid of ethanol with increases in both lymph flow and dietary lipid output that were not as great as those of pair-fed controls. Thus, acute ethanol administration has a marked stimulatory effect both on the formation of intestinal lymph and on the transport of dietary fat. By contrast, chronic ethanol feeding inhibits these acute effects of ethanol, and, in addition, appears to have moderate inhibitory effects on lipid absorption. Decreased absorption is not only confined to lipids, but also affects calcium metabolism. In a study by Krawitt (1975), the effects of chronic ethanol ingestion on duodenal calcium transport were investigated in rats ingesting 20% ethanol. Calcium transport was inhibited by ethanol ingestion, and the defect could not be reversed by vitamin D or 25-hydroxycholecalciferol administration. Ethanol ingestion by vitamin D–deficient rats did not further suppress transport activity, nor did it interfere with an increase in transport induced by vitamin D. The levels of intestinal calcium-binding activity were not suppressed. The results suggest that ethanol interferes with calcium transport by a mechanism at least in part independent of the vitamin D pathway. It was also found, in confirmation of previous findings of Baraona *et al.* (1974) that intestinal alkaline phosphatase activity was suppressed by chronic ethanol ingestion, as compared to ad-lib-fed control animals. This probably represents a non-specific "corrosive" effect of chronic ethanol ingestion on the intestinal mucosa, resulting in a shortening of the intestinal villi, with a decrease of those enzyme activities associated primarily with the tip of the villi (Baraona *et al.*, 1974).

12.5. Acetaldehyde—Its Metabolism and Metabolic Effects

The year 1975 has witnessed a revival of interest in acetaldehyde, the first metabolite of the oxidation of ethanol in the liver. Although the potential toxicity of acetaldehyde has been recognized for a number of years (Truitt and Duritz, 1966), little was known about blood acetaldehyde levels after alcohol consumption. Recently, Korsten *et al.* (1975) showed a difference between the blood acetaldehyde levels of alcoholic and nonalcoholic subjects after comparable ethanol challenges. The blood acetaldehyde and ethanol levels were measured in 11 subjects (6 chronic alcoholic and 5 nonalcoholic controls) after alcohol had been given intravenously. Despite a progressive fall in blood ethanol concentration over a range of 54–33 mM, acetaldehyde did not decrease in any of the 11 subjects. The mean acetaldehyde plateau level was significantly ($P < 0.001$) higher in alcoholic (42.7 $\pm$ 1.2 μM) than in nonalcoholic (26.5 $\pm$ 1.5 μM) subjects

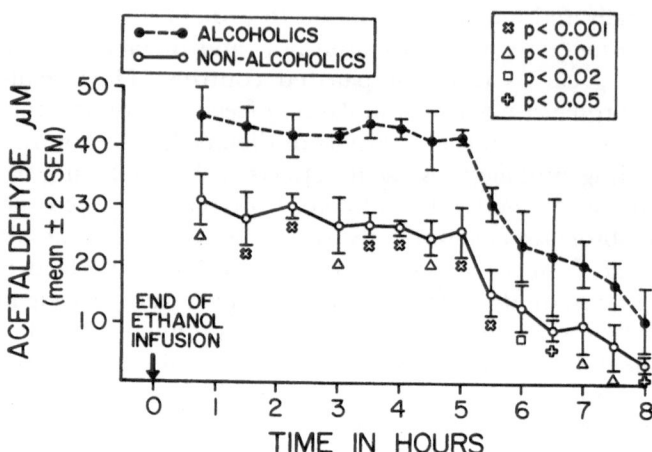

Fig. 2. Comparison of blood acetaldehyde levels of alcoholic and nonalcoholic subjects after intravenous alcohol infusion. The significance level of the difference of the means is noted. (From Korsten *et al.*, 1975.)

(Fig. 2). When the mean blood ethanol concentration reached 24 mM, the acetaldehyde plateau ended abruptly in each subject. The ethanol concentration at which this fall of blood acetaldehyde occurred suggests desaturation of an ethanol oxidizing system other than ADH, and indicates that at high ethanol blood levels, such a system contributes to ethanol oxidation. If it is assumed that during the plateau period of acetaldehyde, production and elimination of acetaldehyde are constant, it follows that either decreased production or increased degradation could explain the decline in acetaldehyde levels at a mean ethanol concentration of 24 mM. Since a sudden increase in degradation is unlikely (Marjanen, 1972; Tottmar *et al.*, 1973), and excretion of acetaldehyde is minimal (Forsander, 1974), it appears that production of acetaldehyde must have decreased. Acetaldehyde production by alcohol dehydrogenase should be unchanged, since this system is fully saturated at ethanol levels associated with the drop in acetaldehyde (Lundquist and Wolthers, 1958; Reynier, 1969; Makar and Mannering, 1970). On the other hand, the MEOS, which has a K_m between 8 and 9 mM, would become desaturated, and its activity would decrease at these ethanol levels (Lieber and DeCarli, 1970; Teschke *et al.*, 1974). Catalase (Thurman *et al.*, 1972) represents another possible pathway of ethanol oxidation, but is limited by the very low capacity of the liver to generate hydrogen peroxide (Oshino *et al.*, 1973; Boveris *et al.*, 1972). Higher levels of acetaldehyde may have been due to decreased catabolism, possibly in relation to alcohol-induced liver damage. Indeed, early structural and functional changes are induced by alcohol in liver organelles (Svoboda and Manning, 1964; Kiessling and Pilström, 1971; Lane and

Lieber, 1966; Cederbaum *et al.*, 1974b). Since these alterations primarily involve the mitochondrion, it is possible that defective acetaldehyde dehydrogenation, which is predominantly intramitochondrial (Marjanen, 1972; Grunnet, 1973), delays acetaldehyde clearance and results in higher concentrations. Indeed, in rats fed ethanol chronically, Hasumura *et al.* (1975a) found that the liver mitochondria had a significantly reduced capacity to oxidize acetaldehyde; this reduction was associated with decreased mitochondrial respiration with acetaldehyde as substrate.

The reduction of acetaldehyde metabolism observed in rats fed ethanol continuously over a long period might result in the accumulation of acetaldehyde in the liver as well as in the blood if the production rate of acetaldehyde is unchanged or increased, as discussed before. The enhanced blood acetaldehyde may in turn explain a number of ethanol-related complications. Indeed, numerous toxic effects have been attributed to acetaldehyde (Walsh, 1971). In addition to the release of catecholamines (Eade, 1959), acetaldehyde has been shown to participate in and favor the condensation reactions of biogenic amines (Davis and Walsh, 1970; Cohen and Collins, 1970). The products of these interactions could have addictive properties if sufficient amounts were generated *in vivo*. Acetaldehyde has also been shown to affect myocardial protein synthesis at concentrations (Schreiber *et al.*, 1972, 1974) comparable to those found by Korsten *et al.* (1975) in the blood. Acetaldehyde has also been shown to reduce the activity of various mitochondrial shuttles involved in the disposition of reducing equivalents, and to inhibit oxidative phosphorylation (Cederbaum *et al.*, 1974a). More recently, Cederbaum *et al.* (1975b) have shown that acetaldehyde depresses the capacity of liver mitochondria to oxidize fatty acids, thereby mimicking the defects of chronic alcohol consumption discussed before (Cederbaum *et al.*, 1975a). The concentrations of acetaldehyde required to achieve the hepatic effects in the mitochondria of normal animals were greater than those seen in the blood. However, the mitochondria of rats fed ethanol chronically were found to have an increased susceptibility to the effects of acetaldehyde; under these conditions, concentrations of acetaldehyde known to occur in the liver were found to depress mitochondrial functions (Matsuzaki and Lieber, 1976). In view of the reactivity of acetaldehyde, a number of other metabolic effects of ethanol could be due to the action of this metabolite of ethanol. For instance, recent studies have indicated that individuals with chronic alcohol abuse frequently exhibited lowered plasma levels of pyridoxal 5'-phosphate, the coenzyme form of vitamin B_6. Veitch *et al.* (1975) found that in rats fed ethanol (36% of total calories), as part of a liquid diet equivalent to the one described by Lieber and DeCarli (1970), there was a significant decrease in the hepatic pyridoxal phosphate content both in animals given a sufficient amount of vitamin B_6 in their diet and in those rendered B_6-deficient. In isolated perfused livers, the addition of 18 mM ethanol lowered the pyridoxal phosphate content of livers from vitamin B_6-deficient animals and decreased the net synthesis of pyridoxal phosphate from pyridoxine by the livers of vitamin B_6-deficient animals. Ethanol also diminished the rate of release of pyridoxal phosphate into the perfusate by the livers of vitamin B_6-deficient rats. These effects of ethanol, *in vitro*, were abolished by 4-methylpyrazole, an inhibitor of alcohol dehydrogenase. Thus, the derangement of pyridoxal phosphate metabolism produced by ethanol is dependent on its oxidation. One interpretation of these findings was that acetaldehyde may be the responsible agent, since in human erythrocytes, it has been shown that acetaldehyde acts to enhance the enzymatic hydrolysis of pyridoxal-5'-phosphate by cellular phosphatase (Lumeng and Li, 1974). Similar observations were also made in isolated rat hepatocytes in preliminary studies thus far published only in abstract form (Veitch *et al.*, 1974). The latter study also reportedly showed that acetaldehyde can displace pyridoxal-5'-phosphate from its protein binding, thereby promoting its degradation. Thus, through a multitude of mechanisms, acetaldehyde may explain a variety of metabolic complications associated with alcohol abuse.

References

Anton, A. H., 1965, Ethanol and urinary catecholamines in man, *Clin. Pharmacol. Ther.* **6**:462.

Baraona, E., and Lieber, C. S., 1975, Intestinal lymph formation and fat absorption: Stimulation by acute ethanol administration and inhibition by chronic ethanol feeding, *Gastroenterology* **68**:495.

Baraona, E., Pirola, R. C., and Lieber, C. S., 1974, Small intestinal damage and changes in cell population produced by ethanol ingestion in the rat, *Gastroenterology* **66**:226.

Baraona, E., Pirola, R. C., and Lieber, C. S., 1975, Acute and chronic effects of ethanol on intestinal lipid metabolism, *Biochem. Biophys. Acta* **388**:19.

Bernstein, J., Videla, L., and Israel, Y., 1975, Hormonal influences in the development of the hypermetabolic state of the liver produced by chronic administration of ethanol, *J. Pharmacol. Exp. Ther.* **192**:583.

Boveris, A., Oshino, N., and Chance, B., 1972, The cellular production of hydrogen peroxide, *Biochem. J.* **128**:617.

Cederbaum, A. I., Lieber, C. S., and Rubin, E., 1974a, The effect of acetaldehyde on mitochondrial function, *Arch. Biochem. Biophys.* **161**:26.

Cederbaum, A. I., Lieber, C. S., and Rubin, E., 1974b, Effects of chronic ethanol treatment on mitochondrial functions: Damage to coupling site, *Arch. Biochem. Biophys.* **165**:560.

Cederbaum, A. I., Lieber, C. S., Beattie, D. S., and Rubin, E., 1975a, Effect of chronic ethanol ingestion on fatty acid oxidation by hepatic mitochondria, *J. Biol. Chem.* **250**:5122.

Cederbaum, A. I., Lieber, C. S., and Rubin, E., 1975b, Effect of acetaldehyde on fatty acid oxidation and ketogenesis by hepatic mitochondria, *Arch. Biochem. Biophys.* **169**:29.

Cederbaum, A. I., Dicker, E., Gang, H., Lieber, C. S., and Rubin, E., 1976, Effect of chronic ethanol feeding on ethanol oxidation by isolated rat liver cells, *Fed. Proc.* **35**:1709.

Chance, B., 1947, An intermediate compound in the catalase–hydrogen peroxide reaction, *Acta Chem. Scand.* **1**:236.

Chance, B., and Oshino, N., 1971, Kinetics and mechanisms of catalase in peroxisomes of the mitochondrial fraction, *Biochem. J.* **122**:225.

Choisy, H., and Potron, J., 1972, Action des vitamines sur le metabolisme de l'alcool, *Rev. Alcool.* **18**:292.

Cohen, G., and Collins, M., 1970, Alkaloids from catecholamines in adrenal tissue: Possible role in alcoholism, *Science* **167**:1749.

Davis, V. E., and Walsh, M. J., 1970, Alcohol, amines and alkaloids: A possible biochemical basis for alcohol addiction, *Science* **167**:1005.

DeCarli, L. M., and Lieber, C. S., 1967, Fatty liver in the rat after prolonged intake of ethanol with a nutritionally adequate new liquid diet, *J. Nutr.* **91**:331.

DeCarli, L. M., Ishii, H., Hasumura, Y., and Lieber, C. S., 1972, Effect of ethanol and a low-fat diet on hepatic microsomal enzymes, in: *Proceedings of the Ninth International Congress of Nutrition*, p. 189, S. Karger, New York.

Domschke, S., Domschke, W., and Lieber, C. S., 1974, Hepatic redox state: Attenuation of the acute effects of ethanol induced by chronic ethanol consumption, *Life Sci.* **15**:1327.

Eade, N. R., 1959, Mechanism of sympathomimetic action of aldehydes, *J. Pharmacol. Exp. Ther.* **127**:29.

Forsander, O. A., 1974, Variations in the acetaldehyde level of some tissues in hyper- and hypothyroid rats, *Second International Symposium on Alcohol Intoxication and Withdrawal*, Section of 20th International Institute on Alcoholism, ICAA, Manchester, England, Vol. 59, p. 139.

Gale, C. C., 1973, Neuroendocrine aspects of thermoregulation, *Annu. Rev. Physiol.* **35**:391.

Goldberg, M., Hehir, R., and Hurowitz, M., 1960, Intravenous tri-iodothyronine in acute alcoholic intoxication, *N. Engl. J. Med.* **203**:1336.

Gordon, E. R., 1977, ATP metabolism in an ethanol-induced fatty liver, in: *Alcoholism: Clinical and Experimental Research*, Vol. 1 (in press).

Grunnet, N., 1973, Oxidation of acetaldehyde by rat liver mitochondria in relation to ethanol oxidation and the transport of reducing equivalents across the mitochondrial membrane, *Eur. J. Biochem.* **35**:236.

Guynn, R. W., and Pieklik, J. R., 1975, Dependence on dose of the acute effects of ethanol on liver metabolism in vivo, *J. Clin. Invest.* **56**:1411.

Harrison, T. S., 1964, Adrenal medullary and thyroid relationships, *Physiol. Rev.* **44**:161.

Hasumura, Y., Teschke, R., and Lieber, C. S., 1975a, Acetaldehyde oxidation by hepatic mitochondria: Decrease after chronic ethanol consumption, *Science* **189**:727.

Hasumura, Y., Teschke, R., and Lieber, C. S., 1975b, Hepatic microsomal ethanol-oxidizing system (MEOS): Dissociation from reduced nicotinamide adenine dinucleotide phosphate oxidase and possible role of Form I of cytochrome P-450, *J. Pharmacol. Exp. Ther.* **194**:469.

Hawkins, R. D., and Kalant, H., 1972, The metabolism of ethanol and its metabolic effects, *Pharmacol. Rev.* **24**:67.

Hawkins, R. D., Kalant, H., and Khanna, J. M., 1966, Effects of chronic intake of ethanol on rate of ethanol metabolism, *Can. J. Physiol. Pharmacol.* **44**:241.

Hillbom, M. E., 1971, Thyroid state and voluntary alcohol consumption of albino rats, *Acta Pharmacol. Toxicol.* **29**:95.

Hillbom, M. E., and Pikkarainen, P. H., 1970, Liver alcohol and sorbitol dehydrogenase activities in hypo- and hyperthyroid rats, *Biochem. Pharmacol.* **19**:2097.

Hillbom, M. E., and Pösö, A. R., 1975, Effects of ethanol on serum electrolytes and respiration in euthyroid and hyperthyroid rats, *Toxicol. Appl. Pharmacol.* **32**:168.

Himms-Hagen, J., 1967, Sympathetic regulation of metabolism, *Pharmacol. Rev.* **19**:367.

Hoch, F. L., 1974, Metabolic effects of thyroid hormones, *in: Handbook of Physiology, Section 7: Endocrinology*, Vol. 3, *Thyroid* (M. A. Greer and D. H. Solomon, eds.), p. 391, American Physiological Society, Washington, D.C.

Ismail-Beigi, F., and Edelman, I. S., 1970, Mechanism of thyroid calorigenesis: Role of active sodium transport, *Proc. Nat. Acad. Sci. U.S.A.* **67**:1071.

Ismail-Beigi, F., and Edelman, I. S., 1971, The mechanism of the calorigenic action of thyroid hormone: Stimulation of $Na^+ + K^+$-activated adenosinetriphosphatase activity, *J. Gen. Physiol.* **57**:710.

Israel, Y., Kalant, H., Orrego, H., Khanna, J. M., Videla, L., and Phillips, J. M., 1975a, Experimental alcohol-induced hepatic necrosis: Suppression by propylthiouracil, *Proc. Nat. Acad. Sci. U.S.A.* **72**:1137.

Israel, Y., Videla, L., Fernandes-Videal, V., and Bernstein, J., 1975b, Effects of chronic ethanol treatment and thyroxine administration on ethanol metabolism and liver oxidative capacity, *J. Pharmacol. Exp. Ther.* **192**:565.

Joly, J. -G., and Hétu, C., 1975, Effects of chronic ethanol administration in the rat: Relative dependency on dietary lipids, *Biochem. Pharmacol.* **24**:1475.

Kalant, H., Sereny, G., and Charlebois, R., 1962, Evaluation of tri-iodothyronine in the treatment of acute alcoholic intoxication, *N. Engl. J. Med.* **267**:1.

Kalant, H., Khanna, J. M., and Endrenyi, L., 1975, Effect of pyrazole on ethanol metabolism in ethanol-tolerant rats, *Can. J. Physiol. Pharmacol.* **53**:416.

Khanna, J. M., Kalant, H., and Loth, J., 1975, Effect of chronic intake of ethanol on lactate/pyruvate and β-hydroxybutyrate/acetoacetate ratios in rat liver, *Can. J. Physiol.* **53**:299.

Kiessling, K. -H., and Pilstrom, L, 1971, Ethanol and the human liver. Structural and metabolic changes in liver mitochondria, *Cytobiologie* **4**(2):339.

Kinard, F. W., Hay, M. G., and Kinard, F. W., Jr., 1962, Effect of tri-iodothyronine on ethanol metabolism in the dog, *Nature*, **196:**380.

Klingman, G. I., and Goodall, McC., 1957, Urinary epinephrines and levarterenol excretion during acute sublethal alcohol intoxication in dogs, *J. Pharmacol. Exp. Ther.* **121:**313.

Korsten, M. A., Matsuzaki, S., Feinman, L., and Lieber, C. S., 1975, High blood acetaldehyde levels after ethanol administration: Difference between alcoholic and nonalcoholic subjects, *New Engl. J. Med.* **292:**386.

Krawitt, E. L., 1975, Effect of ethanol ingestion on duodenal calcium transport, *J. Lab. Clin. Med.* **85:**665.

Lane, B. P., and Lieber, C. S., 1966, Ultrastructural alterations in human hepatocytes following ingestion of ethanol with adequate diets, *Amer. J. Pathol.* **49:**593.

Lefevre, A. F., DeCarli, L. M., and Lieber, C. S., 1972, Effect of ethanol on cholesterol and bile acid metabolism, *J. Lipid Res.* **13:**48.

Lieber, C. S., and Davidson, C. S., 1962, Some metabolic effects of ethyl alcohol, *Amer. J. Med.* **33:**319.

Lieber, C. S., and DeCarli, L. M., 1970, Hepatic microsomal ethanol-oxidizing system: *In vitro* characteristics and adaptive properties *in vivo, J. Biol. Chem.* **245:**2505.

Lieber, C. S., and DeCarli, L. M., 1972, The role of the hepatic microsomal ethanol oxidizing system (MEOS) for ethanol metabolism *in vivo, J. Pharmacol. Exp. Ther.* **181:**279.

Lieber, C. S., and DeCarli, L. M., 1976, Metabolic aspects of alcohol on the liver, *in: Metabolic Aspects of Alcoholism* (C. W. Lieber, ed.), Chapter 2, p. 31, MTP Press, Lancaster, England (in press).

Lieber, C. S., Jones, D. P., Mendelson, J., and DeCarli, L. M., 1963, Fatty liver, hyperlipemia and hyperuricemia produced by prolonged alcohol consumption, despite adequate dietary intake, *Trans. Assoc. Amer. Physicians* **76:**289.

Lieber, C. S., Jones, D. P., and DeCarli, L. M., 1965, Effects of prolonged ethanol intake: Production of fatty liver despite adequate diets, *J. Clin. Invest.* **44:**1009.

Lieber, C. S., Rubin, E., and DeCarli, L. M., 1969, Respective role of dietary and metabolic factors in the pathogenesis of the alcoholic fatty liver: The biochemical basis for the ethanol-induced liver injury, *in: Biochemical and Clinical Aspects of Alcohol Metabolism* (V. M. Sardesai, ed.), p. 176, C. C. Thomas, Springfield, Illinois.

Lieber, C. S., DeCarli, L. M., and Rubin, E., 1975, Sequential production of fatty liver, hepatitis, and cirrhosis in sub-human primates fed ethanol with adequate diets, *Proc. Nat. Acad. Sci. U.S.A.* **72:**437.

Lumeng, L., and Li, T. -K., 1974, Vitamin B_6 metabolism in chronic alcohol abuse: Pyridoxal phosphate levels in plasma and the effects of acetaldehyde on pyridoxal phosphate synthesis and degradation in human erythrocytes, *J. Clin. Invest.* **53:**693.

Lundquist, F., and Wolthers, H., 1958, The influence of fructose on the kinetics of alcohol elimination in man, *Acta Pharmacol.* **14:**290.

Makar, A. B., and Mannering, G. J., 1970, Kinetics of ethanol metabolism in the intact rat and monkey, *Biochem. Pharmacol.* **19**:2017.

Marjanen, L., 1972, Intracellular localization of aldehyde dehydrogenase in rat liver, *Biochem. J.* **127**:633.

Matsuzaki, S., Teschke, R., Ohnishi, K., DeCarli, L. M., and Lieber, C. S., 1976, Acceleration of ethanol metabolism at high ethanol concentrations and after chronic ethanol consumption: Role of microsomal ethanol oxidizing system (MEOS), *in: Proceedings of the Canadian Hepatic Foundation 3rd International Symposium on Alcohol and the Liver,* May 14 and 15, 1976, Toronto, Canada.

Meijer, A. J., Van Woerkom, G. M., Williamson, J. R., and Tager, J. M., 1975, Rate-limiting factors in the oxidation of ethanol by isolated rat liver cells, *Biochem. J.* **150**:205.

Mitchell, H. H., 1935, The food value of ethyl alcohol, *J. Nutr.* **10**:311.

Newman, H., and Smith, M. E., 1959, Triiodothyronine in acute alcoholic intoxication, *Nature (London)* **183**:689.

Ogata, M., Mendelson, J. H., Mello, N. K., and Majchrowicz, E., 1971, Adrenal function and alcoholism. II. Catecholamines, *Psychosom. Med.* **33**:159.

Oshino, N., Chance, B., Sies, H., and Bucher, T., 1973, The role of H_2O_2 generation in perfused rat liver and the reaction of catalase compound I and hydrogen donors, *Arch. Biochem. Biophys.* **154**:117.

Patek, A. J., Toth, I. G., Saunders, M. G., Castro, G. A. M., and Engel, J. J., 1975, Alcohol and dietary factors in cirrhosis, *Arch. Intern. Med.* **135**:1053.

Perman, E. S., 1958, The effect of ethyl alcohol on the secretion from the adrenal medulla in man, *Acta Physiol. Scand.* **44**:241.

Perman, E. S., 1960, The effect of ethyl alcohol on the secretion from the adrenal medulla of the cat, *Acta Physiol. Scand.* **48**:323.

Perman, E. S., 1961, Observations on the effect of ethanol on the urinary excretion of histamine, 5-hydroxyindole acetic acid, catecholamines and 17-hydroxycorticosteroids in man, *Acta Physiol. Scand.* **51**:62.

Pilström, L., and Kiessling, K. H., 1972, A possible localization of α-glycerophosphate dehydrogenase to the inner boundary membrane of mitochondria in livers from rats fed ethanol, *Histochemie* **32**:329.

Pirola, R. C., and Lieber, C. S., 1972, The energy cost of the metabolism of drugs, including ethanol, *Pharmacology* **7**:185.

Pirola, R. C., and Lieber, C. S., 1975, Energy wastage in rats given drugs that induce microsomal enzymes, *J. Nutr.* **105**:1544.

Pirola, R. C., and Lieber, C. S., 1976, Hypothesis: Energy wastage in alcoholism and drug abuse: Possible role of hepatic microsomal enzymes, *Amer. J. Clin. Nutr.* **29**:90.

Raskin, N. H., and Sokoloff, L., 1972, Ethanol-induced adaptation of alcohol dehydrogenase activity in rat brain, *Nature New Biology* **236**:138.

Rawat, A. K., and Lundquist, F., 1968, Influence of thyroxine on the metabolism of ethanol and glycerol in rat liver slices, *Eur. J. Biochem.* **5**:13.

Reynier, M., 1969, Pyrazole inhibition and kinetic studies of ethanol and retinol oxidation catalyzed by rat liver alcohol dehydrogenase, *Acta Chem. Scand.* **23**:1119.

Rubin, E., Beattie, D. S., Toth, A., and Lieber, C. S., 1972, Structural and functional effects of ethanol on hepatic mitochondria, *Fed Proc. Fed. Amer. Soc. Exp. Biol.* **31**:131.

Schreiber, S. S., Briden, K., Oratz, M., and Rothschild, M. A., 1972, Ethanol, acetaldehyde and myocardial protein synthesis, *J. Clin. Invest.* **51**:2820.

Schreiber, S. S., Oratz, M., Rothschild, M. A., Reff, F., and Evans, C., 1974, Alcoholic cardiomyopathy. II. The inhibition of cardiac microsomal protein synthesis by acetaldehyde, *J. Mol. Cell. Cardiol.* **6**:207.

Shaw, S., Heller, E. A., Friedman, H. S., Baraona, E., and Lieber, C. S., 1976, Effect of ethanol on hepatic oxygen metabolism: Is ischemia a mechanism of alcoholic liver injury?, *Gastroenterology* **71**:(in press).

Singlevich, T. E., and Barboriak, J. J., 1971, Ethanol and induction of microsomal drug-metabolizing enzymes in the rat, *Toxicol. Appl. Pharmacol.* **20**:284.

Smith, D. E., Fallis, N. E., and Tetreault, L., 1963, Effect of tri-iodothyronine on rate of alcohol oxidation in dogs, *N. Engl. J. Med.* **268**:91.

Stokes, P. E., and Tasley, B., 1967, Further studies on blood alcohol kinetics in man as affected by thyroid hormones, insulin and *d*-glucose, *in: Biochemical Factors in Alcoholism,* First Ed. (Roger P. Maikel, ed.), p. 101, Pergamon Press, Elmsford, New York.

Svoboda, D. J., and Manning, R. T., 1964, Chronic alcoholism with fatty metamorphosis of the liver: Mitochondrial alterations in hepatic cells, *Amer. J. Pathol.* **44**:645.

Tata, J. R., 1964, Biological action of thyroid hormones at the cellular and molecular levels, *in: Actions of Hormones and Molecular Processes* (G. Litwack and D. Kritchevsky, eds.), p. 58, John Wiley and Sons, New York.

Teschke, R., Hasumura, Y., and Lieber, C. S., 1974, Hepatic microsomal ethanol oxidizing system: Solubilization, isolation and characterization, *Arch. Biochem. Biophys.* **163**:404.

Teschke, R., Hasumura, Y., and Lieber, C. S., 1975a, Hepatic microsomal alcohol oxidizing system: Affinity for methanol, ethanol, propanol and butanol, *J. Biol. Chem.* **250**:7397.

Teschke, R., Hasumura, Y., and Lieber, C. S., 1975b, Hepatic microsomal alcohol oxidizing system in normal and acatalasemic mice: Its dissociation from the peroxidatic activity of catalase–H_2O_2, *Mol. Pharmacol.* **11**:841.

Thurman, R. G., Ley, H. G., and Scholz, R., 1972, Hepatic microsomal ethanol oxidation: Hydrogen peroxide formation and the role of catalase, *Eur. J. Biochem.* **25**:420.

Tottmar, S. O. C., Pettersson, H., and Kiessling, K.-H., 1973, The subcellular distribution and properties of aldehyde dehydrogenases in rat liver, *Biochem. J.* **135**:577.

Truitt, E. B., and Duritz, G., 1966. The role of acetaldehyde in the actions of ethanol, *in: Biochemical Factors in Alcoholism* (P. P. Maickel, ed.), p. 61, Pergamon Press, Elmsford, New York.

Ugarte, G., Iturriaga, H., Pino, M. E., and Pereda, T., 1975, Ethanol metabolism and enzyme changes in alcoholics with and without hepatic damage, *in: Alcoholic Liver Pathology* (J. M. Khanna, Y. Israel, and H. Kalant, eds.), p. 341,

Alcoholism and Drug Addiction Research Foundation, Toronto.

Veech, R. L., Eggleston, L. V., and Krebs, H. A., 1969, The redox state of free nicotinamide–adenine dinucleotide phosphate in the cytoplasm of rat liver, *Biochem. J.* **115**:609.

Veitch, R. L., Lumeng, L., and Li, T. K., 1974, The effect of ethanol and acetaldehyde on vitamin B_6 metabolism in liver, *Gastroenterology* **66**:868.

Veitch, R. L., Lumeng, L., and Li, T. K., 1975, Vitamin B_6 metabolism in chronic alcohol abuse: The effect of ethanol oxidation on hepatic pyridoxal 5'-phosphate metabolism, *J. Clin. Invest.* **55**:1026.

Videla, L., Flattery, K. V., Sellers, E. A., and Israel, Y., 1975, Ethanol metabolism and liver oxidative capacity in cold acclimation, *J. Pharmacol. Exp. Ther.* **192**:575.

Walsh, M. J., 1971, Role of acetaldehyde in the interactions of ethanol with neuroamines, *in: Biological Aspects of Alcohol* (M. K. Roach, W. M. McIsaac, and P. J. Creaven, eds.), p. 233, University of Texas Press, Austin and London.

Ylikahri, R. H., 1970, Ethanol-induced changes in hepatic α-glycerophosphate and triglyceride concentrations in normal and thyroxine-treated rats, *Metabolism* **19**:1036.

Ylikahri, R. H., and Mäenpää, P. H., 1968, Rate of ethanol metabolism in fed and starved rats after thyroxine treatment, *Acta Chem. Scand.* **22**:1707.

Index